THE
PREGNANCY
BOOK

Also by William Sears, M.D., and Martha Sears, R.N.

❖

Parenting the Fussy Baby and High-Need Child

The Discipline Book

The Birth Book

The Baby Book

300 Questions New Parents Ask

Nighttime Parenting

Becoming a Father

Also by William Sears, M.D.

❖

SIDS: A Parent's Guide to Understanding and
Preventing Sudden Infant Death Syndrome

T·H·E

PREGNANCY BOOK

A Month-by-Month Guide

❖ ❖ ❖

WILLIAM SEARS, M.D.,
AND MARTHA SEARS, R.N.,
WITH LINDA HUGHEY HOLT, M.D., F.A.C.O.G.

LITTLE, BROWN AND COMPANY
New York ◆ *Boston*

Little, Brown and Company
Time Warner Book Group
1271 Avenue of the Americas, New York, NY 10020
Visit our Web site at www.twbookmark.com

First Edition

Drawings by Deborah Maze

"When One Becomes Two" by Jacquelyn deLaveaga.
Copyright © by Jacquelyn deLaveaga. By permission of the author.

Library of Congress Cataloging-in-Publication Data

Sears, William, M.D. : a month-by-month guide
    The pregnancy book / William Sears and Martha Sears, with
Linda Hughey Holt.
        p.   cm.
    Includes index.
    ISBN 0-316-77917-2 hc
    ISBN 0-316-77914-8 pb
    1. Pregnancy.   2. Childbirth.   I. Sears, Martha.   II. Holt, Linda
Hughey.   III. Title.
RG525.S3977   1997
618.2'4 — dc21   96–48905

10

Q-FF

Designed by Jeanne Abboud

PRINTED IN THE UNITED STATES OF AMERICA

Contents

Many Thanks

BESIDES THE NOTES we kept during our own pregnancies (eight little Searses and three little Holts), much of the material for this book was provided by mothers who were asked to keep journals during their pregnancy and share them with us: Chris Kurt, Amy Wade, Kristina Marcus, Gwen Gotsch, Cheryl Sears, Diane Sears, Stacy Prince, Sherri Alden, Ellie Halliburton, McCall Gordon, Terri Trierweiler, Lyn Reed, Rebecca Tookey, Gina Bassler, Diedre Jenkins, Jacquelyn Delaveaga, Bonnie Solomon, and Paula Benson. Many thanks to all of them.

Thanks also to our assistant, Tracee Zeni, for her dedicated work in preparing the manuscript. A special thanks to our editor, Jennifer Josephy, and our copyeditor, Pamela Marshall, for their patience and dedication toward repeatedly improving this book. Finally, we wish to thank the many mothers in our obstetrical and pediatric practices who shared their experiences with us to help us focus on the most common physical and emotional experiences and the most common worries pregnant women have. We called these mothers our "board of directors" who kept us focused on the task of providing the most useful information that expectant couples need.

A Word from the Authors

WE HAVE NOT ONLY written this book, we have lived it. We speak to you as professionals, bringing you experience from our respective careers as childbirth educator, pediatrician, and obstetrician. More important, we speak to you as parents, Martha and Dr. Bill as parents of eight, Dr. Linda as the mother of three.

As professionals and parents, we have learned a great deal from pregnant couples — specifically, what worries they have and what information they want. We write to you with the belief that the more you know, the more likely you are to have a safe and satisfying pregnancy and birth. Pregnancy is not an illness to be endured; rather, it is a normal and healthy female function. Pregnancy is more than morning sickness and nighttime trips to the bathroom. It is a personal journey, during which you will make discoveries about yourself, the mysteries of your mind and the marvels of your body. During these nine months you will not only grow a baby, you will grow as a person. Pregnancy will challenge your body, your mind, your marriage, your job, and your whole being, as you experience feelings you've never had before. Each day you will grow millions of new cells that will eventually all come together to form a separate human being who will one day be quite independent of you. Pregnancy can be difficult but, oh, so wonderful.

Everything will change, from making breakfast to making love. Embrace this change. Throughout your body an emotional and physical metamorphosis is taking place that is pretty much beyond your control. It's an experience unique to each woman. Even though intellectually you may understand that billions of women have been pregnant before you, you are the only one to carry your particular child. You are entitled to feel proud and special and part of a miracle. When you consider that you are bringing forth a life in just nine short months, the time you spend and the inconvenience and discomforts that you go through will become secondary.

Although pregnancy is a journey unique to every woman, most women share certain physical and emotional concerns. Throughout this book we have let the experts speak for themselves. You will find helpful hints and actual stories from pregnant women who have traveled a similar road.

We want this to be a reassuring book, informing you about what's normal, what's not, and what to do. Yet we also want this book to be realistic. Pregnancy is neither a constant, ecstatic, cloud-nine state of mind (or body), nor nine months of relentless misery. It is a process to be experienced to the fullest, not just endured. By knowing how to appreciate and work with your body, you can transform pregnancy and childbirth from nine months of worry and complaining into a season of personal growth that will equip you to forge ahead as a parent. As a healthier, more mature and understanding human being, you'll claim your prize — your baby! Here's the whole story about how you and your baby grow.

William and Martha Sears
San Clemente, Calif.
Linda Hughey Holt,
Evanston, Ill.
June 1997

How to Use This Book

TO GET A FEEL for what lies ahead, you may find it useful to read this entire book early in your pregnancy. It helps to know that many of the discomforts you feel at one stage ease during the next, and that the worries of one month can become the joys of the next. We have listed the physical and emotional concerns of pregnancy that most women have in the order that most women have them, from month to month. Yet each pregnancy is different, and some of your concerns are sure to arise during different months from where they appear in the book. If you have a question or concern that doesn't appear in the chapter that discusses the month of pregnancy you're in (or the month you are reading about), consult the index under the heading of your concern.

This book is meant to be read in addition to, not as a substitute for, regular prenatal care by your practitioner. Books can only generalize about what most women experience most of the time. Your pregnancy is as unique as the baby you are carrying. Because you may have special obstetrical needs that lie beyond the scope of this book and require different management from what we recommend, be sure to discuss your concerns with and follow the advice of your practitioner.

To avoid cluttering both this book and the already overwhelmed minds of pregnant women, we have placed the rare conditions in the glossary (see page 407). As writers and parents, we don't want to worry the 99 percent of mothers-to-be needlessly with unusual problems that may occur in the other 1 percent.

THE PREGNANCY BOOK

First-Month Visit to Your Health-Care Provider* (1–4 weeks)

On your first visit to your health-care provider, expect to have:

- confirmation of pregnancy
- a general medical history taken, plus a previous obstetrical history, if you have one
- a general physical exam, including an internal exam
- blood tests: hemoglobin and hematocrit for anemia; blood-typing; rubella titer; hepatitis B screen (HIV screen, venereal disease screen, and sickle-cell screen are optional)
- possible cultures for vaginal infections
- Pap smear for the detection of cervical cancer
- blood test for genetic diseases, if your history warrants it
- urinalysis to test for infection, sugar, and protein
- weight and blood-pressure check
- counseling on proper nutrition and on avoiding environmental hazards
- an opportunity to discuss your feelings and concerns

---

* *The month-by-month schedule of visits to your health-care provider is the one recommended by the American College of Obstetricians and Gynecologists.*

The First Month —
Newly Pregnant

YOU'RE PREGNANT! Congratulations! Ahead of you lies one of the most exciting experiences of your life and one that will bring momentous change. There's much to think about and much to do as you prepare for the birth of your baby — a high point of many women's lives.

Even though you are pregnant, you may not yet feel pregnant. Perhaps your pregnant "feelings" are so far only emotional, or maybe you have begun to feel physically pregnant. You may have eagerly awaited pregnancy and be happily anticipating any signals (beyond a missed period) your body might give you that "this is it." You may be feeling slightly nauseated already, or hungry, thirsty, tired, hot, weak, or dizzy. Maybe you have been caught a bit off-guard by the knowledge that you are pregnant. You may initially have thought you had the flu until your body or your doctor told you otherwise. Perhaps you simply "knew" when you became pregnant, even before you experienced any symptoms.

Whatever your physical symptoms, the fact that you are pregnant is likely to take some adjusting to whether this baby was planned or not. Whether you heard the news in a doctor's office or at home, bent watchfully over a do-it-yourself pregnancy test, you may find yourself feeling happy, scared, relieved, unbelieving, confused, or all of the above. Of course, your initial reaction will depend greatly on whether your pregnancy comes as a surprise or after months of planning and hoping. Even if you are ready to embrace this life-changing experience — one that will affect everything from your diet to your marriage — don't be surprised if you have to let the news sink in a bit before you act on the fact that you are pregnant. Here is an overview of what lies ahead.

HOW YOU MAY FEEL EMOTIONALLY

Happy. The news that you are pregnant may leave you feeling ecstatic, especially if you have been trying to get pregnant for a long time and you have finally succeeded. You may feel complete, fulfilled, and have an overall sense of well-being now that you are what you have wanted to be — a mother-to-be.

Knowing there is a little person growing inside me who is so dependent on me for love

1

and life is not only an awesome responsibility but also a great blessing. It is the most fulfilling experience in my life.

Incredulous. At other times you may wonder, "Am I really pregnant? I don't feel any different." These feelings are especially strong in the early weeks, when you may not experience any symptoms. Or you may convince yourself that the nausea and fatigue you feel only mean you are sick. If you have been longing to get pregnant, you may fear that your body's signals are only wishful thinking, especially since you don't look any different. You may find this early misery disillusioning. Soon your expanding waistline will erase all doubt that someone is growing inside you.

Dr. Linda notes: My own reaction was one of total shock and disbelief. We had not really been planning a family, at least not until some "convenient" time, which I am sure would have been well past menopause. So, when a year out of my residency I realized I was late for a period, I really did not think pregnancy was a possibility. I blamed my long hours and erratic work schedule for my late period. I am always surprised when patients deny the possibility of pregnancy, but somehow for myself, a late period and erratic diaphragm use did not add up to the possibility of pregnancy. My husband was running a lab that did pregnancy tests. I had a friend take my blood sample to his lab as an anonymous sample. When it came back positive I insisted he do it again, as I was convinced there must be some lab mistake.

Ambivalent. While you may think the word "mother" has a nice ring to it, you may also feel overwhelmed with the life changes that come with this title. It's usual to have mixed feelings about being pregnant, especially if your news comes as a surprise. It's normal to be happy about the prospect of becoming a mother, yet feel sad or worried about what you'll have to go through or give up to earn the title. On the one hand, you may be excited, thrilled, proud, and eager to assume this new role and all the responsibilities that go with it. On the other hand, all the changes that will occur in your lifestyle, your marriage, and your body may seem frightening. Many women find it comforting to consider pregnancy a developmental stage, like adolescence. A mother-to-be typically goes through an identity crisis. The realization "I'm going to be somebody's mother" leads to the question "What will happen to the me I am now?" It's normal to feel anxious about giving your life over to such a major change. Even when a pregnancy is planned and longed for, a woman may wonder if she's as ready or as capable as she thought she was. Change is always scary, even when it is positive.

You may feel like a dual-career woman even in the first month of pregnancy. There may be days when you are so excited (or so worried) about the pregnancy that you can't focus on anything else, and fear that if you don't come down to earth soon, you will lose your job. You may be worried about leaving your job, whether on maternity leave or permanently, and about taking on the awesome responsibilities of motherhood. On other days you may be so engrossed in your current life you almost forget you're pregnant (and then feel guilty for forgetting). It's normal to have difficulty staying enthusiastic about your job while pregnant. It's impossible to tune out for long the constant reminders of the little life growing inside you; you do, in fact, have a whole new additional job description: baby builder. Your "real-life" job somehow begins to seem less important. For some women biology takes over, and they come to the realization that they can't work to their full capacity, physically or mentally, at their job. Most women, however, soon settle into both the pregnancy and a slightly altered daily routine.

My mother told me about her first pregnancy, "I got up, threw up, made breakfast, and then your dad and I went to school to teach."

How you feel about your body may also have its ups and downs. You may experience pride in your femininity and fertility, and such delight in nourishing another life within your own body that you can't wait to show or tell about it. You may anticipate glowing, the way pregnant women are supposed to. On the other hand, you may not relish giving over your comfortable, familiar body to the widening and bulging of pregnancy, and you may have heard from friends that they didn't feel very radiant when they were pregnant; in fact, they looked and felt awful! Many women worry about becoming less attractive to their husbands.

Don't be surprised if you find yourself developing a sudden fondness for the way your body looks and feels right now. Even if you are not prone to vanity, you may now enjoy admiring your body in front of a mirror, knowing full well that you won't see this shape again for at least a year. Part of you wonders if you will ever get your "normal" body back. Will you look the same? Feel the same?

Some women, expecting to feel ecstatic when they discover they are pregnant, find much to their surprise, that they don't feel any excitement. And don't be alarmed if you don't yet experience those warm and tender feelings of bonding with your baby. It's not unhealthy or abnormal in the early weeks to feel more like an incubator than a mom. Some women don't feel motherly until they feel the first kick or see the ultrasound picture of their moving baby. Others don't really feel connected until after birth. Getting connected with your baby is a long process, and it works differently for different mothers and babies.

Moody. A completely blissful pregnancy is as rare as a perfect parent. As the initial elation of discovering you're pregnant subsides and the reality of impending parenthood sinks in, it's common to have good days and not so good days. One day you may feel on top of the world, the next day you may feel sad and weepy. There are several reasons for these mood swings. One is the normal emotional letdown that naturally occurs after an intensely emotional experience; in human emotions, lows usually follow highs. Another reason is purely physiological: it's those hormones. The surge of pregnancy hormones that is upsetting your body also accounts for the volatility of your emotions. Of course, feeling depressed may catch you by surprise, especially if this is a long-anticipated pregnancy. And feeling bad that you don't always feel happy doesn't do anything to lift your spirits. Add to these emotional woes the usual nausea and fatigue of early pregnancy, and it's no wonder that most mothers go from glad to sad several times a day. Expect mood changes especially in the first three months, when hormone levels are changing most dramatically, and in the final weeks, when anticipation increases and fatigue sets in.

Filled with doubts. Even though you may be ecstatic about being pregnant, it's normal to have second thoughts. You and your partner may even wonder, "What have we done?"

A child will affect your career, your lifestyle, your marriage, how you spend your time. Even if you already have a child, you may experience doubts about the changes a second or third child will bring to your family. You wonder if you will ever get control of your life. Life after children is never the same as it was before. It's different, and while you may have doubts, you can learn to adapt to the changes.

It's normal to wonder if you will be a good enough mother and to question your ability to pull all this off — to carry your baby to term, to go through the ordeal of labor and delivery, and to care for your new baby. Feeling inadequate goes with the profession of parenthood. A year from now, when your baby gives you an appreciative smile that says, "You're the best mom in the world," you'll feel more confident.

Our lives were just getting back to normal after the birth of our first child, who is now two years old. Now I realize that after having children, my life will never be the same anyway. This is now my "normal" life.

Anxious. It's normal to feel anxious about the unknown. If you have been settled in a childless, adult lifestyle for many years, the prospect of diapers, middle-of-the-night feedings, and a tiny person controlling your life may leave you feeling very anxious. When you close one chapter in your life to open another, it's normal to have some misgivings. When you announce to your friends that you are pregnant, you also invite an army of veterans to share their birth and pregnancy stories. The tales from the front may be interesting, but all these war stories can add to the fears of a first-time pregnant woman. Learn to take these stories with a grain of salt. Your experience will most assuredly be unique.

Fear of the miseries of pregnancy and the pain of childbirth produces its own anxiety, despite the fact that all mothers get through it — and most even choose to do it again. Worries about miscarriage are common early in pregnancy, though the odds against having one are in your favor. Once your pregnancy goes beyond the first month, for most women the chance of miscarrying is less than 10 percent. The longer your pregnancy progresses, the less you need to worry about a miscarriage. Concerns about all the things that might go wrong with the pregnancy may be reinforced if your health-care provider goes through a scary list of what-ifs during your first prenatal visit. A certain amount of worrying is normal during pregnancy, but if you find your worries escalating as your pregnancy progresses, or if anxiety prevents you from living your life as usual, consider seeking professional help.

HOW YOU MAY FEEL PHYSICALLY

Tired. Pregnancy brings a strange fatigue that may be unlike anything you've experienced before, especially in the first trimester, when your body forces you to sleep. There may be times during the day when you feel bone-deep exhaustion. You crave sleep. You can be sitting at your desk and fall asleep in the middle of the morning. When you consider how hard your body is working, it's no wonder you are tired. Nearly every organ in your body is laboring overtime to accommodate your new guest, and every part of you is affected by the hormonal and physiological changes of pregnancy. At the same time, you

Early Signs of Pregnancy

Soon after you suspect you're pregnant, your body will confirm your suspicions. How a woman's body notifies her that she is pregnant and the order in which these signs appear vary from woman to woman. Here are common signs of early pregnancy.

WHAT YOU MAY EXPERIENCE	COMMENT
Fatigue	You no longer have the stamina for usual activities, such as walking up a hill or staying awake after supper. The changes in your body are using huge amounts of energy.
Nausea and vomiting (morning sickness)	Morning sickness may be confused with the flu or feeling like you're "coming down with something." It can range from a mild feeling of nagging unease or queasiness to day-long nausea or dry heaves.
Missed menstrual period	There are also some nonpregnancy-related reasons for menstrual irregularity, such as stress.
Slight staining or spotting	Bleeding or spotting at the time of implantation can be mistaken for menstruation, and a few woman may experience bleeding in the early months of pregnancy at the time when they would otherwise have menstruated.
Aversions to odors, alcohol, and smoke	Baby-protective mechanisms click in. You begin skipping your morning coffee; exposure to cigarette smoke makes you sick.
Food cravings	Maybe you salt everything you eat or you can't get enough orange juice. Mysteriously, you may crave foods that you seldom ate before or previously found distasteful.
Breast changes	The changes are similar to premenstrual feelings in your breasts, only more dramatic: nipples tingle, breasts feel tender and fuller, the areola begins to darken, and tiny glands on the areola enlarge.
Crampy pelvic discomfort	Discomfort may be felt generalized throughout the lower abdomen and pelvis; sharp one-sided pain is not normal and should be reported to your doctor.
Abdominal discomfort, bloating	You may feel gassy and crampy and, as with morning sickness, this symptom may be confused with the beginning of an illness.
Frequent urination	Early on, you will urinate more often due to pregnancy hormones. (Later on, it will be caused by pressure of the enlarging uterus on the bladder.)

Pregnancy Tests

You no longer have to wait until you've missed a period or two to confirm you're pregnant. By the end of the first week after conception, when implantation occurs, the developing placenta begins to produce the hormone HCG — human chorionic gonadotropin. This hormone, detectable as early as one week after conception in your blood and seven to ten days after conception in your urine is the basis of all pregnancy tests.

Urine tests for pregnancy. A urine test performed in your doctor's office or at home (if you properly follow the directions of a do-it-yourself home pregnancy kit) is nearly 100 percent accurate by seven to ten days after conception. Of course, the test is not foolproof. The results of urine pregnancy tests performed in a doctor's office are usually more accurate since the tests are performed by a person used to doing them and whose hands are not trembling. A very early test may register negative if your body has not yet produced enough HCG to be detected, and a repeat test a few days to a week later may come out positive. Also, according to the American Academy of Obstetrics and Gynecology, a few medical conditions and some drugs can produce a false-positive urine-test result, indicating that you are pregnant when you really are not. False-negative test results (showing that you are not pregnant when you really are) may also occasionally occur. False-positive results rarely occur as long as the directions are followed accurately. False-negative results are more common. Waiting for the test result in a home pregnancy kit may be the longest five minutes of your life, and your reaction may be a mix of many emotions.

Regardless of the test results, if you could be pregnant or suspect you are, take care of yourself and your baby as if you were pregnant. If you absolutely, positively have to know, have a blood test done, which is more accurate than a urine test.

The blood test for pregnancy. Performed in your practitioner's office or a laboratory on a few drops of blood, this test is nearly 100 percent accurate (assuming no lab error) as early as one week after conception and will give you the results within a day or two.

By the time you have missed a period, urine and blood tests (barring human error in performing the tests) should be 100 percent accurate in detecting pregnancy. If your period is late, but a pregnancy test is negative, wait a week and repeat either test (urine or blood). You may have conceived later than you thought or the HCG level in your blood or urine may still not be high enough to be detected by the test. If you have missed a period and suspect you are pregnant, yet home pregnancy tests continue to be negative, check with your doctor to rule out an ectopic pregnancy (a pregnancy that implants in a place other than your uterus; see page 28).

No matter how you get the news, whether by a color change on a chart or a phone call from your doctor, make the news-breaking event special. Most women remember the "positive" event as vividly as their baby's birthweight.

My husband froze in his tracks. His mouth was gaping. That day we both walked around in a daze, on a roller coaster of emotions: excited, scared, happy, anxious, crying, laughing.

are making new organs: your uterus is growing a placenta to nourish your baby, and the baby is growing organs of his or her own. All that growth consumes a lot of energy. Add to your tiredness the ravages of morning sickness and the big psychological changes pregnancy brings, and you're bound to be exhausted.

This strange fatigue will subside in the middle trimester. You will regain your normal energy level as your body becomes more accustomed to being pregnant. This is not to say you won't be tired now and then. In the last six to eight weeks especially, you will be very tired because of the heavy load your body carries around, but this is a different type of tiredness. Consider fatigue in early pregnancy to be a signal as well as a symptom. It's your body's warning light, saying "slow down, take time off, pace yourself, refuel." You need to rest because much of your energy is being diverted to the rapidly growing person inside. Refueling yourself so that you'll have fuel for your baby is the key to an energy-efficient pregnancy. Here are some ideas to minimize fatigue:

Consider yourself. Here's a vital principle that will hold true during pregnancy, when you have a new baby, and for years afterward: **take good care of yourself so that you can take good care of your baby.** Managing your fatigue in the first months of pregnancy is good preparation for handling fatigue in the first months postpartum. The first hurdle to get over is recognizing that you need rest. Convince yourself that you need to make changes and that throughout your pregnancy you need to be on the receiving end as well as being the giver.

Being very tired was always the first sign for me that I was pregnant. I would fall asleep on the couch at eight o'clock at night. My husband called it "sleeping for two." It's funny, but it's true.

Change your priorities. You cannot expect yourself to be housekeeper, wage earner, and ever-ready-and-willing lover all the time, even if you want to be; you won't have the energy. You will have days when you feel you are getting nothing done or just barely getting by between naps. Yet you are doing the most important job in the world — growing a baby. As much as possible (and it's more easily advised than done), temporarily shelve obligations that keep you from resting enough. If you are a woman who does too much, don't try to be all things to all people; you can't, and no one should expect you to be.

Dr. Linda notes: I found it helpful to make a list of all the tasks I had to do and divide them into three parts. The first part was things I absolutely had to get done and could only do myself; the second part was tasks that I could delegate — and I really had to delegate these; the third part was tasks that could be ignored, and I crossed them out with a big, red pencil. Whenever I started feeling overwhelmed, I simply asked myself, "What are the consequences of not getting something done?" I discovered that 90 percent of the time, life went on if I simply ignored the tasks.

Sleep like a baby. Make sleep a priority. Go to bed when you are tired, even if it means missing a favorite TV show. (Tape it or watch it in reruns while nursing your baby.) As much as you need some time to unwind at the end of the day, you need sleep more. If possible, wake up naturally when your body

Writing Your Baby's Story

Martha has enjoyed writing journals during our pregnancies — and someday we hope our children will enjoy reading them. You may find, as we have, that your personal pregnancy journal becomes one of your most prized possessions.

Why write. Writing about your baby and about yourself makes this inner relationship more real. This exercise also has therapeutic value. When you are struggling with difficult emotions, putting them into words helps you define and understand what you are feeling. Oftentimes, expressing your problems in writing helps you come up with solutions. When you reread it in years to come, your journal will also help you replay one of the highlights of your life, and it will fascinate your child when he or she is ready to have babies. We are rereading our pregnancy journals as we write this book. When we look up during our reading and see our rambunctious son run across the room, we realize, "There goes that little person whom we used to know only as 'Thumper.'"

I look forward to giving my journal to my children when they become expectant parents. I believe they will be thrilled to read about their lives before they were born, and even during their infancy and childhood. I hope that my journal is just one more way of keeping my children connected to their parents.

What to record. What you write and how you write it is up to you. You might write a very simple chronicle of what you're doing and how you are feeling. Or you may want to write as if you were talking to your baby. Record how you feel each day — your joys, your worries, especially what you did to help yourself feel better. The important point is to get it down; don't get hung up on how you say it. You may want to highlight special occasions, such as discovering you were pregnant, feeling the first kick, making the first baby-item purchase, and experiencing the first twinge of labor. Tell your baby how you <u>felt</u> at these moments.

Recording tips. You can collect your thoughts in an elaborate fill-in pregnancy journal or a simple seventy-five-cent notebook. We have found it easiest to keep a pocket-size tape recorder handy in our

---

is ready, not to the buzz of a preset alarm clock. Steal a nap after work or take a fifteen-minute catnap with your head on your desk at lunchtime. Most pregnant women find they cannot go from sunrise to sundown without taking a nap.

Show and tell. Your spouse and your older children may not totally understand why you are so tired or why you may not be able to do as much as they would like you to do. They need to know why you drift off to sleep while reading bedtime stories, seem to be tuned to another wavelength during a conversation, leave the laundry unfolded, order takeout food three times a week, or take on fewer clients. Few men and no children truly understand the energy-consuming changes that go on in a pregnant woman, especially in the early months. Talk to them. Tell them how very tired you are (and that things will get better in a month or two). Read this chapter together. Use picture books to show your

home and to carry it with us when we go outside. We dictate memorable moments when they happen, sometimes even as they are occurring, such as first kicks. Once you get hooked on recording your baby's story (on paper or on tape) while he or she grows in the womb, you will want to continue this exercise during infancy and childhood. It's best to make short, frequent entries, with longer, more elaborate ones reserved for times of exciting changes in your baby's growth or your feelings. There will be times when you are tired or otherwise occupied and your journal goes without an entry for a few days.

I feel being pregnant is the greatest part of being a woman. During my pregnancy I felt that my life was just about perfect, like I was doing exactly what I'm supposed to do. I never felt better about being a woman in all my life. I wouldn't have traded it for the world. I also have more of an appreciation for my mother. I wish I knew exactly what she felt like when she was pregnant with me and what kind of mom she was when I was little. I wish my mom had written her thoughts down.

If you journalize during each pregnancy, you will be able to compare how you have changed from pregnancy to pregnancy. You will be amazed at how each story is different. Also, encourage your spouse to make entries in the journal. After all, fathers have feelings, too.

During my pregnancy I had feelings that I had never had before and may never have again, and so did my husband. These experiences were too unique to go unrecorded.

This is a valuable story only you can tell (and perhaps only your family will want to read). The time in your womb is a very short time in the total life of your child, but keeping a journal will make these memories last a lifetime.

At the end of each month you will notice a couple of pages to help you create your own pregnancy diary. After your baby's birth, you can photocopy these pages and collate them into a diary that will be treasured by you and your co-star forever.

family how the baby is growing, how the new organs are forming, how you are growing a placenta and your uterus is getting bigger. Once you explain to your mate why you are not able to function at peak capacity with just the help of a soda cracker and a half-hour nap, he is likely to be more sympathetic — and more helpful.

Dr. Linda notes: *With my third pregnancy, I described my early feelings to my older*

children as like having stomach flu and bone-chilling fatigue plus queasiness.

Listen to your body. You will have days when you feel best being busy. You will look forward to going to work or you'll tackle household projects with gusto. You will also have days when your body tells you that you need time off — not just off your feet but time off from social, household, and interpersonal responsibilities — completely off. And, unfortunately, you may not know ahead of time how you'll feel from one day to the next. Try not to agonize over your body's unpredictability; accept that there just isn't enough energy to go around to continue your prepregnant lifestyle. Don't let yourself get overtired; that way you'll have some energy reserved for things that must get done. You may need a day or two of "sick leave" now and then. If you have a demanding job, you may also need to negotiate easier working hours. (See the related discussion, "Working While Pregnant," page 134.)

Keep a peaceful home. The pregnant mind needs rest just as the pregnant body does. Favor the factors in your environment that give you peace and minimize those that don't. Arrange for a sitter or for a few hours of preschool for any restless little charges. Try classical music, relaxation tapes, or a warm soak. (Avoid getting too hot, though; see page 56.) Now is a good time for your mate to learn the fine art of massage. Do not feel guilty about the time you spend relaxing. You need it and your baby needs it.

Enjoy the great outdoors. A change of scenery is good for a tired mind and body. During times when your body is willing, treat yourself to exercise (not too strenuous): a long walk in the park, a shopping trip, a relaxing swim. The change of scenery will be as good for a weary mind as the moderate workout will be for your body. Know that there will be days when the mind is willing but the body is not, and listen to your body. There's no reason a bike ride can't wait until tomorrow. (See the related discussion, "Exercising Safely While Pregnant," page 169.)

Eat to your body's content. Not eating enough can lower your energy and aggravate fatigue. Choose nutritious food and nibble frequently throughout the day. (See suggestions for eating well when you don't feel well and on maintaining good nutrition while pregnant in "Eating Right for Two," pages 87 to 102.)

Notice that the suggestions outlined above incorporate the mainstays of anyone's well-being: eating right, sleeping enough, relaxing, and exercising. While pregnant you need an extra dose of these energy replenishers.

Sick. The nausea, queasiness, vomiting, and general abdominal discomfort that many pregnant women endure can sour the sweet feelings about being pregnant. It is hard to feel good about growing a baby when you feel so lousy yourself, especially when "morning sickness" extends to all hours of the day. While a perfectly settled stomach is rare during early pregnancy, there are many things you can do to relieve digestive discomforts. Here are common questions pregnant mothers ask about morning sickness:

I am newly pregnant and I feel fine, but I dread the morning sickness I hear other pregnant mothers complain about. How might I feel?

The intensity and duration of morning sickness is as individual as a mother's weight gain. You may experience some or all of the symptoms mentioned in the next answer. Fortunately, few mothers suffer all of these miseries all the time.

The two big miseries of morning sickness are hypersensitivity to odors and aversion to certain foods. Certain smells may "go right to your stomach," triggering instant nausea. Some women find strong odors, such as garlic, fish, or coffee, particularly offensive, whether or not they minded them before. Others complain that typical household odors that didn't bother them prepregnancy become intensely unpleasant. The family dog may smell more "doggy." A favorite perfume may send a woman running outdoors to retch. Even favorite foods may now be inedible because the smell sets off a gag response. Some women find even the normal masculine odors of their beloved mate repulsive.

Aversion to foods can also take many forms. Sometimes women are unable to eat certain foods (meat, greens, milk) without gagging. At other times, only a few foods are palatable. We suspect that the stereotypical pregnant woman's "cravings" are actually hunger for the few things she can stand to eat. It is not uncommon for women to feel that nothing tastes good. So why eat? Not eating can actually aggravate the cycle of nausea: a woman feels too nauseated to eat, waits too long between snacks or meals, ends up eating too much, and throws up.

While much of morning sickness revolves around food — even the thought of preparing a meal sickens many pregnant women — sometimes it seems to come out of nowhere. Some mothers find they have regular periods of queasiness; others feel ill all day long. Nor is it uncommon for a mother who is feeling fine one moment to be hit by a sudden urge to throw up, with no apparent trigger in sight (or smell).

Some women are able to refuse to vomit, using mind over matter. More seem to get relief from throwing up, so they let it happen. (Many women who feel sick all day wish they could throw up, but they can't.) Some want to sleep more because, for them, sleep makes morning sickness go away.

There is no "right" way to have morning sickness. Whether you experience slight queasiness, feelings of breathlessness, dizziness, a sense of being suffocated, or have the dry heaves or the full-blown whoopsies, you've joined the club.

Do all pregnant women experience morning sickness?

No. A few women coast through early pregnancy with never a twinge of nausea. Some experience no stomach upset, and others suffer only occasional queasiness. But these lucky women are the exceptions rather than the rule. If you're pregnant, expect to feel pregnant. Around 80 percent of pregnant women experience nausea, retching, vomiting, or all of the above at some time during their pregnancy.

I feel sick to my stomach in the evening. Could this be morning sickness?

The term "morning sickness" is misleading. Morning sickness, afternoon sickness, evening sickness, midnight sickness — call it what you want. We have heard this malady called "pregnancy sickness," but we do not like the term. Pregnancy is already regarded as an illness in some circles, and using this term simply fosters that misconception. Pregnancy is a normal and natural state. While it is more common to feel nauseated early in the day and early in pregnancy, the intestinal upsets of pregnancy can occur at any time of the day or night and in any month of your pregnancy. The term "morning sickness" was probably coined by men who remember their wives' being most miserable in the morning but weren't around the rest of the day.

If pregnancy is so great, why do I feel so miserable?

It is biologically correct to blame your mood swings and your morning sickness on those hormones. It helps to think of pregnancy hormones as a miracle drug that is necessary for maintaining the well-being of mother and baby. Yet these hormones, like all drugs, have a few unpleasant side effects, namely intestinal upsets. For example, the same hormone that supports your pregnancy (human chorionic gonadotropin, or HCG) also unsettles your stomach. Levels of the hormone cholecystokinin also increase in pregnant women. This hormone increases the efficiency of digestion by making better metabolic use of food within the mother's system. The unpleasant side effect is that while increasing the body's ability to store energy, this hormone also contributes to low blood sugar, nausea, dizziness, delayed emptying of the stomach, and the after-meal sleepiness many pregnant women experience. Rising estrogen and progesterone levels also contribute to nausea by their direct influence on intestinal hormones. You are likely to feel the worst when hormonal changes are the greatest — in the first trimester. By the end of the third month, when the blood level of some of these hormones levels off or starts to decline, so (usually) do the intestinal maladies caused by these hormones. Expect to have more than your fair share of morning sickness if you are carrying twins; you are producing more hormones, so you may feel "more pregnant" than a woman who is growing just one baby.

Pregnancy hormones also slow the action of your intestines, causing accumulation of stomach acids, indigestion, and heartburn. All these contribute to morning sickness. The slowing of your intestines plus their competition with the expanding uterus for room to work may leave you feeling constipated, another addition to your long list of intestinal upsets.

I know I'm supposed to gain weight, but I'm afraid I'll lose weight since I feel so sick.

Don't worry about losing weight during periods of sickness. In fact, most women continue to gain weight quite well even during these weeks or months, probably because in order to feel better, they are eating small meals frequently. Surprisingly, many women end up eating more food during periods of morning sickness, not less. Even those women who do lose weight make up for it by gaining weight quickly once the sickness subsides.

When should I worry about vomiting so much? Will all my nausea and vomiting hurt my baby?

No. The good news is your baby doesn't share your misery. While it's not literally true, preborn babies are often dubbed "the perfect parasite." For most nutrients, when there isn't enough for two, baby will get what he or she needs, and mother's needs will suffer.

In most cases of morning sickness your body chemistry is not affected, you don't lose weight, and you eventually feel better. Less than 1 percent of pregnant women suffer a severe form of persistent vomiting called "hyperemesis gravidarum" (Latin for excessive vomiting in pregnancy). In this condition, the body is unable to compensate for the relentless vomiting. It loses valuable body salts, called "electrolytes," and body fluids; in other words, the mother becomes dehydrated. If unrecognized and untreated, this severe vomiting can make you very sick, which may, in turn, compromise your baby. With treatment, even babies of mothers with severe hyperemesis stay remarkably healthy.

Here are signs that you are becoming de-hydrated and should call your doctor:

- The vomiting is not getting better.
- You're urinating less and your urine appears darker in color.
- Your mouth, eyes, and skin are feeling dry.
- You are feeling increasingly tired.
- Your mental acuity is lessening.
- You are feeling increasingly weak and faint.
- You haven't been able to keep any food or drink down for twenty-four hours.

In addition to preventing dehydration, you need to prevent a condition called "starvation ketosis." When your body is starved for nutrition, especially carbohydrates, your tissues begin to break down, and an excess of ketones (an organic compound) is produced in your blood, which aggravates nausea. To keep this from happening, try drinking salty fluids, such as chicken broth, and oral electrolyte solutions (e.g., Pedialyte, available over the counter).

Because of the uncertainties surrounding the safety of antivomiting medications, most practitioners prefer (and most women welcome) twenty-four to forty-eight hours of intravenous therapy to combat dehydration. The fluids and salts that were lost are replenished, and feelings of well-being quickly return. Unless seriously dehydrated, most pregnant women suffering from dehydration or ketosis can receive intravenous therapy in the comfort of their homes.

I've always felt that there's a naturally good reason for the way my body acts and feels. Does this reasoning apply to morning sickness?

Yes. In this case there *is* logic to the biologic. Think of morning sickness as a protective mechanism, forcing you to retreat from substances or situations that may not be good for you or your baby. Most noticeable is the hypersensitivity to potentially harmful odors, such as paint, gasoline fumes, and tobacco smoke. One time Martha knew she was pregnant when the smell of coffee made her sick; in another pregnancy, a less-than-inviting glass of champagne was the telltale sign. Nausea and aversion to odors may be nature's way of warning mothers to watch what they breathe or consume. Some mothers dub this sharpened sense of smell "radar nose." Biologists theorize that an enhanced sense of smell allows pregnant animals to smell dangers before they see them. Pregnant women, of course, are not always impressed with this system. At times, it seems that mother nature is being overprotective.

My obstetrician told me that my nausea is a sign of a healthy baby, but I have my suspicions I am being told this just to make me feel better.

If your misery needs some scientific consoling, it may help to know that the high levels of pregnancy hormones that contribute to nausea also suggest a well-implanted embryo. In fact, statistics show that the more nausea a mother has, the more likely she is to deliver a healthy baby. In obstetrical jargon, "the sicker the mother, the better the outcome." In some women, low pregnancy-hormone levels reflect a pregnancy that isn't developing normally and that has an increased risk of miscarrying. This does not mean, though, that if you don't feel sick, you won't deliver a healthy baby. Many mothers coast through pregnancy with a minimum of morning sickness and are blessed with healthy babies.

There are days when I feel so sick, the only thing that makes me feel better is giving in to my cravings, but I worry that I'm not eating a balanced diet.

When you are feeling sick, the last thing you think about is the nutritional content of what you are eating. You just want to eat what helps you feel better — and that's what you should do. Remember, any food (except those known to be unhealthy or unsafe) that helps mother feel better by staying down and giving her energy will be good for baby. There may be days when you seem to overdose on carbohydrates, other days when you consume megadoses of protein, and days when you simply eat or drink anything that will stay down. You may be surprised to find that the variety of food cravings you experience over a month leads you to a diet that is not so unbalanced after all. When nausea is at its worst, forget about a balanced day's nutrition. Shoot for a balanced week instead.

During stomach upsets there is no such thing as a good or bad food. Eat whatever appeals to you and helps you feel better. (We know one mother, previously a vegetarian, who lived on roast beef sandwiches, orange juice, and tomatoes for two months. She suspected her body was crying out for iron and vitamin C, necessary for the metabolism of iron, but it really didn't matter: she just couldn't eat anything else.) If your nausea is constant, keep a tray full of feel-better foods at your bedside and chairside — and nibble away. Strive for a more balanced diet on days when you are better able to tolerate it.

I am pregnant for the second time. With my first pregnancy I felt "green" for four months. Will I feel better or worse this time?

Odds are you will feel better. Like labor, morning sickness is usually easier to endure once you've been through it. You can anticipate how you might feel and you have already developed coping strategies. Yet, because the hormonal surges of each pregnancy are different, the duration and intensity of the morning sickness they engender may be different, too. Martha found that her last two pregnancies caused her to feel much sicker, and stay that way longer, than her first three. The middle two were somewhere in between. Once past sixteen weeks, though, she loved being pregnant those last two times as much as the other five times.

My husband isn't very sympathetic to my feeling sick. He thinks it's all in my head.

Those who say morning sickness is all in the head have never had a baby in their uterus or don't even have a uterus. Your husband needs a clear picture of what you are going through. If he has ever been seasick or carsick (those who have will never forget that feeling), tell him to imagine feeling like that most of the day. And then tell him it's all in *his* head. True, emotional upsets can aggravate morning sickness, but your body, not your mind, is where you feel the effects. Lovingly remind your husband that it's your body that changes during pregnancy, not his. Many men feel helpless when they don't understand why their mate is miserable and feel even more frustrated when they can't fix it. It's hard for them to stand by and see the person they love hurting. Let your husband know how he can help ease your discomforts (see suggestions, page 19). It's great practice for his later role as labor comforter.

There is, however, sometimes an emotional

component to morning sickness. Women in our culture are preprogrammed to expect to feel sick. The attitude of "I'm pregnant, therefore I'll be sick" contributes to a self-fulfilling prophecy. Our family hobby is sailing. One of the laws of the sea is never to talk about feeling sick, especially around novice sailors. Just the thought of feeling seasick can be contagious. By the same token, it's probably a good idea morning sickness support groups aren't very popular.

For most women, morning sickness begins toward the end of the third week and eases toward the end of the third month. But don't count on the end of the first trimester bringing an end to your morning sickness. Some women continue to experience nausea and vomiting of varying degrees well into the second trimester, though most report it eases slightly as the months go on. A few rare but unfortunate souls endure nine months of nausea and are delivered of this malady only when they deliver their baby.

Dr. Linda notes: I could identify no rhyme or reason to my own morning sickness. I had very little with my first pregnancy, a boy, and almost none with my third, a girl, but was violently sick practically all of the first few months with the middle pregnancy, which was a girl. This was completely unrelated to my stress level, which was consistently high during all these pregnancies.

How long will this miserable feeling last?

Many mothers are rewarded with "well windows" — hours of the day or even whole days when they feel well enough to function normally. As your pregnancy progresses, keep your perspective. The good days will get bet-ter, and there will be fewer and less intense bad days. Morning sickness, like labor, sooner or later will pass.

Seventeen Ways to Ease the Discomforts of Morning Sickness

There are as many remedies for morning sickness as there are for infant colic. Most women have found the following to be successful — at least some of the time.

Detect the trigger and avoid it if you can. After a couple of weeks of living with nausea, you will probably have a mental "misery list" of sights, sounds, and scents that set off queasiness. Most women find their hypersensitivity to certain odors the most unsettling. While odor-free living is as unreasonable an expectation as pain-free childbirth, there are things you can do to identify and remove the triggers. Compare your good and bad days. What was different about the day when you seemed constantly sick versus the day when you felt relatively comfortable? As much as humanly possible, design your day to avoid the known triggers. If your mate's morning breath gives you the dry heaves, delay the morning kiss. If the smell of wet dog or the litter box gets to you, inform your mate that he'll have a new job for a while. (*Note:* Pregnant women must avoid cat feces anyway, because they may contain toxoplasmosis bacteria, which can cause serious damage to the baby. See page 57.) To some extent, identifying those odors that irritate you will keep you busy while the problem naturally gets better.

Of course, if your trigger is dog food and there's no one else around to feed the dog, you're going to have to find a way to cope. Most pregnant women become adept at mouth-breathing, holding their breath for a

Food Cravings

Veteran pregnant women find that the best way to handle food cravings, especially during periods of morning sickness, is to give in to them. Treating your stomach to what it's asking for may make the difference between a queasy day and a comfortable one. Cravings during pregnancy may actually reflect the wisdom of the body: many nutritionists who study food cravings conclude that several common cravings actually serve vital nutritional needs during pregnancy. Consider two common cravings: pickles and potato chips. These foods are high in salt, which your body needs, and they stimulate thirst, so you drink more water. Perhaps your body knows that it will need a lot of extra fluid to fill up baby's amniotic swimming pool. Some women even yearn for foods they never liked before, perhaps because their changing body has nutritional needs that it didn't have before they were pregnant. Most women find that their cravings change throughout pregnancy, perhaps in keeping with their changing nutritional needs. And as with morning sickness, food cravings don't seem to be as extreme in the later months of pregnancy.

Dr. Linda notes: I noticed severe cravings for steak and hamburger early on in pregnancy, a somewhat unusual response. My husband was shocked, since he had rarely seen me eat any meat other than lean chicken or fish. I'm sure it was my body's way of getting extra minerals and iron, since my diet tended to be somewhat low in these.

Your wants and your body's needs may not be all that far apart, but don't rely on your cravings to be 100 percent nutritionally correct. Today, with fast-food restaurants, packaged foods, and high-power advertising, a pregnant woman's wants are influenced by many outside messages as well as by her baby's needs. Feeling your life won't continue unless you get your nightly hot fudge sundae is more likely to be an emotional need than a nutritional one. If you absolutely, positively must have that late-night Chinese takeout (even if it means your spouse must risk his life on a wintery night to get it), give in and consider it a biological need rather than an emotional want. But if you feel your crave control is getting out of hand, take a closer look. List them, the amounts you eat, and the frequency with which you consume these favored foods. Consult your health-care provider or nutritionist for help in determining whether these cravings are in your and your baby's best interest. But, as a general rule, when it comes to food cravings during pregnancy, consider what you want to eat to be what you need, unless the food you are craving is clearly unhealthy.

I look at sweets in magazines and actually start drooling. My big craving is Gummy Bears. I just love them. Unfortunately, I don't think it's healthy for my two-year-old to see Mommy sitting there wolfing down Gummy Bears and then telling her they're not good for her. I wish I could be more like my friends and crave healthy things, like fruits and salads.

few seconds or holding their noses to avoid the smells. (Doing chores with one hand now is great practice for when the baby comes.)

Give your day a comfortable start. Waking up suddenly with an acid-filled, hungry stomach is a surefire setup for morning sickness, and, as many women note, if you start the morning off sick, you are likely to stay sick all day. Give your queasy stomach a fighting chance. Eat something before you go to bed so your stomach won't be so empty at 7:00 A.M. Put a tray of easy-to-digest favorites at your bedside. When you trek to the bathroom in the middle of the night, treat your stomach to a nibble. A good rule is to put food into your mouth before your feet touch the floor. Continue to munch all morning, carrying your nibble tray around with you if necessary.

Sudden transitions often trigger nausea. And what could be more unsettling than being abruptly awakened by an inconsiderate alarm? Ease into your day. Try awakening to soothing music from a clock radio. At least one company manufactures a noiseless alarm light, which gradually increases brightness at a preset time. If you don't have to awaken at a set time, don't. If your mate must, get him his own noiseless alarm, perhaps a pager that clips onto his clothing and vibrates at a preset time.

If possible, begin your day with a non-stressful, enjoyable activity, such as walking, meditating, or reading. Preprogram your body for the kind of day you want it to have.

Graze to your stomach's content. Low blood sugar, which can trigger nausea, can occur upon awakening or anytime you go many hours without food. The traditional eating pattern of three squares a day is not meant

for pregnant women. A more digestible pattern is six smaller meals. Try this especially when your stomach thinks it doesn't want anything at all. Grazing on *nutritious* snacks throughout the day keeps your stomach satisfied and your blood sugar steady.

I felt like I was always hungry, always thinking about my next meal. As my stomach got empty, I would just get sick, so I had to keep my stomach not just partially full, but full all the time. Right after breakfast I would think, "What am I going to eat for lunch?" My days revolved around food and what I was going to eat next.

Nibble on stomach-friendly foods. Some foods are just naturally harder on stomachs than others. High-fat, spicy, and some high-fiber foods are hard to digest. Try to follow these easy-on-the-stomach eating tips:

- Consume rapid-transit foods: foods with nutrients that are easily digestible and pass through the stomach quickly, such as liquids, smoothies, yogurts, and low-fat, high-carbohydrate foods. Avoid hard-to-digest fatty foods and fried foods, such as premium ice cream, french fries, and fried chicken.
- Try nutrient-dense foods, those that are packed with a lot of nutrition for each calorie: avocados, kidney beans, cheese, fish, nut butter, whole-grain pasta, brown rice, tofu, and turkey. If peanut butter doesn't appeal to you, try a milder-tasting butter, such as almond or cashew butter. Spread it *thinly* on crackers, bread, apple slices, or celery sticks; a large glob of it may be slow to digest due to its high fat content.
- To help avoid dehydration, which aggravates nausea, eat foods that stimulate your

thirst. You might try the three P's: pickles, potato chips, and pretzels.
- Avoid letting your saliva hit an empty stomach. An empty stomach is hypersensitive to saliva, and nausea will soon follow. Most women produce an excess of saliva while pregnant, and even thinking about food can stimulate you to salivate. Lining your stomach with milk, yogurt, or ice cream before eating a saliva-stimulating food (such as salty or dry foods, such as crackers) may keep saliva-induced nausea from striking. Many pregnant women claim peppermint candy or gum helps nausea, but it's best not to use either on an empty stomach, as these foods increase saliva production but put no bulk in the stomach.
- If your prenatal vitamins trigger nausea, try taking them with your biggest meal.
- Foods with a high water content are not only easy on your intestines but also prevent the dehydration and constipation that aggravate nausea. Try melons, grapes, frozen fruit bars, lettuce, apples, pears, celery, and rhubarb.
- Determine which all-day suckers (Lifesavers, lemon drops, etc.) work for you, and tote around a pocketful.

Whenever we went to a restaurant, I couldn't even look at a menu without nausea coming on. Sometimes just thinking about food made the nausea worse. I learned to open a menu and quickly select the very first thing I glanced upon.

I learned to stay away from anything that could cause heartburn. For me, heartburn and morning sickness were a drastic duo I didn't want.

Eat high-energy foods. Complex carbohydrates (grandmothers called them "starches") act as time-release energy capsules, slowly re-leasing energy into your bloodstream and helping to keep your appetite satisfied. The main food group represented here is grains (rice, corn, wheat, oats, millet, barley), found in breads, cereals, pastas, and crackers. The whole-grain versions of these foods are even more nutritious and satisfying.

Stick to feel-better favorites. Within a few weeks of trying to manage morning sickness, you will have compiled a list of those foods that help you feel better — or at least don't aggravate your nausea. But don't be surprised if a favorite food suddenly loses its magic. Go ahead and switch to whatever works, even if it is less healthy. Chances are the foods you crave are those that will help you feel better.

Make yourself eat. There may be days when you don't want to eat or drink anything. But you are likely to feel worse if you don't eat or drink something. Don't set yourself up for a day in the bathroom by allowing yourself to get an acid-filled stomach and low blood sugar. Eat something. Anything.

Get out. Just as you may have days when you don't feel like eating but you must, there will be days when you have no motivation to get off the couch. Do it anyway. Fresh air, a change of scenery, even visiting friends or going to a movie may provide a stomach-settling distraction. If you feel better being active, be active. If you feel better resting, by all means rest. But try not to do all your resting in the same place. If you work in an office, don't eat lunch at your desk. Go out, even if only for a few minutes.

Dr. Linda notes: *Even when I felt like not going to work, I was actually better off at work. I felt awful anyway. At least while I was working I had less time to think about how awful I felt.*

Drive, don't ride. If riding in a car bothers you, volunteer to drive. When your mind is actively engaged and your eyes are anticipating the stops and starts ahead, you may have less of a problem. (This, by the way, explains why the helmsman on a boat is the least likely to get seasick.)

Delegate, delegate, delegate. Stay in bed until both your stomach and the household settles. Let your mate get the older kids off to school or the little one fed and occupied before he starts making mom the target of his toddler-size demands. This prepares your spouse to take over the morning duties at least in the first few months after birth. Keep in mind the list of what triggers your nausea and use your household help — spouse and older kids — to do the jobs that unsettle you. Delegate feeding the dog or cleaning his dish. You deserve to wake up to a clean-smelling kitchen. Have the trash taken out and the dishes done the night before. Let your comfort needs be known. Post a list of things that bother you and things that make you feel better. Your spouse's job description may change as your body does: there will be days when he becomes a gofer, doing the shopping and running errands; on other days he'll be a caterer, serving you snacks or meals. Don't feel guilty about asking for cereal in bed. Remember that you're growing a baby for both of you. If a special food (even one requiring a trip to the grocery store), a foot rub, or relief from a problem chore (such as doing laundry in a musty basement) would help, speak up. You may have to cook simpler meals. If the entire family eats cheese and crackers and carrots for a few meals, they will survive. If your spouse complains, let him cook.

Dr. Bill notes: Martha had a craving for zucchini, and I would often make midnight treks to the supermarket to satisfy her cravings for before-bed zucchini pancakes. One night as I was going through the checkout counter with a foot-long zucchini, the clerk concluded, "Your wife must be pregnant."

As you become hypersensitive to your environment, your spouse needs to become extra sensitive to your needs. Some women find the smorgasbord of aromas in supermarkets intolerable, at least in the early months of pregnancy. Consider your options: send your mate shopping, hire a teen to fetch your groceries, or choose a store that delivers.

I loved my before-dinner naps while my husband cooked. We then enjoyed having dinner together.

Plan ahead. If you know what triggers your nausea, try to arrange for detours around those things. If cooking odors bother you, consider precooking and freezing foods on days when you feel well. Or lower your standards temporarily and buy more convenience foods. If you are invited to another home for dinner, offer to bring a dish you know you'll be able to eat. When you're at work or doing errands, be sure to carry your reliable edibles with you; when a hunger surge hits, the nausea is sure to follow if you don't have a tried-and-true tidbit handy.

Reduce stress. Morning sickness is in your body, not your mind. Yet mind and body are connected. Your brain and stomach share nerves, so when you are upset, your stomach can be, too. Many mothers get stuck in a stress-nausea cycle. The worse they feel, the more stressed they become, and then they feel worse.

You may have to make major lifestyle and career changes while pregnant. Prenatal researchers feel it's better for a baby in utero to be spared a steady barrage of stress hormones. If your job is giving you lots of stress and little satisfaction, you may need to negotiate some changes in hours or responsibilities or do whatever makes your mind and body feel better. Spouse and kids excluded, rid your home of unnecessary stressors. Learning to reduce stress now is good practice for maintaining serenity as a new mother. Remind yourself that WHAT YOUR BABY NEEDS MOST IS A HAPPY, RESTED MOTHER, BOTH BEFORE AND AFTER BIRTH.

Pregnancy for me was a chance to retire from the rat race. It was a time for me to get

Favorite Comfort Foods

During spells of morning sickness, there is no such thing as a good or bad food, only foods that help you feel better. Here are some stomach-friendly foods, including several that are natural remedies for nausea:

- ginger, available in many forms: root extract, fresh-ground, capsules, tea, sticks, crystals, pickled, or snaps
- lemons: for sucking on or sniffing
- raspberry leaf tea
- mints, peppermint
- potato chips
- potatoes (baked, boiled, mashed)
- salted sunflower seeds
- papaya juice
- chewing gum
- watermelon
- yogurt smoothies
- frozen yogurt
- rice cakes
- grapes
- pickles
- puddings
- chamomile tea
- carbonated mineral water with a twist of lemon
- avocado
- applesauce
- rhubarb
- sorbet, sherbet
- soda crackers
- pears
- celery sticks
- carrot sticks
- lemon drops
- bananas
- licorice
- zucchini
- bagels
- pasta
- cereal
- tomatoes
- oatmeal

   A food or drink that eases nausea in one woman may trigger vomiting in another. By trial and upset, you'll compile your own list of tummy-settlers. Stick to these foods during the first trimester. As your intestines become less selective, increase your menu. Also, keep your list of six or so personal best comfort foods and nibble on these during labor. These will help combat the nausea you may experience.

out of the high-pressure profession of stock-brokering, where I was surrounded by the effects of male hormones; now I could get into my female hormones and be comfortable with it.

Try acupressure. Both Eastern and Western medical practitioners describe a pressure point about two inches above the crease on the inner aspect of the wrist that, if stimulated, may relieve nausea and vomiting associated with pregnancy and other conditions (such as seasickness). Acupressure bands, available without prescription at pharmacies and marine stores, are meant to be worn around one or both wrists. Each band contains a button that presses on the nausea-sensitive pressure point. A study published in the reputable journal *Obstetrics and Gynecology* compared the incidence of morning sickness in pregnant women who wore the real band with that of women who wore a placebo band, one on which the button had been blunted so as not to exert pressure on the adjacent point. Around 60 percent of women felt better during the three days they wore the actual acupressure bands, while only 30 percent in the placebo group felt better. The physicians who organized the study concluded that this method of acupressure was both safe and effective.

Dress comfortably. Wear loose clothing. Many pregnant women find that anything pressing on their abdomen, waist, or neck is irritating and nausea-triggering.

Position yourself for comfort. As if nausea and vomiting were not enough, many women experience heartburn as part of the morning sickness package. This burning feeling, which is caused by reflux of stomach acids into the lower esophagus, occurs more frequently during pregnancy (thanks to hormones, again, which relax the stomach walls) than at other times. For heartburn, gravity will be your best remedy; any position that keeps the outlet of your stomach lower than the inlet will lessen reflux. Keep upright or lie on your right side after eating. Lying on your back is more likely to aggravate heartburn. (For further suggestions, see page 71.)

Sleep it off. It's fortunate that the increased need for sleep coincides with the morning sickness phase. At least you can count on sleep to bring blessed relief. Martha remembers craving sleep for this one reason alone — to escape from nausea. So precious is this rest that you will want to ensure that sleep goes on for as long as possible. For some women, bed rest doesn't help. They need to do something mind-absorbing to get their focus anywhere but their stomach.

If you have a toddler running around, you

Usual Discomfort Foods

- fried foods
- greasy foods
- high-fat foods (read labels)
- sausages
- fried eggs
- spicy foods
- foods containing monosodium glutamate (MSG)
- onions
- sauerkraut
- cabbage
- cauliflower
- caffeine-containing beverages, such as coffee and colas

may not have the luxury of staying in bed or sleeping in. To avoid waking up sick, before retiring, eat one last light meal, preferably of fruit and long-acting complex carbohydrates (grains and bland pasta), which will slowly release energy into your bloodstream throughout the night yet be unlikely to keep you awake. Along with this snack, eat natural antacid foods, such as milk, ice cream, and yogurt to neutralize upsetting stomach acids as you drift off to sleep. Some women find it helpful to take their daily required dose of chewable calcium tablets before retiring; others find it more helpful to take them upon awakening. (Chewable calcium tablets act as an antacid.)

The old saying "She got up on the wrong side of the bed" has some psychological basis. It usually means that she went to bed on the "wrong side." If you go to bed stressed, you are more likely to awaken in the same state. A sleepless night is likely to be followed by a day of vomiting and nausea. To avoid entering sleep with unsettling thoughts on your mind, read or do something relaxing before going to bed. Many couples enjoy using this time to talk about the joys of upcoming parenthood or to practice what we call "laying on of hands": you and your mate put your hands on your abdomen and begin talking to and blessing your preborn child. Pregnant women report this is a very relaxing thought to carry into their sleep.

Be positive. Choose the people with whom you share your misery. Mothers who have been there and felt it will understand. Others won't. Especially try to emphasize the positive parts of pregnancy to your children. When you're having a day when you can't keep anything down, keep your eyes on the prize.

I felt fine in the morning because I had had a good night's sleep, but I felt miserable in the afternoon when the kids came home from school. They would see me only tired, grumpy, and needy. The poor kids didn't get too many decent meals either. One time our fourteen-year-old heard me complaining and groaning and asked, "Mom, are you sorry you're having a baby?" That made me stop and realize that I had better soft-pedal my complaining a bit and try to present a more positive attitude around the children. I didn't want to model all that negativity to my daughters.

My daughter was worth every moment of morning sickness.

HOW YOUR BABY IS GROWING (1–4 WEEKS)

All the time you are working, walking, relaxing, and sleeping there is a miracle going on inside your body.

One week: Egg meets sperm, fertilization occurs. As soon as a sperm cell penetrates the egg, fertilization occurs, usually high up in one of the fallopian tubes. At the moment of fertilization the baby's gender is determined (some sperm produce males, others produce females). Right at the start, the fertilized ovum contains a full complement of genetic codes: twenty-three chromosomes from mom and twenty-three from dad. Occasionally two eggs are fertilized by two sperm, resulting in fraternal twins. Less commonly, one egg is fertilized by one sperm and then divides into two, with identical twins the result. Each day during the four-inch, four-day trip down the fallopian tube, these cells di-

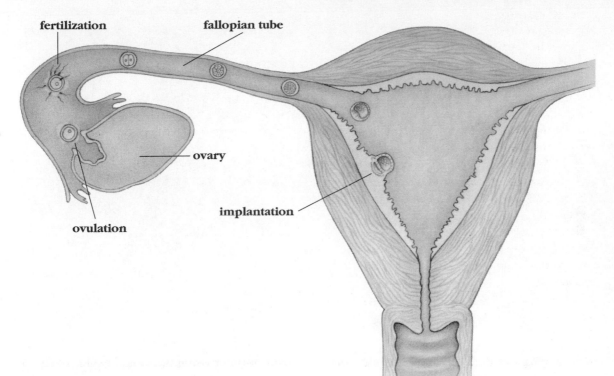

fertilization

fallopian tube

ovary

ovulation

implantation

Week one: from fertilization to implantation.

vide and double in number, so by the time this bundle of baby-to-be reaches the uterus, he or she is at least sixteen cells large. For the first eight weeks, these cells are called an "embryo" by scientists, but most of the moms and dads we know prefer the term "baby."

Two weeks: Implantation occurs. By day seven the embryo, now resembling a microscopic raspberry, searches out a spot to land and implants into the lining of the uterus, usually settling in the upper third or near the top of its new home. As baby burrows into the blood-rich lining, a few drops of bleeding or spotting may occur. This blooming ball of life, called a "blastocyst" — meaning "sprout pouch" — begins to organize into groups of several hundred cells each. Some of these

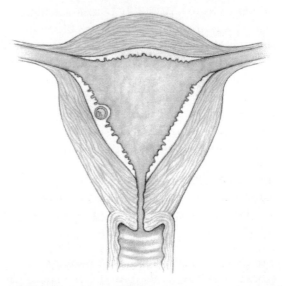

Implantation of the embryo.

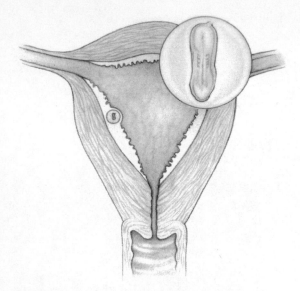

Embryo at 3 weeks.

Embryo at 4 weeks.

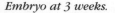

cells take root in the plush uterine lining; others arrange themselves in clusters and cavities, each with a different destiny. The uterus, responding to the presence of the embryo, begins to form a primitive placenta, which transfers nutrients from mother's blood into the developing baby and facilitates disposal of the baby's waste products. As the placenta develops, it begins to produce human chorionic gonadotropin (HCG), a hormone that keeps the uterine lining in place and stimulates its growth by keeping the levels of estrogen and progesterone high. HCG is released into the mother's bloodstream at an increasing rate as the placenta develops. By the end of the second week, a pregnancy test will be able to detect HCG in the mother's urine.

Three weeks: Placenta and baby grow, hormones surge. By now the menstrual period is late. A woman may suspect she is preg-

nant, and her rising hormone level is likely to cause her to begin feeling pregnant. Pregnancy hormones notify the ovaries not to ovulate again, and the ovaries, via hormonal messengers, notify the pituitary gland in the brain to no longer stimulate menstruation. Within three weeks, what started out as a single cell has grown to millions of cells that now begin to differentiate into three types of cells: those that will become the nervous system, skin, and hair; those that will make up the gastrointestinal tract; and those that will form the circulatory, genito-urinary, and musculo-skeletal systems. By the end of the third week, a rudimentary heart tube begins to beat and circulate blood.

Four weeks: Baby takes shape. During this week, baby grows to the size and shape of a curved grain of rice. An umbilical cord containing three distinct blood vessels appears. Along the outer rim of baby's tiny body, blocks of tissue stack up to form the back-bone. Tiny buds, soon to become arms and legs, emerge from the body. The ball-like heart divides into chambers and pumps blood into already formed major vessels. Specialized ultrasonic equipment can even detect a regular heartbeat. Tiny pits now present in the baby's head mark the spots where eyes and ears will form. Lobes of baby's brain and a primitive spinal cord develop. Rudiments of future organs such as the trachea, esophagus, stomach, mouth, liver, gall bladder, thyroid, and urinary system appear. Amazingly, by the time most mothers-to-be attend their first prenatal checkup, most of their baby's major organs are well on their way.

CONCERNS YOU MAY HAVE

As your baby grows, so do your concerns. With something so new and different happening to your body, there's lots to learn and lots to think about. Here are some issues you may be considering for the first time.

Due Date

Like so many aspects of preparing for parenthood, your baby's birth day is not perfectly predictable. That's because babies grow at different rates prenatally, just as they do postnatally. Your health-care provider will calculate your due date by taking the first day of your last normal menstrual period, or LNMP, adding 266 days or thirty-eight weeks (the length of the average pregnancy from the date of conception), plus another fourteen days (the average number of days from the first day of the LNMP to the time of next ovulation). From a due-date calculator, your health-care provider will come up with an estimate for when your baby will be born. And that's all a due date is — an estimate. The actual medical term is "estimated date of delivery," or EDD (you may also see EDC, "estimated date of confinement"). Try this do-it-yourself calculation for determining your due date:

- take the first day of your LNMP (e.g., January 1)
- add one year (January 1 of next year)
- subtract three months (October 1)
- add seven days, and you have your EDD (October 8)

You may notice that your own EDD differs by a couple of days from the one given by your health-care provider. That's because you use months in your calculations (and not all months have the same number of days) while your practitioner uses an EDD chart, which calculates gestation in terms of days. If you are absolutely certain of the day you conceived, add 266 days to this date, and your accuracy will probably beat the charts. Realize, however, that only about 5 percent of babies arrive on their predicted due date, though most mothers give birth within two weeks before or after their EDD.

You can understand why the calculation of the due date is not an exact science if you consider the many uncertainties. A woman may be uncertain of the date of her last "normal" menstrual period. Women who have recently stopped taking birth control pills may experience irregular cycles for a while, making it difficult to pinpoint when normal menstruation resumes and ovulation occurs. Some women have irregular periods for other reasons, so that the time between the start of their period and ovulation may be more or less than fourteen days. Even if you are very regular, the length of your menstrual cycle matters, too: the closer you are to the average twenty-eight-day cycle, the more likely you are to deliver close to your estimated due date. With a long cycle, you're more likely to deliver after the due date, and with a short cycle, you are more likely to deliver before the due date.

For some women and in some obstetrical situations, an accurate due date is important. If your due date and how your baby is growing aren't matching, your health-care provider will look for other signs that you have a special pregnancy (such as multiples or a problem with baby's growth). The good news is that the further your pregnancy progresses, the more accurately your practitioner will be able to estimate your due date. That's why by using the following information, you are likely to get an updated due date as you and your baby grow:

- During your prenatal visits, your practitioner will measure your uterus to see if your baby is growing as anticipated. (The average uterus will have grown to the level of the navel by around twenty weeks.)*

- Using a Doppler ultrasound device, your practitioner will usually be able to hear your baby's heartbeat by twelve weeks.

- Most mothers first feel their baby move by sixteen to twenty weeks. (Second-timers may feel the little flutters earlier because

The "weeks" your practitioner uses to date your pregnancy are measured from the first day of your last normal menstrual period (not when conception occurred) and are therefore approximately two weeks longer than the actual number of weeks you have been pregnant. Be aware that in describing baby's growth throughout this book, we will be using the actual age in weeks from conception. You may want to use this same way of describing your baby in your own journalizing.

they know how to distinguish them from intestinal rumblings.)

- If necessary, your doctor will perform one or two ultrasound examinations between the sixteenth and twentieth week and use this information to update the due date.

Ultrasound is particularly helpful for estimating the delivery date for women with confusing or irregular menstrual periods. The accuracy of ultrasound varies with different stages of pregnancy. During the first twelve to thirteen weeks of pregnancy, ultrasound dating will be accurate to within a few days of baby's actual age. At sixteen to twenty weeks, the margin for error is a week to ten days. By the third trimester, ultrasound estimates of baby's age may be as much as three weeks off.

It's very helpful for obstetrical management to establish an accurate date during the early months of pregnancy. Obstetricians usually stick with that date unless there is overwhelming and consistent evidence that the dating was wrong in the first place. In many instances, if a mother knows the exact day she conceived, her history is more accurate than either menstrual dates or ultrasound dates. Obstetricians usually take the mother's menstrual date to be accurate if the ultrasound dates are within the range of menstrual dates. If repeated ultrasounds point to a different date, your obstetrician may issue a different EDD. Ultrasound dating can be wrong due to both normal biological variations and problems in the pregnancy.

Numbers are nice, but the fact remains that babies determine their own birthdays. *Pencil in* the EDD on your calendar; as the clues come in, you may need to erase one EDD and write in another. In fact, to avoid being disappointed during that last "I can't wait to hold my baby" (or "I can't stand being pregnant any longer") week, you might move the EDD down one week on your calendar. That way, you may be delighted when your baby comes "early." This will also help you avoid those "are you still pregnant?" phone calls that start to come in one day after that elusive due date passes. Another strategy for avoiding this kind of harassment (and it will seem like harassment if your tummy is huge, your baby is late, and your mood is turning sour) is to tell everyone your due date is "early January" instead of January 2, "mid-January" instead of January 10, "late January" instead of January 20, or "early February" instead of January 29. Instead of a due date think a "due week."

Sharing the News

When should you tell friends and family that you are pregnant? You may not be able to keep silent any more than you can later conceal your telltale abdominal bulge. Within minutes after discovering you are pregnant, the urge to tell everyone you know may be overwhelming. And you may not want to hide your pride. Or, you may choose to wait for a while before telling friends and family. No matter whom you tell and when you tell, this is a very special announcement.

Breaking the news to your mate should be a special event. Sharing such life-changing news deserves more than a phone call. Be sure to tell your mate face-to-face. You don't want to miss seeing your spouse's reaction. Especially if this is your first baby, tell your mate in private. He deserves your special attention. You may want to make the announcement over a private candlelit dinner. To have more time to absorb this relationship-changing news, you may want to take a day, a weekend, or a week's vacation as a special

time to let the realities of pregnancy sink in and to share the many feelings and decisions that come with it.

Dr. Bill notes: Ten years later, I still vividly remember the setting in which Martha told me she was pregnant with our sixth child, Matthew. On Christmas Day she gave me a gift-wrapped box that contained the results from an early-pregnancy kit. I still remember opening the package and seeing the purple ring, revealing a positive test. I especially enjoyed reading her attached love note.

Using the maritally correct phrase "*We're* pregnant!" lets your mate know right from the start that something exciting has happened to him, too, and not just to you. Don't be taken aback if your mate does not initially share your excitement, especially if the news comes as a surprise. Your spouse's reaction may not be in sync with yours. You have already had a little time to experience your feelings, and it may take your partner a while to adjust. Don't take negative reactions personally. Your mate may need to work through his concerns: "Is the timing right?" "Can we afford a baby at this time?" "How's this new person going to affect our marriage?" Some new dads-to-be need a bit of time before the reality sinks in and they can get excited about becoming a father.

Decide together when to tell others. You may choose to wait for a while before telling friends and family. You may feel you are not yet ready to be on the receiving end of a barrage of questions and advice about pregnancy and baby care, so you may elect to tell only a chosen few. You may wish to share the news with your nearest and dearest first. If you are private types, you may wish to keep this delicious secret to yourselves at first. If you have had a previous miscarriage or fear you may have one, you may be nervous or superstitious about sharing the news until you feel confident that this pregnancy will go the distance. You may not yet want to tell anyone that you will have to "untell" if you miscarry. Be prepared to be on the receiving end of "stupid things people say to pregnant women," such as, "Was it a mistake?" "Why would you want another baby? You already have a girl and a boy!" Just take this as preparation for parenting, when you will become the target for more unwelcome and unhelpful advice.

Once you tell your children, expect the whole town to know. Different ages and different personalities need different approaches, so how and when you talk to your children will vary with their level of interest and understanding. Most little ones like picture books about pregnant mommies and new baby siblings. You may introduce the subject to older children by showing them the how-baby-is-growing pictures in this book. Even fairly young children will sense that something is different about their mommy, so you do need to talk to them, especially if they're hearing snatches of adult conversation about the pregnancy. They'll be proud to be among the first to know. Be sure they understand that you are going to need more rest, more help, and more understanding. Explain to them why you may have grouchy days and sick days, but also reassure them that you will be fine and that you will continue to love and take care of them. This may be the first time in their little lives that your children get the message that someone else's needs are as important as theirs. Use age-appropriate explanations, such as, "Baby uses a lot of mommy's energy to grow, so mommy is feeling tired and needs a lot of rest. Mommy needs you to be as quiet as a mouse so mommy can rest and the new baby can rest."

When to break the news to your employer may be an exercise in career strategy, especially if you are concerned about how your pregnancy may affect your job description or job security. Legally, you can't be discriminated against because you're pregnant, but you may want to think carefully about your plans for returning to work after the baby is born before you tell your supervisor about your pregnancy. That way you'll be ready to handle the questions that are sure to follow. This may put you in a better bargaining position if you are looking for an extended maternity leave or part-time or flexible hours when your baby is young. (See the related section, "Working While Pregnant," page 134.)

I knew my company would start mommy-tracking me as soon as I told, so I waited. Sure enough, they gave me a huge raise when, unbeknownst to them, I was two months along, and then they were shocked when I announced, at four months, I was going to have a baby.

When to go public with your news is a personal decision. Even if you say nothing, sooner or later your body will give your secret away. (See "Working Out the Right Maternity-Leave Package for You," page 138.)

Ectopic Pregnancy

An ectopic (literally, "out of place") pregnancy occurs when the fertilized ovum implants outside the uterus. Ninety-five percent of such pregnancies occur in one of the fallopian tubes, which is why the condition is also known as a "tubal pregnancy." Ectopic pregnancies also occur in the ovary, abdominal cavity, or cervix, but these cases are rare.

Only about one in one hundred pregnancies occurs ectopically. If you haven't had any symptoms of an ectopic pregnancy by the time you suspect you are pregnant, you are likely to be past the stage when you might worry, since symptoms of ectopic pregnancy usually appear in the first week after fertilization. Some women, however, may not experience signs of an ectopic pregnancy until after they realize they are pregnant.

Why ectopic pregnancies occur. Most of these abnormal pregnancies occur because of some blockage in the fallopian tube, either a developmental defect in the tube or scar tissue from a previous infection. This defect or scarring prevents the normal passage of the fertilized ovum into the uterus, and the embryo begins growing in the tube (or another place outside the uterus). Some ectopic pregnancies occur for no apparent reason. As you might expect, some women are more at risk than others for ectopic pregnancy. Risk factors include the following:

- *A previous ectopic pregnancy.* A woman who has had one ectopic pregnancy has approximately a 10 percent chance of subsequent pregnancies being ectopic.
- *Previous surgery on or near the fallopian tubes.* Surgery may leave residual scar tissue that blocks the tubes. Having had a reversal of a previous tubal ligation or an unsuccessful tubal ligation increases the chance of ectopic pregnancy.
- *A history of pelvic infections.* Pelvic infections such as pelvic inflammatory disease or sexually transmitted infections may damage the tubes.
- *Endometriosis.* Tissue resembling the uterine lining (endometrium) grows in various

locations other than the uterus throughout the pelvis.
- *Exposure to DES.* Daughters of women who took diethylstilbestrol (DES) during their pregnancy have an increased risk of abnormalities of the reproductive system, including an increased chance of ectopic pregnancy.
- *Infections associated with an IUD.* An infection caused by an IUD, used either previously or when conception occurred, increases the likelihood of ectopic pregnancy.

If you have any of these risk factors, be sure you discuss with your doctor the possible symptoms of an ectopic pregnancy. Early diagnosis and treatment of an ectopic pregnancy are important, not only to preserve your chances of a normal subsequent pregnancy but also possibly to save your life; a pregnancy that grows in the fallopian tube gradually enlarges and pushes through the tube, causing permanent damage to the tube and rupturing blood vessels that could lead to a life-threatening hemorrhage.

When to worry. Any of the following symptoms may signal ectopic pregnancy, and when all are present, ectopic pregnancy is confirmed.

- *Pain.* Nearly 100 percent of ectopic pregnancies are associated with pain, which varies from generalized lower abdominal pain to a pain on one side of the lower abdomen near the site of the ectopic pregnancy (similar to the pain of appendicitis, but in this case it may be on either side). If a tubal pregnancy has ruptured or is about to, a woman may experience sudden, severe, crampy, stabbing lower abdominal pain, which sometimes radiates to the shoulder on the side of the pain. Any lower abdominal pain that becomes more severe, localized, and rapidly changes characteristics should be reported to your doctor immediately.

• *Bleeding.* Bleeding in itself is not a symptom of ectopic pregnancy. (Around 75 percent of women who experience some vaginal bleeding during pregnancy go on to deliver healthy babies.) Before an ectopic pregnancy ruptures, there may be little or no bleeding. If there is bleeding, the blood may be light or heavy, a bit of brownish staining, or a dark red flow. Bleeding may precede the pain or begin after the pain does.

• *Nausea, vomiting, and dizziness.* As the pain increases in severity and becomes more localized, and the bleeding becomes heavier and more red, the woman experiences nausea, vomiting, and dizziness. She may feel faint and notice an increasingly rapid pulse.

• *Severe pain during a pelvic examination.* Another clue is severe pain when the cervix is moved during a pelvic examination.

• *Tenderness over the tube.* Mild to severe tenderness may be present over the site of the pregnancy. The doctor may even be able to feel the embryo.

Sometimes it is difficult to tell the difference between a miscarriage and an ectopic pregnancy. But generally, the pain of a miscarriage tends to be milder and more toward the middle of the abdomen — more like menstrual cramps. The pain of a tubal pregnancy tends to be severe and localized — more like appendicitis. The bleeding of a miscarriage is usually heavier and contains blood clots, while that of an ectopic pregnancy that has not yet ruptured tends to be less heavy and darker.

What to do if you suspect that you are having an ectopic pregnancy. Seek medical attention immediately if you are experiencing pain. If you are experiencing any of the above signs and symptoms, and a pelvic exam suggests a tubal pregnancy, your practitioner will probably perform a specialized ultrasound, which, in the case of an ectopic pregnancy, will show either an empty uterine cavity or the presence of a tiny pregnancy outside the uterus. If the ultrasound fails to diagnose a suspected ectopic pregnancy and there are no signs of rupture, your doctor may follow the HCG hormone levels in your blood for a few days, which will either fall or not increase if a pregnancy is ectopic. If an ectopic pregnancy is still suspected but remains unconfirmed, a laparoscopy may be performed in order to view the tubes directly. Use of this procedure, in which a flexible telescope-like tube is inserted through a tiny incision around the navel, lessens abdominal scarring and improves postoperative recovery. During the surgery, every attempt is made to preserve the tube and therefore future fertility. With the use of such specialized medical technology, most ectopic pregnancies are now diagnosed and treated before they have a chance of rupturing. Even if the tube has already ruptured and is severely damaged by the ectopic pregnancy, new microvascular surgical techniques sometimes make it possible for the tube to be repaired. If the ruptured tube cannot be repaired, your other tube will still be fine, and you will probably be able to complete other pregnancies. A recent innovation is treating suspected tubal pregnancies with medications rather than surgery.

Experiencing an ectopic pregnancy is like experiencing a miscarriage — a pregnancy that ends before its time. Expect to feel similar emotions. (See page 81.)

Choices in Childbirth

The '90s are a great time to birth a baby. At no other time in history have expectant couples had so many choices about how and where to bring their baby into the world. Yet all these options have their price; with choice comes responsibility, possible confusion, and often a good deal of pressure to have the "perfect" birth. We wish to guide you through the selection process to a choice that's right for you. Once, when we had a discussion with a group of obstetricians, nurses, and midwives about how some women are more prepared for their births than others, these birth attendants all agreed that the more informed women are, the easier they birth. As you explore your options by reading books and magazines and by talking to friends and professionals, you will discover that having a baby in the '90s may differ drastically from how your mother had you.

A historical perspective. To better understand where obstetrical practices are today, it helps to understand where they have been. Thirty years ago birthing was still treated as a surgical event; a woman delivering a baby might as well have been having her appendix removed. Mother was a medicated patient, shaved and prepped for the "operation," then placed on her back on a surgical table, with her feet strapped into stirrups. After the baby was extracted, mother recovered from the "operation" of birth while experts cared for baby, often feeding baby an artificial product called "formula." Even after mom took her

baby home, she had to contend with baby-care pundits who warned of the hazards of spoiling and allowing the baby to manipulate the parents. "Let your baby cry it out" and "feed on schedule" advice and a low-touch style of parenting became the standards in baby care.

Throughout the twentieth century, medical and technological advances have made birth safer for mothers and babies. By the late '60s, reform-minded women were asking that it also be more satisfying. A new philosophy of birth began to emerge, and many women began attending childbirth classes to learn about it. "Choice" and "alternatives" became birthing buzzwords. Over the next decade, roles in the birth ritual began to shift: the birthing mother took centerstage, and many doctors came to realize that it was in the best interest of mother and baby to let the pregnant woman work *with* her body to control pain during childbirth instead of trying to escape it through heavy sedation. Mothers then became participants in their birthing decisions.

Shaving is now a thing of the past (research showed it increased the risk of infection), and stirrups and episiotomies are no longer routine. Mothers stand, lean, sit, or squat to give birth. Along with the new positions for birth have come new members of the birthing team. For at least the last two decades dads have been present in the delivery room to support moms and to experience the joy of seeing their children come into the world. A women-helping-women network of professional labor assistants is also now emerging.

As the monetary costs of having a baby have risen and the birth rate has fallen, it has become an economic fact of hospital life that those who bear the babies and pay the bills want their consumer's voice heard in the baby-business decisions. Hospital marketers, eager to attract this new breed of birth-savvy consumers, have changed their slogans from "We do it all for you" to "Have it your way." Obstetrical wards have been transformed and remarketed as "family birth centers." Delivery tables have become the more comfortable and labor-friendly "birthing beds." Taking a shower during labor has been upgraded in many hospitals to immersion in a "labor tub." Hospital maternity units now advertise in the family pages of the Sunday newspaper. The doctor no longer "delivers" the baby; he or she "attends the birth." (Martha goes ballistic if Bill says he "delivered" their babies, even though he actually caught three of them — two because the official birth attendant didn't get there on time, and one because he wanted to. She is quick to point out that since she did all the work, she delivered her babies. (Bill was there as "birth attendant," a title he feels is loftier than "baby-catcher.")

Along with changes in childbirth, bonding, breastfeeding, and babywearing have become the three B's of baby care in the 1990s. Instead of whisking drug-groggy babies away from groggy moms and having them cared for by nurses, healthy babies are now handed right to the mother, and they stay with her. Doctors and midwives have come to agree with researchers that "from mother's womb to mother's room" is the best way for mother and baby to start off their relationship. This practice of bonding is simply a scientific re-construction of what a mother would natu-rally do anyway. Breastfeeding, a way of nurturing as well as transmitting nutrients, has largely replaced artificial feeding in the early months. Babywearing, carrying babies in a sling instead of pushing them in strollers, is becoming the mother-baby attachment scene for the modern pair.

There are many more choices in birth philosophies, birth attendants, and birth places than ever before: midwife or doctor, unmedicated or epidural, high-risk, high-tech, or hands-off. Women can now make informed choices, but they realize that every option has a price. Fewer drugs may mean more pain. More drugs mean less pain but also less control. High-tech labors and pain manage-ment can lead to more complicated births. Home birth is lovely and gives the mother more control but poses risks in an emer-gency. The list of trade-offs goes on. In some ways birth has never been simpler or safer; in other ways it has never been more compli-cated.

What's ahead? Birth reform will continue as women educate themselves about the birth process and take responsibility for their births. Malpractice reform, should it come to pass, will restore the art of decision making to what's best for mother and baby instead of what's less risky for the doctor. Economic re-form will cause managed-care insurers to ask what is the best birth buy and to question whether today's high-priced help and high-tech equipment are routinely necessary for a safe and satisfying birth.

As you progress through this book month by month, we will guide you through the full range of choices, including many of the newer alternatives available to pregnant women, so that you can make the choices that are right for you. New is not always bet-ter, at least not for every woman. We will also try to steer you away from risky alternatives that have not been proven safe by the test of time yet may have received a lot of media at-tention. As you explore the myriad of birth choices available to you, you will discover many questions you never thought of and many procedures you never thought to ques-tion. You will also discover that making birth choices sometimes seems like selecting items from a menu, and you have to balance each choice against the next to produce a satisfying "meal." Depending on where you live and what, if any, medical insurance you have, some items on the menu will not be available to you. What you learn by doing the choosing is as important as what you choose. Approach your birth team and your birth place prepared with the knowledge of alternatives and the confidence you need to get the birth you want. You never have to feel apologetic for wanting the best medical care for yourself and your baby.

Assembling Your Birth Team

With the privilege of pregnancy comes the responsibility for making wise decisions. One of the first issues you must decide is who will be your birth attendant. Whom will you trust to help you have a healthy pregnancy and a safe birth? Before you interview birth attendants, do a little soul-searching yourself. It helps to know what is truly important to you and what you really need before you set out to get it.

Interview yourself. Searching for a health-care provider who shares your birth philosophy presupposes you have a birth philosophy. But if this is your first pregnancy, you may not yet know what type of birth you want or what "philosophy" to have. Ideally, you would be all studied up, having read and explored all the alternatives of birthing and the risks and benefits of procedures, tests, and technologies. Realistically, you may have only a vague sense of what you want your baby's birth to be like, and your knowledge may come from family and friends or from what you've seen in movies or on TV. Many first-time mothers are not able to work out their birthing needs in detail before they must begin the process of selecting a birth attendant. For most women, a birthing philosophy evolves throughout pregnancy, often with the input of a health-care provider. As your pregnancy progresses, so will your knowledge of birthing alternatives and the needs of your particular pregnancy.

Nevertheless, you need to pick a caregiver now, one who will work with you as your pregnancy and birth philosophy evolve. If this is your first baby or your first major relationship with the medical system, you may find doctor-choosing somewhat unsettling. How can you know ahead of time what you'll want at delivery? You may think you know the type of "patient" you will be, but yet this knowledge may not be entirely helpful, since pregnancy, for most women, is not an illness, and you are not a patient. You are not sick. Even if you have had a previous need for hospital care — say, to have your appendix removed — there was little philosophy involved. You just wanted your inflamed appendix out as quickly as possible, by skillful hands, and at a competent hospital. Your present needs are a bit more complex. Yes, you want to have a healthy pregnancy and deliver a healthy baby, but you also want to cope with pain in appropriate ways, take advantage of relaxation techniques, and enjoy an emotionally satisfying beginning to your parenting career.

Even if this is not your first pregnancy, you still may be going through the caregiver selection process. Perhaps you were unsatisfied with your previous birth experience or birth attendants and want to do it differently this time. Perhaps your first practitioner retired or you moved away. You now know the questions to ask and may have resolved to be more assertive about your birth wants. You may also be more willing to be flexible and listen to the wisdom of your advisers.

In determining what you want from a health-care provider, it may help to ask yourself the following questions:

- Do I have a specific vision of what I want for the birth? Can I articulate it to others?
- Do I want a doctor or a midwife? Or both?
- Do I like to be in control in a high-energy situation or to cede control to someone more authoritative?
- Do I want to manage my pain with medication or through self-help techniques?
- How comfortable am I with hospital procedures?
- How will I react if I have to have a cesarean?
- What am I scared of?
- Do I care if my practitioner is male or female?
- Do I want to learn everything I can about pregnancy and delivery or just enough to get through it?
- How involved does my partner want to be in the pregnancy and delivery? What do I expect of my partner?
- Will my partner be a good advocate for me if things don't seem to be going as planned?

Talk to your friends about their birth experiences to get an idea of what giving birth is really like. Ask like-minded friends what they would do differently next time around, and what they were happy with. Read all you can on birthing alternatives. Have a good sense of what you want *before* you visit your health-care provider.

After interviewing yourself, you are ready to interview birth attendants, the people who will care for your health during your pregnancy and be with you during delivery. If you have your heart set on being both the leading lady and director in the drama of birth, most practitioners are happy with the role of consultant, provided you have studied your part. If, on the other hand, you want to keep the starring role and have the birth attendant as director, you may feel in the best hands by choosing an authority-figure type, usually a doctor, not a midwife. Whatever mother-professional partnership you construct, we hope you take responsibility for your birthing decision. The very fact that you are reading this book probably means you want to.

The best combination for a safe and satisfying birth is a woman in charge of what she does best plus a birth attendant in charge of what he or she does best. In this type of give-and-take relationship, each partner gives advice and expresses preferences, respecting the wisdom of the other's experience. Good communication from the start helps you avoid the "my way versus doctor's way" clash that can arise at crucial moments during your pregnancy and delivery. Even in this early doctor-shopping and birth philosophy–building stage, remember that as you grow in knowledge and experience, you may find the roles in the drama of birth less well defined than you imagined, and oftentimes they change on opening night when the plot takes an unexpected turn. There is, after all, no rehearsal for the drama of birth.

Seeking Doctor Right

Ask for doctor recommendations from like-minded friends or health-care professionals. Obstetrical nurses are excellent resources, having seen many local obstetricians in action. Narrow the list down to several candidates and call to make an appointment to interview these physicians. (If your insurance plan limits your choice of obstetrician, you can still interview several birth attendants.) Be sure to tell the receptionist that your visit is for an interview only, and if you are on an insurance plan that limits your choices, be sure to ask the receptionist if the prospective doctor accepts your plan. If the receptionist has time, you may even want to run your most important concerns by her or one of the nurses before you make an appointment.

Ideally, visit the doctor at a time when both you and your partner can attend. Don't be offended if the doctor does prenatal interviews only once a week or if on interview

---

Take Your Time

It's early, so try not to be overwhelmed by the many choices available to you. Where to birth your baby, what childbirth class to take, and what pain relief to use are decisions that you can easily postpone. Now you may just want to concentrate on getting through these early months of fatigue and nausea. Focus on what's going on inside your body and on taking care of yourself. Birthing choices can be put on the back burner for a while. Do, however, choose your health-care provider as early as possible in your pregnancy, as good prenatal care can't wait. (You can switch health-care providers mid-pregnancy if necessary.) Make other decisions gradually. As your pregnancy progresses, you can sort out your options and, together with your birth attendants, develop a birthing philosophy and solidify your birth plan.

---

day you are bumped because the doctor is at the hospital attending a delivery. His or her first allegiance is to the patients (something you'll appreciate if you become one of them).

Make a list of important questions you must have answered. Keep your list with you at all times and jot down concerns as they occur to you. (You won't forget to mention them this way if you are one of those women who suffer from forgetfulness as a side effect of pregnancy.)

Interviewing the office. Arrive early and browse around the office a bit. Introduce yourself to the office personnel. Are they friendly? Accommodating? You'll be spending a lot of time on the phone with these people if you choose this practice. Many of the important facts that you need to know you can learn from the office staff even before meeting the doctor: the doctor's call schedule, vacation plans (in case it is during your due week), accepted insurance plans, fees, hospital affiliations, and, if the doctor is in solo practice, who covers for him or her. If you ask the office personnel these questions, the doctor will appreciate your respect for his or her time, and you'll be able to concentrate during your interview on the specifics of your pregnancy and birth. If you can, chat with other clients in the waiting room. "Interviewing" other expectant moms can give you a sense of the doctor's birthing philosophies. But remember, the qualities one mother absolutely feels she must have in a birth attendant may be just the ones you don't want.

Conducting the interview. The main purpose of the initial interview is to determine if this practitioner can deliver the birth experience you want. If this is your first baby and your first interview, you may not know yet what your birthing options are or have decided the type of birthing experience you want. Share where you are in your homework stage with your prospective doctor. Perhaps this practitioner can discuss your options with you, guide you through some of the decision-making process, and help you make informed choices. The doctor's ability and willingness to have a give-and-take discussion tells you whether or not this is a person you can comfortably work with through your pregnancy and labor.

You want to come away from this interview with two pieces of information: how this doctor *approaches* birth and how this doctor *manages* birth. Try to get a sense of what the doctor's birthing philosophy is. Does he or she approach pregnancy and birth as primarily a normal and healthy process, yet one that needs surveillance and sometimes intervention when the process doesn't go as desired? Or, do you get the feeling that this doctor is rigid and, even though he or she may give lip service to your birth wishes, might click into his or her way of doing things midway through your labor, when you are in no physical or emotional state to negotiate?

Most women today look for a doctor whose philosophy is one of informed partnership. Ideally, he or she would say something like, "I regard the typical pregnancy and birth as a healthy and uncomplicated process, and I do my best to help nature take its course. Yet sometimes pregnancy and birth don't go according to plan or desire, and I may have to suggest some alternatives to you. I'll do what I do best, which is to safeguard the health of both you and your baby, and I'll help you do what you do best, which is to grow and birth a healthy baby. That's what a partnership is all about."

After you get a feel for how a prospective doctor approaches birth, determine how he or she manages birth. This is where your birth wants and your doctor's practices will either mesh or clash, and you want to find out about this before the first contraction. Even though you have probably not completely worked out your own birth-management plan, ask questions that give you a general impression as to how this doctor supports a mother during labor and delivery. Look for a balance between natural methods of pain control and medical management, as well as a supportive presence. Here are some questions that will help you get a feel for the doctor's birth-management philosophy:

- How do most mothers in your practice cope with pain in labor?
- In what position do most mothers in your practice give birth?
- What percentage of mothers in your practice have an epidural?
- What percentage of mothers in your practice have an episiotomy?
- What percentage of mothers in your practice have a cesarean?
- What percentage of your previous cesarean mothers have their next baby vaginally?
- What percentage of mothers in your practice have an induced labor?

The doctor's answers to these questions will give you a clue to the mind-set he or she will bring to your delivery. One of the best indicators of a doctor's birthing philosophy is whether he or she views you as a *participant* or a *patient* during birth. Another is whether or not this doctor realizes the value of a woman's laboring in different positions at different stages of birth to alleviate pain and enhance progress. All too many doctors are still members of the "horizontal woman attended by the quarterback baby-catcher" school.

Convey to your prospective doctor that having a safe and satisfying birth experience is a top priority in your life. In so doing, you are telling him or her that you care enough to choose the best, which puts the ball in the doctor's court, generally making him or her want to impress you with the fact that he or she can deliver (as much as is humanly possible) the birth experience you want. Remember, your doctor is wondering about you just as you are about him or her. Tell the doctor the type of person you are, what type of client you are, and the birth needs that are most important to you. As we've mentioned, it's unlikely that you've formulated a complete birth-management plan within a few days of a positive pregnancy test, but you at least want to give the doctor a clue as to what you need. You in turn will have an opportunity to see how attentively and empathetically the doctor listens and how willing he or she is to help you work out a birthing philosophy. How carefully does the doctor explain tests, technology, and other medical options? Do you feel comfortable sharing your birth wishes with this doctor and taking the advice he or she offers?

Don't be put off if, after you have presented your birth wish list, your doctor hedges a bit. This experienced professional knows that birth does not always go according to plan. If you are like many of today's prepared expectant parents, you have probably decided that you will have an ideal birth. You need to construct this mind-set because if you don't set up an ideal, you won't know the steps to take to get it. A perceptive doctor, on the other hand, knows by experience that birth seldom goes according to plan, and you should be prepared to receive an answer somewhat like this one: "I respect your desires completely but I must, in the best medical interest of you and your baby, reserve the right to intervene medically should the need arise, and I ask you to trust my judgment." The doctor is asking of you the same respect and flexibility that you are asking of the doctor.

A few notes on interview etiquette: Negative openers do not make good first impressions, so don't begin with a barrage of "I don't want's" ("I don't want an IV, electronic monitoring, stirrups, and so on"). Ease into your interview with positive statements about the birth experience you want. You don't want to come across as a wet-behind-the-ears recent graduate of the school of birthing books that unfairly portray all doctors as adversaries. Even if your mind is made up as you enter your doctor's office (though few first-time pregnant women are so exceptionally educated this early in their pregnancy), you owe it to yourself and your baby to open your mind to viewpoints you may not have considered. Your doctor has had the benefit of perhaps thousands of birth experiences. On the other hand, you don't want to assume that the course of action the doctor recommends must be better than any decision you might make for yourself. Taking no responsibility for your birthing decisions devalues both the power of your own individuality and the specialness of your birth.

Dr. Linda notes: One of the problems I often note during interviews is mother rigidity. These women come in with inflexible expectations for a "good" birth, and their rigidity may be setting them up for a bad experience. Good birthing experiences may require a little flexibility on the part of the woman and a little bit of a "go with the flow" attitude.

Marge, a first-time mother, empowered herself with all the tools she could find to increase her chances of a satisfying birth experience. She told us how her partnership with her birth attendant worked:

I wanted to be in complete control of my faculties — no drugs or intervention unless there was a need. But I also wanted the security of a doctor's knowledge. And I wanted to know from the nurses and doctors what was going on at all times and why. I didn't want to be left out of the decisions, but at the same time I didn't want the sole responsibility for making them.

This mother took the best from herself and the best from her birth attendants and had a satisfying birth experience.

Choosing a Midwife

Obstetrical and technological advances have made having a baby now safer than ever. At no other time in history has a mother with pregnancy complications been more likely to deliver a healthy baby. Today's pregnant woman now has one more option to choose to make her pregnancy and birth even more satisfying — a midwife.

Around 95 percent of mothers deliver their babies into the hands of obstetricians or family physicians, but a growing and vocal contingent of moms swear by their midwives. Most modern midwives practice in hospitals and birth centers, though some attend home births. Certified nurse midwives hold a graduate degree in midwifery. Direct-entry midwives receive their training in other ways and, depending on local laws, may or may not be licensed. Martha and Bill had some of each: three deliveries by an obstetrician, one birth attended by a family physician, and four midwife-attended births. We took the roles of each professional literally.

"Obstetrician" means "one who stands by," and "midwife" means "with woman." They are different professionals with different birth philosophies, different training, and different roles. One is not better than the other, but one may be more appropriate than the other for your particular birth situation. Remember that the obstetrical mind-set is, as it should be, to take no chances. This is the philosophy with which obstetricians are trained. This is what you pay for. You can't expect obstetricians to think like midwives. They are not supposed to, and they have not been trained to do so.

Depending on the hospital or obstetrical practice you choose, you may be able to have the best of both worlds; a midwife *and* a family physician or obstetrician — a nurturing professional woman to attend you during labor and birth and obstetrical care from someone who knows you, in the unlikely event a complication occurs. Physicians and midwives work together in many European countries, and these countries show high patient satisfaction and excellent birth outcomes. Many U.S. health maintenance organizations (HMOs) are now employing this model in their obstetrical services, and you may even find this system available within some private obstetrical practices. If you are fortunate enough to have access to such an HMO or a private practice, you will be attended during your pregnancy by both a midwife and a physician, and which of them you have as a birth attendant will depend upon your individual obstetrical needs.

Why choose a midwife? Many women report satisfaction with the medical model of birth, especially if they had or were at risk of having a complication during pregnancy or delivery. Some women also welcome the medical pain relief a physician can provide

Questions to Ask Your Doctor

Though you certainly can't expect to get the answers to all these questions on your first prenatal visit, you will need to ask them sometime during your pregnancy. Bring them up as your birthing philosophy and your relationship with your practitioner evolve.

- What hospital(s) is your doctor affiliated with? The doctor and the birth place often come as a combined package, but some doctors deliver at more than one hospital. After working out your birth wishes, which birth place would your doctor suggest? Some hospitals are high-tech, others are high-touch, still others are both. Find out which one is right for you.

- Ask about your doctor's call schedule. Who covers for your doctor, how often, and what are these physicians' birthing philosophies? If your doctor is part of a group practice, will you meet each of his or her colleagues during your prenatal visits?

- What exercises are safe to do during pregnancy? How often should you do them? Should you stop them as your abdomen gets heavier?

- What would be a healthy rate of weight gain for you during your pregnancy? Does the doctor provide nutritional counseling?

- What prenatal screening tests does the doctor advise and why? If he or she suggests routine tests, ask the doctor to be more specific about what and why, since you don't consider your pregnancy to be "routine."

- What childbirth classes does your doctor advise you to take?

- Does your doctor agree with your wishes if you choose to employ a professional labor support person for your birth, and does the office provide referrals?

- What is the doctor's recommended schedule of prenatal visits?

- How does your doctor feel about birth plans, and of what assistance can the doctor be in helping you create one?

- What are your doctor's views concerning walking and changing positions during labor? Will he or she help you improvise labor and birthing positions, such as standing, squatting, and side-lying? You'll want to have a good idea of whether or not your doctor uses the force of gravity during labor or if his or her birthing philosophy is stuck in the horizontal position. Does he or she welcome your active participation during labor?

- What about pain management? What are your doctor's views on the epidural, pain relief by injection, use of labor tubs for pain relief, and how to find a balance between natural and medical pain relievers during birth?

- Find out what procedures are routine during labor and delivery, such as the use of ultrasound, intravenous fluids, and electronic fetal monitoring.

- What are your doctor's views on episiotomy? Routine? As needed? What alternatives to episiotomy does he or she suggest and use at delivery?

- If you have had a previous cesarean section and wish to try a VBAC (vaginal birth after cesarean), what is your doctor's VBAC success rate, and what specific measures will he or she offer to increase your chances? Does your doctor believe you can have a VBAC?

- Questions for office staff: fees, insurance plans, doctor's vacation schedule, payment plans.

and feel safe in the technology-oriented hospital birthing scene. Other women, however, need or want a less medically managed birth.

The most appealing aspect of a midwife-attended birth is that, ideally, a midwife provides hands-on labor support from early contractions through the final push. Your obstetrician, on the other hand, will check you periodically during labor, but may not stay with you until your delivery is imminent. A midwife not only delivers a baby but also acts as a labor support person. She patiently blends into the birth scene, sometimes with watchful waiting and at other times giving hands-on support that eases the discomfort or accelerates the progress of labor.

With the midwife, the mother is the star and director of the show, and events proceed at her pace. The midwife assumes that the birth will go well, because most of the time and with the right support it does. Yet she is also trained to look for complications and work together with a physician, if necessary, to ensure the safety of the mother and baby. Because of her training and her philosophy, a midwife sees labor as a natural process requiring little intervention other than informing and comforting the mother and helping her to work with her body. An obstetrician, on the other hand, often has a "what-if" mindset, looking for things to go wrong. Both of these mind-sets can serve a pregnant woman well, depending on her circumstances. Interestingly, we have found that one of the main assets of the midwife is her belief that fear is enemy number one of the pregnant and laboring woman because it increases the pain and slows progress of delivery. An experienced midwife is a valuable person to have around an otherwise fearful birth scene because practitioner attitudes are contagious; her calmness can be catching.

If the obstetrical system in your community is not set up for midwife-attended births, you can still enjoy this "best of both worlds" approach by having an obstetrician-attended birth and employing a professional labor assistant. (For how these professionals work, see page 273.)

Is a midwife for you? If your pregnancy begins low-risk and remains that way, and if you prefer a high-touch, low-tech birth, a midwife-attended birth may be for you. Of course, the decision will depend upon your overall health, your knowledge of the birth process, your ability to handle pain, and your attitude about where the risks lie in the birthing process. It will also depend on what kinds of midwife services are available in your community. If you have delivered a baby before, your decision may depend in large part upon your previous birth experience.

Your decision will also depend upon what you want to get out of your birth experience. Most women want not only to enjoy a healthy pregnancy and deliver a healthy baby; they also want a satisfying birthing experience. Ask yourself what you really hope to achieve. Your chances of having the birth you want may be greater if you have a physician and a midwife with physician backup.

Interviewing yourself. Before you consider interviewing a midwife to care for you during pregnancy and birth, ask yourself these questions:

☐ Are you currently in good health, and is your pregnancy uncomplicated? Or do you have a pregnancy complication that requires medical attention, such as diabetes or high blood pressure?

☐ Do you have any reason to anticipate special medical needs at the time of delivery, such as a premature baby, maternal diabetes, or toxemia?

☐ Is the medical system in your community set up for midwife-attended births? Not only should your midwife be professionally trained and licensed but shc should also have a regular working relationship with qualified doctors who can act as her backup should an unforeseen emergency arise.

Interviewing a midwife. If you decide to interview midwives as part of your health-care provider selection process, ask them the same questions you would ask a doctor (see page 36), along with these:

☐ Where did you receive your education in midwifery? Are you also a nurse? Are you certified and by whom? Are you licensed? (Some states do not license midwives.)

☐ How long have you practiced? Approximately how many births have you attended? Would you give me the names of a few mothers as references?

☐ Who is your backup doctor? What percentage of the time is he or she called in? How long will it take the doctor to get to me? At what point is the backup doctor generally called in? Will I have a say in the decision? Will I have a chance to meet the backup doctor ahead of time? Who covers for the doctor if he or she is busy with another delivery? Is the doctor's fee included in the fee I pay you? Are you allowed to

stay with me if we have to call the doctor? May you stay if I have a cesarean? Call the backup doctor or doctors to confirm their relationship with your prospective midwife.

☐ Who covers for you if you are on vacation or are occupied with another mother in labor? Are your backup midwives also certified and licensed, and what is their experience?

☐ Do you carry a pager?

☐ At what point in my labor will I go to you (or you to me)? How long will it take you to get to me? Will you stay with me during my whole labor if I want you to?

☐ What kind of testing, if any, do you routinely recommend for pregnant women of my age? If I am found to be "high-risk," can you and a specialist co-manage my care?

☐ Do you provide childbirth education or work with someone who does? Do you recommend a particular birthing method (e.g., Lamaze, Bradley)?

☐ What arrangements do you have to transfer a home-birthing mother or baby to the hospital if needed? Do you have an arrangement with the hospital that allows you to attend or co-manage my birth in the hospital?

☐ Are you certified in newborn resuscitation? What resuscitation equipment do you bring to the delivery?

☐ Are you experienced at manually turning a baby who is presenting in a posterior position? Do you perform perineal massage? Episiotomy?

☐ What are your fees? (Some states mandate insurance coverage of licensed midwives, but be sure to check with your insurance provider about whether your chosen midwife is covered.)

☐ Do you offer postpartum care? What postpartum services do you provide?

Do not assume that, just because someone is a midwife, her birth philosophy and man-

agement techniques are best for you. Spell out your wishes to her just as you would to a doctor.

If you are interviewing both midwives and doctors, be sure to interview several of each. The difference between individual practitioners can be as great as or greater than those between the midwifery and obstetrical professions.

Additional Questions You May Have About Midwives

Won't the labor nurses give me all the support I need during labor and delivery?

Probably not. We have heard women rave about their delivery room nurses, but it's the luck of the draw. You could get an experienced, supportive nurse who has had good childbirth experiences herself or a new, impatient one with a negative attitude toward the whole process. It's also quite likely that a nurse you come to trust will end her shift before you're ready to deliver. Also, you never know whether you'll deliver on a slow day, when the nurses have lots of time, or on a busy night, when you may be left alone for great chunks of time. Midwives are generally there for you, and only you, during your entire labor. They follow your lead, giving you attention when you need and want it and leaving you alone when you don't.

I was told that having a midwife lowers dramatically my chance of having a cesarean. Is this true, and is it a good enough reason to use a midwife?

Statistics claiming that cesarean rates among patients of midwives are lower may be misleading since mothers who are attended by midwives are low-risk and less likely to need

---

To Find a Midwife

To obtain a list of midwives in your community, try the following resources:

The American College of Nurse Midwives (ACNM)
818 Connecticut Avenue NW, Suite 900,
Washington, DC 20006
202-728-9860

MANA (Midwives Alliance of North America)
600 Fifth Street
Monett, MO 65708

ICAN (International Cesarean Awareness Network)
1304 Kingsdale Avenue
Redondo Beach, CA 90278
310-542-6400; fax 310-542-5368

An informative booklet is "Midwife Means 'With Woman,'" by Elizabeth Hallett and Karen Ehrlich, published in 1991 by the California Association of Midwives (CAM), PO Box 417854, Sacramento, CA 95841 (800-829-5791).

a cesarean anyway. But it stands to reason that the use of any labor support person (a midwife or someone else) who can help you work with your body and make informed choices during labor will lower your chances of needing a cesarean section.

Will a midwife be angry with me if I decide I need medication during labor?

Most midwives take a "no drug" stance in general, but if you're on the fence about a medicated labor, ask any midwife you interview about her feelings toward and experience with medicated births. No practitioner should be angry with you, no matter what your birth preference, but most midwives will offer alternatives to discourage you from choosing medication in a moment of desperation. If you decide you want drugs for pain relief during labor, the responsibility for your care will probably shift to a physician, since midwives usually do not manage medicated labors without the assistance of a doctor.

I have a friend studying to be a midwife — she has four kids herself — who has offered to attend me. I trust her totally. Can I use her?

No. She's probably a terrific person, but unless she's had a good deal of experience as a midwife (not as a student, apprentice, or birthing mother) and has a backup obstetrician, you'd do better to have her there in a nonprofessional capacity (say, as a labor support person) while you are attended by a more experienced caregiver. If it will make her feel better, you can tell her that your health insurance company will not cover any emergency care if you use an attendant who is not licensed.

I've heard that midwives are into empowering women. How do they feel about husbands?

Great! Midwives tend to be family-centered, and part of empowering a woman to do what she needs to do in birth is allowing her the full support of her mate. A good midwife is very careful not to usurp the father's position, and she will work at showing him what his role is if he seems hesitant. Midwives tell us they like nothing better than seeing a family — mother, father, sometimes even grandparents and children — share a birth experience. (See the related section "Choosing a Home Birth," page 241.)

CREATING A HEALTHY WOMB ENVIRONMENT

You now have another person to consider in every decision you make regarding your body, and that little person can be far more seriously affected by your habits than you are. Parenting this little one begins even before birth as you strive to create a healthy womb environment for the child you are growing.

If you are in doubt about what you should eat or drink or about a particular substance, consult your health-care provider. It's equally important to rely on your common sense. Any substance that affects your body is likely to affect your baby's even more because your baby's immature liver and kidneys are not able to process and eliminate substances as quickly as your organs can. What's good for mother is likely to be good for baby; what's harmful for mother is likely to be even more harmful for baby. During pregnancy your baby shares your habits, via your blood. (Via hormones you two may share even what's in your mind; see page 224.) It's healthiest for you and safest for your baby if you refrain from using or consuming any substance that unnaturally alters your bodily functions.

The doctor confirmed that you are alive and growing inside of me. How exciting! Take all you need, my child. I will try to eat all you need and stay away from whatever would harm you.

Thank You for Not Smoking

Suppose you and your preborn baby are about to enter a room, but you see a warning sign on the door that says, "This room contains the poisonous gases of approximately 4000 chemicals, some of which could kill or damage your baby and increase your risk of miscarriage." "Why, I certainly wouldn't take my baby into that room," most mothers would insist, but that's exactly what happens when a pregnant woman smokes or when she inhales someone else's cigarette smoke.* Among the many poisonous gases in cigarette smoke are nicotine (an addictive drug known to narrow blood vessels), carbon monoxide (an oxygen robber), benzene (a potential carcinogen), ammonia, hydrogen cyanide (used in rat poison), and formaldehyde. The harmful effects of cigarette smoke on mother and baby increase with the number of cigarettes smoked each day. Also, new research shows that smoking causes more

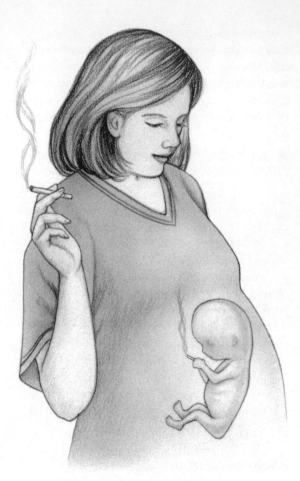

When mommy smokes, baby smokes.

lung damage in women than in men, presumably because women's lungs are smaller.

Smoking robs babies of nourishment. Many studies have shown that infants of mothers who smoke have lower birthweights than infants of mothers who don't smoke. Nicotine passes from the smoke a mother inhales into her bloodstream. The poisonous nicotine narrows uterine blood vessels, thus reducing blood flow to the baby in the womb. Baby depends on this blood flow for

---

* *Nearly everything we state about the health hazard of smoking also applies to breathing secondhand smoke. For a detailed and scientific discussion of the harmful effects of cigarette smoking on babies before and after birth, consult* SIDS: A Parent's Guide to Understanding and Preventing Sudden Infant Death Syndrome, *by William Sears, M.D. (Little, Brown, 1995).*

healthy growth — less blood flow means less nourishment and therefore less growth. As a general rule, bigger babies are healthier and less likely to need special care in the days after birth.

New studies refute the theory that the placenta may act as a barrier, preventing the toxic cigarette chemicals in mother's bloodstream from reaching her baby. When researchers examined the cord blood of newborns whose mothers either smoked or were exposed to secondhand smoke during their pregnancy, they found the presence of cancer-causing chemicals. The newborns received around 50 percent of the carcinogens that were in mother's blood, and the greater the maternal exposure to smoke, the higher were the levels of these poisons in baby's blood.

Smoking robs babies of oxygen. Besides restricting blood flow to the womb, maternal cigarette smoking and breathing secondhand smoke decreases the amount of oxygen available to the baby from that blood. The level of carbon monoxide in the blood of pregnant women who smoke is 600 to 700 percent higher than in those who don't smoke. Carbon monoxide is an oxygen blocker, meaning it prevents blood cells from carrying a full load of oxygen. Researchers equate carbon monoxide levels in cigarette smoke to those in automobile exhaust; in effect, smoking partially smothers the baby in the womb. Lack of oxygen can affect the development of every organ in the baby's body.

Smoking injures little brains. New studies suggest that the developing baby's brain is injured not only by lack of oxygen but also by the chemicals in cigarette smoke, which may be directly poisonous to developing brain cells. Children of mothers who smoked during pregnancy, especially those of mothers who smoked more than one pack a day, were found to have a smaller head circumference as infants, decreased mental performance scores at age one year, reduced IQs, more behavior problems, and diminished academic performance scores in school in controlled studies that compared them to the children of mothers who did not smoke.

Even passive smoke hurts babies. New research shows that when pregnant mothers are exposed to cigarette smoke from other people's cigarettes, their babies are also exposed. These babies are at risk of having lower birthweights and show an increased risk of Sudden Infant Death Syndrome (SIDS), just as the babies of smoking mothers do. If father and mother both smoke, the risk of SIDS is nearly double that incurred when only mother smokes. The risk of SIDS if father smokes but mother doesn't is still greater than if no one in the family smokes. Insist that your husband, relatives, friends, and co-workers respect the life inside your womb and not smoke in the same room with you. If your job requires working in a smoke-contaminated environment, you have grounds for a reassignment; pregnant women have a legal right to work in a smoke-free environment.

What about public places frequented by smokers? "But we always sit in the no-smoking area," you rationalize. No-smoking areas in public places are a step in the right direction, but many still contain significant levels of airborne pollutants. Trying to create a no-smoking area is like trying to chlorinate half a swimming pool. Pollutants travel through the air. To be safe, stay as far away from cigarette smoke as you can.

Kicking the Smoking Habit

The earlier you stop smoking, the healthier you and your baby are likely to be. Best of all would be to quit smoking as you prepare to become pregnant. While the harmful effects of smoking seem to be greatest in the first trimester of pregnancy, even babies of "late stoppers" seem to fare better than infants whose mothers continue to smoke throughout their pregnancies. While there are few hard-and-fast rules in this book, this is one of them: quit. Don't smoke.

Of course, this is more easily said than done. Smoking is not a habit, it's an addiction. Habits are things you can break fairly easily, especially when you are motivated by a little person growing inside you. Addictions are harder to kick. You are accustomed to feeling the strong physiological effects of smoking. Nearly every system in your body is affected by nicotine. You may also be psychologically addicted to the pleasant oral sensation of smoking. It may take a while for your body to get used to feeling right without that hit of nicotine. Quitting will be one of the hardest things you'll ever do. This is a tough addiction to break, but you must give it a try. Here are some suggestions.

Advance Warning

If you are planning to get pregnant, trying to, or in that window of fertility that occurs just a couple of days each month, it is best to avoid alcohol and other drugs — just in case. Consider it "birth-defect control." Also, if you smoke or drink alcohol, cutting down before getting pregnant makes it easier to stop when you have to.

Convince yourself of the dangers. If you are still asking, "Will smoking really harm my pregnancy and my baby?" you are looking for reassurance that no responsible health practitioner can give. Look at it this way: had the evidence against cigarettes not been overwhelming, the government could not have successfully battled a very powerful tobacco lobby and insisted that cigarette ads contain warning labels about smoking during pregnancy. *Statistically, chances are higher that your pregnancy will be more complicated and your baby less smart and less healthy if you smoke while pregnant than if you don't.* It's just not fair to yourself or your baby to gamble.

Try stopping cold turkey. The best moment to extinguish your last cigarette is the moment your pregnancy test shows a positive result. Some women can do that. Others find that sudden physical and emotional withdrawal from cigarettes makes them extremely anxious, and this may not be good for baby either. For these women, a gradual weaning may make more sense. Some "lucky" women find that a natural aversion to the smell of cigarette smoke forces the issue.

Try goal setting. If you can't quit on the first day you know you're pregnant, set a goal for tapering off, say by Day 10. Plan to reward yourself on that day. Calculate how much money you will save in a year of not smoking and spend it on something special for yourself or your baby.

Choose your poison more carefully. Switch brands. Some brands are higher in nicotine and carbon monoxide than others.

Cut down on how much poison you inhale. Take fewer puffs. Smoke only the first half of the cigarette. (More poisons are concentrated toward the end of the cigarette.) Better yet, don't inhale. This can cut down your nicotine dose by half.

Make it inconvenient to smoke. Buy only one pack at a time. Leave the pack somewhere inconvenient, say, in the garage.

Fill the void. Think about what led you to start smoking. Once you identify the psychological factors that may have led to the physiological addiction, it might be easier for you to stop or at least to find a safer substitute habit.

Try healthier substitutes. If you need to hold something and keep your hands busy, try writing, drawing, painting, or working crossword puzzles. If you need something in your mouth, try chewing on carrot or celery sticks, cinnamon sticks, or straws; try sucking on ice, frozen fruit juice bars, or hard candy. Nibble on sunflower seeds or granola. Chew gum. If you smoked for relaxation, try listening to soothing music or reading, or pay for an occasional massage. Take a walk. Go swimming. If you smoked for pleasure, indulge yourself in fun at a no-smoking place: go to a movie or a no-smoking restaurant, go shopping, or visit a non-smoking friend.

Try healthier associations. If you associate smoking with a particular person, place, or pleasure, seek healthier choices. For example, if you associate smoking with restaurants, go only to no-smoking ones. If you enjoy a cigarette with your morning coffee, switch to juice or herbal tea.

Create unpleasant associations. Addictions thrive when they are associated with pleasant thoughts or events. Try associating the desire to smoke or the act of smoking with an unpleasant image. When you get the urge to smoke, for instance, imagine your baby gasping for air inside your womb.

Try scare tactics. Compose your own anti-smoking warnings, such as "Each puff could cost my baby another brain cell" or "Smoking could damage or kill my baby," and hang these reminders in places where you are most likely to want to smoke. Wrap these warnings around your cigarette packs, too.

Get a stop-smoking buddy. If your quitting needs company, enlist the help of a friend or your mate. When you feel the urge to light up, call this person or share in an activity that you both enjoy.

Give yourself credit. Rather than losing hope when you occasionally give in and smoke, pat yourself on the back for each puff you resist. Resolve to do better each day.

Get professional help. If after two weeks you have made no progress on your own, contact a local quit-smoking resource or seek professional help. If you are feeling anxious about quitting, chances are you have some deep issues that might be successfully addressed in psychological counseling. The cost of counseling may be covered by your health plan. Regardless, it will be money well spent.

Feel good about your choice. Mothers who smoke during pregnancy are likely to continue smoking after birth, further increasing the risk of health problems for their infants. Respiratory infections, ear infections, and Sudden Infant Death Syndrome are all more common in the children of smokers.

Furthermore, studies show that mothers who smoke have lower levels of prolactin, the hormone responsible for both milk production and calm "maternal" behavior. Mothers who smoke are likely to have more breastfeeding problems and to wean earlier (probably because of inadequate prolactin). Babies of breastfeeding mothers who smoke tend to have nicotine in their blood, suggesting that they receive tobacco chemicals through their mother's milk (although it is still better for a mother who smokes to breastfeed than to give her baby artificial formula). Quitting now rewards your baby thrice: first, because she is spared toxins in utero; second, because she will not be exposed to them as an infant and child; and third, because she will not learn the harmful habit of smoking from you.

Dr. Bill notes: *During the writing of my book on SIDS, I finally realized why women still smoke during their pregnancy despite their knowledge of the research showing how smoking can harm their baby and themselves. Normally a pregnant mother would do absolutely nothing that could harm her baby. Why is smoking during pregnancy such a hard habit to kick? The fact that a woman continues to smoke during pregnancy is evidence that it is truly an addiction, and such a strong addiction that it overrides her protective maternal instinct. Many women who continued to smoke during their pregnancy told me they really weren't impressed by their doctor's warning that smoking could harm their baby. They were given information such as, "It might lower your baby's birthweight." That vague warning was not enough to override their addiction. It would be better for caring friends and professionals to be less wimpy and tell it like it is:"Smoking may kill your baby, either by a miscarriage, by complications of birth or prematurity, or by Sudden Infant Death Syndrome after birth." In my book* A Parent's Guide to Understanding and Preventing Sudden Infant Death Syndrome, *I told the "smoking during pregnancy" story like it should be told. As a result of reading this, many women immediately stopped or drastically reduced their smoking during pregnancy and after delivery. If your addiction is overriding your intuition during your pregnancy (or if this is happening to a friend of yours), please read this book and learn why you should quit and how to do so.*

Thank You for Not Drinking Alcohol

The harmful effects of alcohol on the developing baby were recognized in the early 1900s, when physicians observed an increase in the number of malformations occurring in babies born nine months after certain European drinking festivals. Unfortunately, any alcohol you drink will get into your baby's blood, just as it does into yours — and at the same levels.

Heavy alcohol consumption during pregnancy can cause babies to be born with fetal alcohol syndrome (FAS), a disorder encompassing a variety of abnormalities. FAS babies weigh less, are shorter, and have smaller brains than normal babies. Sometimes their brains are malformed, and they may suffer from mental retardation. Babies born with fetal alcohol syndrome have unusual facial characteristics: their eyes appear smaller than usual, their nose is short, and their upper lip is thin. They may also have abnormalities of the hands, feet, and heart. Alcohol consumption is most harmful in the first trimester. Studies show that maternal alcohol consumption can also cause pregnancy complications, such as miscarriage, low birthweight, and prematurity. As is true with smoking, alcohol's most harmful effects are on brain development.

Besides directly damaging the developing baby, alcohol is full of empty calories and robs nutrition from the mother. The effects of maternal drinking on the baby have been dubbed "a lifelong hangover."

Questions You May Have About Alcohol

I enjoy an occasional glass of wine with dinner. Is that likely to harm my baby?

Probably not. However, how much is too much is a question no one has satisfactorily answered. Every potentially harmful drug seems to have a "threshold effect," a point at which the drug begins to cause harm. In the case of alcohol, we know that a lot of the drug harms the baby a lot, and a medium amount causes less harm. Whether a very little amount causes very little damage is not known, and perhaps never will be. Could the babies of teetotalers be just a slight bit smarter and bigger than babies of occasional social drinkers? Studies demonstrate that both binge drinking (five or more drinks on one occasion) and regular drinking (an average of two drinks per day throughout pregnancy) definitely harm babies. ("Drink" means 1 ounce of hard alcohol, one 8-ounce glass of wine, or one 12-ounce glass of beer.) Obviously it's riskier to drink an alcoholic beverage during the first trimester than at thirty-six weeks, when your baby's organs are fully formed. An occasional, single glass of wine or beer in the last month is unlikely to harm your baby.

I had a few glasses of wine several times before I knew I was pregnant. Could this drinking have hurt my baby?

Probably not. There is reason to believe that alcohol consumed in very early pregnancy (before implantation occurs) is not harmful to the fetus, as the placenta has not yet begun to form. Folk wisdom holds that the two weeks (on average) between conception and a missed period are sort of a dietary grace period. If you had more than a few drinks at a time, or have been drinking every day since conception, discuss your worry with your doctor. If not, relax.

From now on, however, rely on your common sense as well as scientific studies. Refrain from drinking alcohol during your pregnancy. Subtle effects from small amounts of alcohol have not yet been detected, but it is best to be safe. An occasional glass of wine is *unlikely* to harm your baby, yet no one knows for certain when it comes to alcohol if there is such a thing as a "safe" drink. If you're at social gatherings where alcoholic drinks are served, drink like a child, because you are carrying one. Order your drink "virgin" — your usual drink but without the alcohol. (If this means tomato or orange juice, you'll even come out ahead nutritionally.) Or treat yourself to something else special — extra hors d'oeuvres or dessert.

If you feel you need a drink to unwind now and then, talk to your doctor or midwife about safe, nonalcoholic alternatives (a warm bath, warm milk, chamomile tea, meditation). Soon you may find the fatigue of pregnancy makes sleep the most enticing way to relax!

Thank You for Not Taking Illicit Drugs

Heroin, cocaine, crack, LSD, and PCP.
When a mother takes a drug, so does her baby. When a mother is addicted, so is her baby, and after birth this baby suffers symptoms of drug withdrawal (extreme irritability and jitteriness). Infants of mothers who used addicting drugs during pregnancy are more difficult to care for after birth and may show lifelong effects from their mother's drug use.

Drugs affect a baby throughout pregnancy but are most dangerous in the first trimester. Possible effects of addictive drugs on the developing baby are stillbirth, miscarriage, reduced birthweight, mental retardation, prematurity, and an increased risk in Sudden Infant Death Syndrome. (The risk of SIDS may be increased as much as twenty times in infants of opiate-abusing mothers.) Researchers believe that drugs such as opiates and cocaine also harm developing babies indirectly by constricting blood vessels in the placenta and thus reducing the oxygen supply to the preborn baby — a suffocation effect similar to that caused by nicotine. Cocaine confuses baby's brain, contributing to the hyperirritability of a "crack baby."

Marijuana. Until recently, maternal marijuana smoking during pregnancy was not proven to be harmful to babies. Newer studies, however, suggest that marijuana can harm the fetus in all the ways mentioned above, due to its active ingredient THC.

Amphetamines (speed). Amphetamines are also harmful to the developing baby and increase the chances of prematurity and intrauterine growth retardation. Newborns of speed-addicted mothers show typical speed-withdrawal symptoms (increased heart rate and rapid breathing) immediately after birth.

The Wisdom of the Body

Bodies have a way of telling their owners what's not good for them. Many women develop an aversion to harmful substances while they are pregnant, such as cigarette smoke, alcohol, caffeine, and noxious fumes. Even though these potential poisons lose their appeal, don't rely wholly on what your body tells you. Nature's own protective message is not a perfect one. It's safest to avoid these dangerous substances even if they don't make you nauseous.

If you are addicted to drugs, make an appointment with a professional counselor or enroll yourself in a drug-withdrawal program the day you discover you are pregnant. Even better, start these programs as soon as you decide to get pregnant.

Caffeine

During pregnancy you may want to give up or at least cut back on coffee and switch to pick-me-ups that don't cross the placenta. The concerns about caffeine in pregnancy stem from research that showed that the offspring of pregnant animals given caffeine had a higher incidence of malformations. This statistical finding has yet to be proven in humans, but to be on the safe side, the U.S. Food and Drug Administration (FDA) advises that pregnant women should eliminate or limit the consumption of products containing caffeine — coffee, colas, tea, cocoa, chocolate, and some over-the-counter remedies, including medicines for headaches. Recent research suggests that caffeine use during pregnancy may cause more problems than originally suggested by the early animal studies. Caffeine has now been implicated in miscarriages and low birthweight.

The harmful effects of caffeine revealed in these studies were the result of high doses of caffeine (the equivalent of six to ten cups of coffee a day), but new studies suggest that drinking three or more cups of coffee or tea daily during the first trimester of pregnancy may double the risk of miscarriage. Caffeine does increase the heart rate and metabolic rate in babies, just as it does in adults. Furthermore, caffeine may remain in the baby's bloodstream longer and at higher levels, because baby's immature liver cannot get rid of the caffeine as quickly as can mother's. Caffeine raises levels of the stress hormone adrenaline and, at least theoretically, could reduce the blood flow to the uterus, thus lessening the supply of oxygen and nutrients to the baby.

Whatever the possibility of harm for baby, caffeine use during pregnancy is not all that good for mother. Women process caffeine more slowly when pregnant, allowing this stimulating chemical to remain in their bloodstream longer. Caffeine also drains calcium from a pregnant woman's body by increasing the amount of calcium she excretes in her urine. Caffeine also has a diuretic effect, which may contribute to underhydration and increase the frequency of urination, already a nuisance for pregnant women. Caffeine also interferes with the absorption of iron, an important nutrient during pregnancy.

If your body is used to a daily caffeine lift, here are some ways to wean yourself (and your baby) off this chemical jolt onto a more natural pick-me-up:

• Don't percolate coffee or steep tea too long. A tea bag steeped one minute releases half the caffeine as one steeped for five minutes. In general, the longer coffee and tea are brewed and the darker the chocolate, the greater the caffeine content.

• Try herbal teas that are caffeine-free. Decaffeinated teas and coffees still contain a slight bit of caffeine. If you must drink coffee, use water-processed decaffeinated coffee, since chemically processed decaffeinated coffee contains harmful chemicals.

• Read soda-can labels, or inquire about the caffeine content of a soft drink before you decide to consume it.

• If the warmth of the beverage is what satisfies you, try hot water (you can add lemon), warm milk, hot apple cider, or herbal tea.

• If you find you can't begin your day without the morning caffeine jolt you had been used to, cut down gradually. Brew your coffee using half-decaffeinated and half-regular coffee, and gradually decrease the proportion of caffeine coffee. (Even a small amount of caffeine will relieve the headache that sometimes accompanies caffeine withdrawal.)

Environmental Hazards

Feeling "protective" comes with motherhood and begins at conception. Once her attention is directed to her child within, a world full of pollution, radiation, and chemical agents is bound to worry an expectant mother. Many chemicals that adults use without thinking (bug sprays, household cleaners, building materials, and the like) contain known or suspected teratogens — substances that can cause birth defects. You don't need to be overly concerned, though — statistics are on your side. If you refrain from the "big bad three" (harmful drugs, alcohol, and smoking) and take good nutritional care of yourself, you have a greater than 95 percent chance of delivering a healthy baby.

When to take the most precautions. There are certain high-risk periods in your baby's development when your infant is especially vulnerable to environmental hazards. In general, the greatest danger from environmental toxins comes in the first trimester. During the two weeks after fertilization, your uterus is being readied for implantation. At this time, certain toxins that interfere with how baby "takes root" may increase your chance of miscarriage. However, it's also likely that in the first couple of weeks, before a complete placental and umbilical blood flow is established, the baby is relatively safe from teratogens that enter mother's bloodstream. After the baby begins establishing secure "roots" and the placenta starts developing comes a very vulnerable period: the ten weeks during which the major organs develop.

This is the time when environmental toxins are most likely to cause harm to major organs. By the end of the first trimester all the major organ systems are in place and working, and the risk of major defects decreases as the pregnancy progresses. The second and third trimesters are mainly a period of growth for the already present organ systems; exposure to a harmful substance then is more likely to cause diminishing growth of an organ system rather than a major defect. For example, early exposure to poisons such as drugs, smoke, and alcohol could cause major defects in an infant's brain. Exposure later on in pregnancy is likely to have more subtle effects, such as minor disturbances in mental or motor function.

An environmental substance that causes

Correlation Does Not Mean Causation

The desire to do what's healthiest for your baby and yourself during pregnancy will make you especially sensitive to all the warnings about things that could go wrong during pregnancy. It may relieve you to know that many obstetrical studies show only statistical links between birth defects and suspected teratogens. For example, concerns over caffeine consumption and VDT use were based upon studies that showed that babies whose mothers were exposed to these potential hazards had more developmental problems. Other factors that may have been related to the issue being studied, such as mother's overall lifestyle and just plain genetic bad luck, were not taken into account. In other words, these studies do not prove that exposure actually caused the defect, only that the two things seem to go together, for unknown reasons. Furthermore, a small increase in harm in a large population does not mean that harm will befall every individual exposed to the risk. Remember, the results of one study are often contradicted by the results of another. Statistical studies simply alert us to possible correlations and give us the chance to avoid unnecessary exposure.

little harm to mother can still harm her baby a lot. Toxins remain in baby's bloodstream longer and at higher concentrations than in mother's. Early in pregnancy the baby's liver (which breaks down toxins) and kidneys (which eliminate them) are not developed enough to protect baby. Later in pregnancy these organs are mature enough to be of some help.

Fortunately, what's in the room does not always get into the womb. Just because you are exposed to occasional auto exhaust, gasoline fumes, cigarette smoke from a passerby, and other pollutants of modern life does not mean your baby will be harmed. If you're taking care of yourself, your developing baby is also becoming quite a hearty little person. So try not to worry about the effects of unavoidable pollutants on your baby's development. The stress of worrying may be more harmful than what you're worrying about. Whether you're pregnant or not, avoid unnecessary risks. It doesn't make sense to drive for a mile behind the exhaust fumes of a bus if you can safely pass the bus or take another route. But don't feel that you must pack up and move to someplace where automobiles are outlawed in order to have a strong and healthy baby.

X Rays and Radiation

The word "radiation" conjures up frightening images for many people, yet there is little need to worry about danger from X-ray procedures during pregnancy. First, a quick lesson in the two types of radiation, ionizing and nonionizing. The low-energy waves of nonionizing radiation, which are emitted by radios, televisions, microwave ovens, ultrasound equipment, power lines, and the sun, are considered harmless by experts. Ionizing radiation includes X rays, and these radiation waves have a much higher energy level than nonionizing radiation waves. Repeated exposure to high doses of this kind of radiation could cause tissue damage, but most medical procedures involving radiation use such low dosages that there is little cause for concern. Here's why:

Consider the source. Diagnostic X rays are most unlikely to harm your baby. Medically speaking, X rays are divided into diagnostic radiation (e.g., chest and dental X rays) and therapeutic radiation (e.g., that used in cancer treatment). The unit of measurement for radiation exposure is a "rad." Radiation authorities and the American College of Radiology state that doses under 5 rads do not threaten the well-being of a developing fetus, and that no single diagnostic procedure should pose any threat to the well-being of a fetus. Diagnostic X rays applied to areas outside the abdomen show very little radiation exposure to the baby; for example, the radiation dose in a chest X ray is less than 0.05 rads. Modern radiology equipment produces very little radiation "scatter." The X-ray beams are pinpointed to the necessary area, and X rays do not "go systemic" by entering the bloodstream and spreading throughout the whole body.

Even diagnostic X rays with exposure to the abdomen are well below the worry range for rads: an X ray of the lower spine or abdomen may expose the fetus to around 0.4 rads. However, certain diagnostic procedures may approach a danger range for rads because of the multiple X rays involved. If you need diagnostic X rays that could potentially produce harmful doses, your doctor will recommend an alternative diagnostic procedure, such as ultrasound, if possible.

A CAT (or CT) scan, meaning "computerized tomography," employs multiple X rays, taken in "slices" in a certain area of the body and then put together to form a three-dimensional image. Because multiple X rays are taken, CAT scans are not used in pregnancy unless absolutely necessary. Because of the concern for radiation safety, most high-dose radiation diagnostic procedures have been replaced by ultrasound. More than thirty years of experience with ultrasound scanning has failed to demonstrate any harmful effects on the fetus.

Radioactive dyes are not used in pregnant women because of the possibility of damage to the fetal thyroid. Some radioactive materials, such as xenon, are considered safe during pregnancy and can be used if this type of diagnostic procedure is absolutely necessary.

Consider the timing. Suppose you had an X-ray procedure, even one of the high-dose ones, before you realized you were pregnant. With a single exposure, and especially with the doses previously mentioned, there is unlikely to be any harm to your baby. As a precaution, if there is even a remote chance you could be pregnant, be sure to inform the X-ray technician beforehand so that you can wear a lead apron to shield your pelvis or so that an alternative procedure can be used. In high doses, X rays are considered to be most harmful to the baby during the period of organ development — the first trimester.

Weigh the risks and the benefits. If your doctor recommends a diagnostic X ray during pregnancy, discuss the risks and benefits. If the risks are uncertain or the benefits doubtful, omit or postpone the X ray until later in your pregnancy, or, better yet, until after the baby's birth. On the other hand, if an

X ray is necessary to identify or rule out a problem, and it might influence your doctor's choice of treatment, not having the X ray could be risky. Ask whether the procedure can be modified (by lowering the dose of radiation and being careful to minimize scatter) and whether alternatives, such as diagnostic ultrasound, are available.

You need the X ray; baby doesn't. Reputable radiology laboratories will ask if you are or could be pregnant before doing an X ray. They will also use a lead apron to shield your abdomen and pelvis. If there is even a remote chance you could be pregnant, inform the X-ray technician and follow these precautions. In fact, to reduce potential damage to your eggs, women should always wear a lead apron to shield the pelvis when having an X ray. (Shielding is not quite so important for men, since new sperm are being made constantly; a baby girl already has all the eggs she will ever produce.)

If you work around X rays. If you are an X-ray technician or work near X-ray machines, be sure to wear a lead apron when the machines are operating. Also be sure to wear the required X-ray dosage badge, and have it read at least once a month.

VDTs (Video Display Terminals)

Are VDTs hazardous to a preborn baby's health? Early studies suggested a possible link between extended VDT usage (more than twenty hours a week) and miscarriage. However, recent studies have not confirmed this link. The radiation emitted from VDTs is of the nonionizing type, which, in clinical trials, has not been shown to have the harmful effects on dividing fetal cells that ionizing radiation (e.g., X rays) does. In fact, the amount of radiation emitted from a VDT may be less than you're exposed to next to a television set or even the sun in the great outdoors. But even though newer studies fail to show a cause-and-effect relationship between working around VDTs and pregnancy problems, safety questions remain. Two simple precautions can minimize the risk. If possible, decrease your exposure to less than twenty hours a week and avoid exposure to the back of the terminal, where more of the controversial waves are emitted. Theoretically, you will be exposed to more radiation from the terminal on your co-worker's desk behind you than you will from your own. (Time to move some furniture!)

Household Hazards

You probably never considered your home, sweet home a hazardous environment. Nevertheless, things that you commonly use for "better living" can actually be potent poisons. Now that you are pregnant, you need to take a serious look around and take action on what you can do to improve the quality of the air you breathe and the water you drink — for yourself and your baby. Here's where you can find the most common toxins:

Tap water. In most cases the tap water you drink — and you should drink a lot of water during your pregnancy — is safe. It is always a good idea, however, to have your water (even well water) tested periodically for hazardous chemicals, such as PCBs and lead, by your local Environmental Protection Agency (EPA), health department, water department, or a private water-testing laboratory. In older homes with lead pipes, tap water can pick up lead when it stands in pipes for several hours. When a faucet has not been used for six hours or longer, let the water run for at least two minutes before using to minimize lead levels. Use only cold water for drinking and cooking. In areas where the water quality is marginal (ask your health-care provider), you would be wise to drink bottled or filtered water. Many of the water filters available today do a very good job of filtering lead and other unwanted chemicals from tap water. Even if you opt for one of the more expensive systems, it'll still be cheaper than buying bottled water throughout your pregnancy.

Cleaning products. Avoid all aerosol sprays, stove and oven cleaners, and especially cleaning products with overpowering odors, such as ammonia and chlorine. Never mix chlorine bleach with ammonia, vinegar, or other cleaners because a chemical reaction will occur and produce poisonous gas. Instead of chemically produced cleaning compounds, you might consider "green" cleaning solutions: baking soda, vinegar, and lemon juice.

Grooming products. Chemicals that help you look your best may not be safe for baby. While you are pregnant, avoid hair salons. The fumes from the hairdressers' chemicals and the manicurists' solvents and polishes make for air no human (big or small) should breathe. If possible, have your hair cut in your home or in a salon during hours when no perms or manicures are being done. Avoid the use of permanents and hair dyes while pregnant. While the research is inconclusive about the safety of dyes and perms, enough studies suggest a possible link between these chemicals and birth defects to make it pru-

Getting Too Hot: Baths, Spas, and Saunas

You don't have to give up your hot soaks while you are pregnant, but you may have to lower the temperature a bit and shorten your time in the tub, especially early in pregnancy. Studies show that prolonged, elevated body temperatures of 102°F (39° C) or higher in the first trimester of pregnancy can increase the risk of spinal cord defects in a developing baby. The risks of high temperature harming baby are highest near the end of the first month of pregnancy. How much heat is likely to harm your baby is not known for certain; research is based upon experiments with animals and statistical analyses of pregnant mothers' exposure to heat. Prolonged maternal body temperature of 102° F or higher is suspect.

Suppose you just love relaxing in a warm bath and were accustomed to doing so before you realized you were pregnant. Don't worry — most women automatically get out of hot water as soon as they become uncomfortably hot and long before their body temperature reaches 102° F. Recent studies have shown that a pregnant woman can stay in a bath with a water temperature of 102° F for fifteen minutes without her body temperature rising to harmful levels. Other studies show that during vigorous exercise, a pregnant woman's body temperature is unlikely to reach 102° F for at least forty-five minutes (an unlikely length of time for a pregnant woman to exercise vigorously). These studies are the basis of the recommendation that pregnant women limit their exercise to a maximum of thirty minutes, especially in hot, humid weather.

Saunas also seem to be safe if used wisely. In the cases that make the headlines, women had been in the sauna more frequently, longer, and at much higher temperatures than occur with average use. In Finland, where saunas are common, pregnant women limit their sauna time to around ten minutes, and there is no increased incidence of high temperature–related fetal malformations in that country. You should also know that, despite anecdotes to the contrary, studies show no relationship between the use of electric blankets and fetal malformations.

If you find saunas and/or soaking in the bath or hot tub relaxing during your pregnancy, enjoy yourself, but take the following precautions:

• Get out of the heat as soon as you begin to feel uncomfortable. (As a rough guide, if the temperature of the water is uncomfortable, it's too hot.)

• Limit hot baths or hot-tub soaks to fifteen minutes, and keep the water temperature 101° F (38° C) or below. Limit sauna bathing to ten minutes, and keep the temperature no higher than 100° F (38° C). Because of the cooling effect of evaporation and convection while in the sauna, the body is less likely to get overheated than it could in a hot tub.

• Short, frequent dips in a hot tub are safer than prolonged immersion. Sitting in the tub with much of the top of your body exposed will also lessen the risk of overheating.

• Limit strenuous exercise to no more than thirty minutes at a stretch, even less in hot, humid weather.

dent not to take the risk. At home, use pump instead of aerosol hairspray and hold your breath so you don't draw it into your lungs. Ventilate your grooming area well, especially when applying nail polish. It's best to paint your nails next to an open window or even outside.

Microwave ovens. A quick zap to thaw or cook food is a boon to busy parents. It seems like space-age magic, and you can still use this modern convenience while you're pregnant. Scare stories about microwaves were based upon experiments that showed that developing fetal tissues may be damaged by exposure to radiation. Yet newer experiments show that the amount of radiation emitted from a microwave is so small that it would be very unlikely to damage maternal tissues, let alone those of the fetus inside. Questions have also been raised about possible chemical changes produced in foods exposed to microwave heating. These also have never been shown to be harmful. To be on the safe side, avoid standing in front of the microwave oven while it's on.

Family pets. The family dog poses no health risk to a mother-to-be. Cats can be a problem, but pregnant women can live safely with them too, provided they follow a few safety rules. Of concern is the parasite toxoplasmosis, which is carried by some cats and can infect the pregnant woman, be transmitted through the placenta, and infect the developing baby. Fetal damage from toxoplasmosis is very rare in humans. Most humans are exposed to this germ at some point in their lives and are therefore immune, and most cats don't transmit the germ they carry to humans anyway. However, if you have a cat and you

are the anxious type, ask your health-care provider to order a blood test to see if you are immune to toxoplasmosis. If you are, you do not need to worry. As a second precaution, you can have your veterinarian test your cat for active toxoplasmosis infection. If possible, have someone else take over care of the litter box, since toxoplasmosis is transmitted via cat feces. If you must do the honors, wear disposable gloves when changing and cleaning the litter box.

It is also a good idea to minimize both the ways that the cat can get this parasite and the ways the cat can share it with you. Since cats contract toxoplasmosis from eating infected mice, raw meat, or birds, consider domesticating your free-roaming cat during your pregnancy. Wear disposable plastic gloves when handling soil or sand in the garden or sandbox where neighborhood cats might deposit feces. Better yet, cover sandboxes when they're not in use. To further reduce your risk of toxoplasmosis, don't eat undercooked meat or drink unpasteurized milk.

Insecticides. During pregnancy it's safer to live with insects than to use potentially harmful chemicals to kill them. If you ask exterminators whether a certain pesticide is safe for you and your baby, you are likely to get "I don't know" for an answer. But let's face it: if the chemical is strong enough to kill a bunch of bugs, it's probably not safe for a developing baby. Exterminators wear masks for a reason. If you absolutely must treat your home for insects, plan to be away from home for at least a few days. If an adjacent apartment or the next house upwind is being sprayed, vacate your premises at least until you can no longer smell the fumes. Flea-extermination products applied to your carpet may be sim-

Breathing Clean Air

While it is true that your placenta and your lungs filter some of what gets into your baby, they are not perfect. While we do not want you to be paranoid about every breath you take, consider some precautions you can take to reduce the chances of air pollutants reaching your baby.

- If you live near busy traffic interchanges, factories that emit pollutants into the air, or in a generally smog-filled area, now is the time to consider moving, for the sake of your developing baby and the child he or she will become. Pregnancy is a good time to make healthy lifestyle changes.
- Stay indoors, preferably with the windows closed and the air-conditioning on when the smog level is high.
- Whenever possible, avoid driving on congested streets and idling behind high-exhaust vehicles such as trucks and buses.
- Avoid filling your gas tank. This is another task that you can delegate while pregnant.
- Keep the family car as exhaust-free as possible. Have the exhaust system checked for leaks. Don't idle the engine in the garage.

Keep the tailgate window closed while driving. When driving in heavy traffic, close the windows and air vents and turn on the air-conditioning.

- If you have a coal-burning stove or gas appliances, have them checked for gas and exhaust leaks.
- Avoid strenuous exercise on days when the smog level is high. The heavy breathing that results from aerobic exercise increases the amount of pollution you inhale.
- Insist on a cigarette-free and cigar-free home and workplace.

Remember, humans and their offspring have lived in various levels of pollution for decades, and the majority of babies are born quite healthy. So don't lose precious sleep over the state of the world around you; take reasonable precautions and relax.

Resources for the latest information on substances potentially harmful to pregnant women are Reproductive Technology Center (202-293-5137) and Care Northwest (900-225-2273).

---

ple salt-based products, which are not toxic to humans, even developing ones.

Pesticides, herbicides, and fertilizers. Little is known about the harmful effects of these chemicals on the developing baby. GRAS (Environmental Protection Agency jargon for "generally regarded as safe") guidelines for levels of pesticides are given for adults only. These "safe" levels are not intended to apply to the vulnerable tissues of developing babies, whose cells may be more sensitive to pesticides and whose organs are not developed enough to get rid of them. To be safe, avoid using pesticides in your yard or garden.

When grocery shopping, be informed, but not paranoid, about what you buy to eat and drink, then follow a few simple precautions: thoroughly wash produce with an environmentally safe, nontoxic product, and peel fruits and vegetables. Buy organically grown, pesticide-free fruits and vegetables whenever possible, and buy only domestically grown produce (the pesticide content of imported food is less regulated).

Paint and solvent fumes. Ignore the urge to strip and repaint an heirloom crib or cradle for your baby. Substances to be particularly avoided during pregnancy are old paints containing lead or mercury (both of which substances have been taken off the market), paint removers or thinners, and any spray paints, especially those containing polyurethane. Using new latex paint in a well-ventilated room is considered safe for pregnant women, but even these fumes can trigger nausea. Even if you persuade someone else to strip and repaint the family heirloom cradle, stay away from the area yourself to avoid exposure to lead paint dust; all paint before 1978 contained lead. If possible, paint furniture outside or in a well-ventilated garage or basement. In the final weeks of pregnancy, suppress the overwhelming urge to paint baby's nursery, even when you might experience a strong "nesting" instinct to do so. (Besides, pregnant women don't belong on ladders.) A safe alternative, yet one that may satisfy your urge to create a nice place for your baby, is to design and decorate the nursery but let your partner do the painting. You may as well get used to the art of delegating now. Be out of the house while painting is being done, and air out the freshly painted rooms. Solvents, furniture polishes, and sprays are also dangerous. Go somewhere else while they are being used, and don't reenter your home until the fumes subside. If your hobby is art and you just can't give up painting while pregnant, try to be satisfied with water-based inks and paints. Also, avoid using markers that emit a pungent and possibly toxic odor.

Lead. Lead can cross the placenta and damage the nervous system of your developing baby. Common environmental sources of lead are old plumbing, leaded gasoline, contaminated water, old or imported pottery, construction materials, miniblinds that contain lead, wood preservatives, solders, storage batteries, and old paint. In 1978 the government banned paint containing lead, and homes painted after 1980 are required to use lead-free paint. Houses or apartments built after 1980 should, by law, be free of paint containing lead, but older homes and renovated homes may contain lead paint under newer paint. Best is simply to avoid sanding and repainting while pregnant. If you must renovate an old home or baby's room while you are pregnant, be out of the house during paint-stripping time, and have your contractor use a liquid paint stripper or a HEPA vac (high-efficiency, particulate, air-filtered vacuum) to remove leaded paint dust from the renovated area. As mentioned earlier, have your tap water tested, especially if you drink well water or live in an older home where the pipes may have been soldered or made with lead. Drink bottled water or filter your water if the lead content is high. Don't eat out of pottery that is imported or more than twenty years old.

Besides lead, another potentially toxic metal is mercury. Avoid eating fish from mercury-contaminated waters.

Workplace Hazards

Be as vigilant about the air you breathe at work as you are about your home environment. If you are a hairdresser, become knowledgeable about the often toxic aerosols, dyes, and solvents that you use. Transportation workers should be especially cautious around the carbon monoxide and other gases in exhaust emissions. Workers in print shops and photographic studios should avoid exposure to lead, solvents, and dyes (and their fumes). Assembly-line personnel should be careful about asbestos, formaldehyde, and industrial chemicals. Janitors and cleaning personnel should avoid breathing in fumes from cleaning products. Health-care workers should be careful of radiation exposure and fumes from laboratory chemicals. By law, pregnant women have a right to a safe workplace (see page 138).

THE FIRST MONTH

❖   ❖   ❖

First hints I might be pregnant (e.g., breast changes, morning sickness, tiredness): _____
_____
_____
_____

My first thoughts: _____
_____
_____
_____

My last menstrual period began on: _____

My most likely date of conception: _____

Memories of conception: _____
_____

Date of positive pregnancy test: _____

My reactions: _____
_____

Dad's reactions: _____
_____

Others' reactions: _____
_____

My top concerns: _____
_____
_____

My best joys: _____
_____
_____

My worst problems: _____
_____
_____

Lifestyle changes; habits to break _____
_____
_____

VISIT TO MY HEALTH-CARE PROVIDER

Questions I had; answers I got: _____
_____
_____
_____

My previous gynecological/pregnancy/birth history: _____
_____
_____
_____

My previous medical history: _____
_____
_____
_____

My first physical exam. What I felt: _____
_____
_____
_____

Tests and results; my reaction: _____
_____
_____
_____
_____
_____

My blood type: _____
My weight: _____
My blood pressure: _____
My estimated due date: _____
What I imagine you look like: _____
_____
_____

What I would say if you could hear me: _____
_____
_____
_____

photo at one month

(Include a side view of yourself every month to appreciate how your body is changing. You could also include an ultrasound photo of your developing baby if a photo is medically indicated.)

Comments: _____

_____

_____

_____

_____

_____

_____

_____

_____

_____

_____

_____

_____

_____

_____

Second-Month Visit to Your Health-Care Provider (5–8 weeks)

During this month's visit to your health-care provider, expect to have:

- an examination of your abdomen
- an examination of the size and height of your uterus
- a hemoglobin and hematocrit check for anemia
- nutritional counseling
- weight and blood-pressure check
- urinalysis to test for infection, sugar, and protein
- an opportunity to discuss your feelings and concerns

The Second Month — Feeling Pregnant

DURING THE SECOND MONTH of pregnancy (from the fifth through the eighth week), most women report that they definitely "feel pregnant." Even women who experienced few pregnancy symptoms in the first month are likely to feel at least a bit nauseated and tired now. From here on in, your body will remind you every day of the miracle taking place inside. By now the hormone levels necessary for growing your uterus and your baby are causing an emotional and physical metamorphosis that is pretty much beyond your control. Embrace these rapid changes. You are entitled to feel proud, special, and part of a miracle. Remind yourself that your experience is unique; although millions of women have been pregnant before you, you're the only one to carry this particular child. When you consider that you are creating another life in just nine short months, the inconvenience and discomfort become secondary.

HOW YOU MAY FEEL EMOTIONALLY

Your mind and body will tell you that you're pregnant long before anyone else notices. It's normal to be preoccupied with a pregnancy no one else knows about. During these early months you may become more introspective as you consider the miracle going on inside you and the changes ahead. It's easy to feel preoccupied even at work, especially if this is your first pregnancy. For weeks now you've had something so monumental going on inside you that everything else you're involved in pales by comparison.

Many of the emotions you felt in the first month intensify during the second month and continue to be as unsettled as your stomach. Adjusting to the idea of a pregnancy invading your body takes time. The ambivalence you felt during the first month may peak in the second. It is normal to feel both happy about growing a baby and anxious about the toll pregnancy takes on your mind, body, and lifestyle. Many mothers report feeling some antipathy toward their babies for making them so sick. It's nothing to feel guilty about. (You won't still hold it against your baby when he's born.) No matter how much you love your baby now, you're bound to hate feeling nauseated.

Emotionally I'm feeling at odds with myself. One day I feel excited to be pregnant, the next day I'll almost forget I'm pregnant. One day I'm happy looking at the new maternity fashions, the next day I feel melancholy about losing my figure.

Touchy. With your mind preoccupied with all the issues of pregnancy, little things that didn't bother you previously now set you off, and you may find yourself overreacting to trivial nuisances. Where you previously tolerated quirks in your mate's personality, there may be days when you just can't stand some of the things he does. Or you may go to pieces if he is ten minutes late getting home from work. A dog barking or the doorbell ringing may startle you. If an older child is having a demanding day, you may just want to run away and hide. Daily tasks can seem mountainous when you're tired, nauseous, and awash in ambivalence. Take this touchiness as a signal from your body, telling you to do whatever you can to clear your environment of things that disturb your peace. Of course, you can't tell your mate or your three-year-old to move out for a few months, but you can certainly try to get enough rest, to spend time each day relaxing your body and mind, and to ask for peace and quiet when you need it.

Upset with your mate. As the excitement and novelty of the pregnancy begin to wear off and you settle into the reality of pregnant family life, you are likely to feel less tolerant of the normal upsets of family living. At the same time, your mate may become less understanding. The pregnancy may not seem very real to him yet, so he may not understand that you no longer have the energy to do what you did two months ago. Your sexual desire is waning; it's hard to feel sexy when you're tired, nauseated, and concerned about your changing body. This may further

frustrate your spouse, making matters between you worse. Remind him (tactfully, if possible) that you are pregnant, and even though he can't see the changes in your body, you can certainly feel them. Also, tell him that there's hope: "The book says" you'll be feeling better in another month or two.

My husband is used to my having lots of energy, but ever since I've been pregnant I've been sick and tired and need lots of rest. He seems to think this is all an act so that I can get out of working, doing things around the house, or making love. He makes snide comments like, "Oh, let me guess — you can't make the bed because you're pregnant." I want to strangle him. I want so much to make him understand.

Dependent. Prior to being pregnant you may have been used to a relatively independent lifestyle at work and at home. Perhaps you are used to doing things for everyone else and being on the receiving end of the thanks and the strokes from others. Now you are the one who needs to be cared for, and being on the needy end of a relationship may trouble your self-esteem.

I've been so tired that my mother flew in to help me take care of my other children for a few weeks, and I feel so guilty about it. How come other mothers can do it all, and I can't even get out of bed to take my child to nursery school? I hate being so dependent. How can I ever thank my mother enough, especially since she'll be coming again when the new baby is born?

Remember that you and your body are hard at work preparing to be a mother. Now is a time to let others pamper you and to fill up your inner reserves, so that you will be ready for the challenges ahead. "Mothering the mother" is a good investment for husbands, grandparents, older children, and friends to make. You can make this investment in yourself as well. The long-term beneficiary will be your new baby.

HOW YOU MAY FEEL PHYSICALLY

The pregnancy symptoms you experience in your second month can be a constant reminder of the important changes occurring in your body. Here are the typical physical effects of pregnancy most women experience during the second month.

Nauseated. The nausea and morning sickness that probably began last month often peak in the second month. As you're wondering why you ever got yourself into this, a friend or your doctor offers the cheery dismissal, "Oh, that's just your hormones. Nausea is a sign that your baby is healthy." True enough, perhaps, but not much comfort when you feel seasick around the clock.

Fatigued. The occasional bouts of tiredness you experienced in your first month may now give way to total exhaustion. Last month you wanted to rest; now you *must.* The fatigue of pregnancy may be unlike any other tiredness you have ever experienced, and your hours of rest must increase. Many women describe their tiredness as "bonedeep." This feeling is nature's way of compelling a busy woman to slow down and direct her energy where it is needed. You may find that you have to walk more slowly and that you get out of breath more easily, even during normal walking. Don't fight this fatigue — you can't win. For your own sake

and your baby's, listen to your body's message and rest as much as you can. If you have a demanding job, a demanding spouse, or a demanding toddler, you may not have the luxury of staying in bed or sleeping in, but there will be days when your body simply forces you to get the rest it needs. If the time is not spent sleeping, at least get off your feet. Leave work early, order takeout, or plug in your toddler's favorite videos and sack out on the couch.

I found it helpful to stock up on easy-to-prepare meals my husband could cook. For the first few weeks, I wasn't sure what my name was let alone what was going to be for dinner.

My heart rate is accelerating to a higher rate than usual during my workouts. This must be a sign that my body's getting used to the changes and I need to slow down. I'm surprised this happened so early. My sleep patterns have changed, too. I'm dog-tired in the early afternoon and crash in front of the TV. Then I find myself tossing and turning and staring at the ceiling at 2:00 A.M.

Aware of breast changes. Your breasts will declare that you are pregnant long before your abdomen does. They are likely to feel slightly sore and swollen at first; the earliest sensations are similar to those you may be used to feeling in the second half of your menstrual cycle, only stronger. The buxom look of pregnancy begins. Your breasts are noticeably larger. Breasts typically increase one cup size during the first trimester and another cup size during the rest of the pregnancy. (The most dramatic increase in breast size will occur between two and four days postpartum, when, due to the surge of milk-producing hormones and swelling in the tissues, your breasts will seem to grow overnight!) Breast changes alone typically account for 2 pounds of your weight gain during pregnancy. Small-breasted women will notice these changes more, and first-time pregnant women may notice them more than they do in subsequent pregnancies. The tenderness in your breasts is most noticeable during the first three months and, like most discomforts of pregnancy, becomes less bothersome after that.

Breast changes are caused, as you might expect, by a surge of hormones that stimulate the growth of milk glands and increase the blood flow to the breasts in order to nourish these glands. As the hormones are doing their work, you may notice throbbing sensations throughout your breasts. Your breasts may feel tingly, sore, warm, fuller, or more sensitive to touch. You may experience occasional shooting pains in your breasts that occur off and on for five minutes. You'll probably notice that your areolae (the darker areas around the nipples) enlarge and darken, and that the tiny glands on the areolae that secrete lubricating, antibacterial oil become more noticeable, resulting in a more bumpy look. The veins on your breasts may also become more noticeable, like rivers with tributaries branching out over your breasts to deliver increased blood.

Although the rest of your body will eventually return to normal after pregnancy, your breasts will never be quite the same. They will acquire a different shape, perhaps going from your previous upward curviness to maternal, soft, global fullness. It's impossible to predict what your breasts will look like a year from now. A bit of your pregnant buxomness may linger while you are breastfeeding. Bear in mind that the changes your breasts undergo are due to pregnancy, heredity, and gravity, and will occur whether or not you breastfeed. Be kind to your breasts during pregnancy. Enjoy the comfort of frequent, warm showers and a breast massage if that helps. If you are concerned about sagging, you can help the skin and muscles around your breast tissue by wearing a supportive bra throughout your pregnancy, even at night if you need it (see "Choosing the Right Bra," page 145).

Itchy. Dry, itchy skin is common later in pregnancy, especially on an expanding abdomen (see page 164), but many women report this symptom in their second month. Some experience overall dryness; others mention specific itchy areas, such as the palms of the hands and soles of the feet. If you experience uncomfortable skin symptoms, avoid strong soaps and cleansers that rob your skin of natural oils. You might also try bathing instead of showering, as the constant pounding of hot water against skin may be irritating and drying. On the other hand, some mothers prefer showering because spending too long in bath water can also rob the skin of natural oils. (See page 166, "Pregnancy Skin-Care Basics.")

My stomach was continually itchy wherever fabric touched it, so I typically wore my waistband low to reduce the discomfort.

Urinating frequently. Now would be a good time to pretty up your bathroom, since you will be spending a lot of time there in the months to come. Your growing uterus resides next to your bladder and definitely makes its presence felt on a regular basis. Though you will continue to urinate more frequently throughout your pregnancy, the increased urge to urinate is typically most noticeable during the first three months, before your uterus grows higher out of your pelvis; uterine pressure on even an empty bladder may trigger the urge to go. You can diminish this urge somewhat by emptying your bladder as thoroughly as possible when you do urinate (bear down three times — see "Kegel Exercises," page 176 — and lean forward as you do).

You may also notice that it takes you longer to urinate. Be sure not to confuse the symptoms of cystitis, a bladder infection that many women are prone to during pregnancy, with the normal need to urinate more frequently. Signs of cystitis are a noticeable change in urination pattern accompanied by an increase in frequency, painful urination, an accelerated urge to urinate (whether it's necessary or not), and occasionally a fever. If you suspect you may have a bladder infection, your doctor will need to check your urine for bacteria. Call your doctor's office and ask for instructions on how to do a clean-catch midstream urine sample, what type of sterile container to use, and where to take the sample.

Mouth watering. The composition and volume of saliva change during pregnancy. You may notice that your saliva tastes different and that there is more of it. Some women experience an annoying relationship between morning sickness and saliva production. For some, the increase in saliva triggers the nausea; for others, the nausea triggers the saliva. This excess salivation usually subsides by the end of the third month. If the taste bothers you, try sucking on a mint.

Thirsty. The need to urinate more frequently when pregnant means you'll have to drink more fluids to keep from becoming dehydrated. Thirst is your body's normal signal that you and your baby need more fluids. The increased water you drink helps your kidneys rid your body of the extra waste products produced by the baby. In addition, you need more fluids because your blood volume increases 40 percent when you are pregnant. Your baby also needs fluids to fill his or her growing swimming pool (the amniotic sac). Drink whenever you're thirsty, and then have an extra glass of water for good measure. Do not purposely limit the amount of fluids you drink in order to reduce the number of your trips to the bathroom; you and your baby both need adequate hydration to stay healthy.

You will need to drink at least eight 8-ounce glasses of fluid a day, preferably water or vegetable juice (which is more nutritious than fruit juice). Avoid caffeine-containing beverages, which have a diuretic effect and may interfere with your sleep. If nausea prevents you from gulping down a big glass of any fluid, try the "sips and chips" method: take frequent sips of whatever fluid you can keep down, or suck on ice chips or juice bars. Indulge in high-water-content foods, such as lettuce and melon.

Constipated. Most women are prone to constipation throughout their pregnancy. Early in pregnancy you can again pin the rap on those pregnancy hormones, which slow the movement of food through your intestines. In physiological jargon this change is called "decreased gastrointestinal motility." The slower passage of food and fluid allows more water to be absorbed (perhaps another one of nature's ways of ensuring you get the necessary fluids into your system). The combination of slower movement and harder stools contributes to constipation. In later pregnancy, the pressure of your enlarging uterus on the large intestine further hinders the passage of stools. The good news is you can outwit this uncomfortable effect of your hormones by eating foods that increase the water content of your bowel movements and foods that naturally travel faster through your intestines.

Here are ways to combat the discomfort of constipation:

- *Increase your fiber.* Fiber ("roughage") passes through your intestines undigested and acts like a sponge, soaking up fluid. Increased fluid helps your stools move faster. It also helps you to pass them more easily. Try fruits, especially prunes, pears, figs, and apricots; vegetables, especially crunchy vegetables, such as carrots, zucchini, cucumbers, and celery; psyllium, a natural branlike stool softener, available at nutrition stores; whole grains, such as whole wheat and multigrain baked goods; and legumes and corn. To get the most fiber from your fruits and vegetables, eat them raw or slightly cooked and with the skin left on. To avoid ingesting pesticides, buy or grow organic produce.

- *Increase your fluids.* If you increase the fiber in your diet, you must also increase the volume of fluids; too much fiber and too little fluid can actually aggravate constipation by making your stools even firmer. If you love juice, switch to nectar (prune, pear, apricot), which is not only high in water content but higher in fiber than plain juice. But make sure to drink an additional six to eight glasses of water a day as well. Avoid caffeine-containing beverages.

- *Increase your exercise.* Getting your whole body moving gets your intestines moving. Regular exercise keeps all your physiological systems more regular, and your intestines are no exception.

- *Obey your urges.* One of the conveniences of modern living is that people are seldom more than a few steps from a bathroom, but busy pregnant women may not always take the time to empty their bowels when their intestines tell them to. As with most

of your body's communication systems, however, unanswered signals soon lose their communication value. When you need to go, *go;* otherwise, your intestinal muscles will get lazy, the signals will get weaker, and your constipation will get worse.

(For further intestines-friendly eating habits, see "Eating Right for Two," page 87.)

Gassy and bloated. The same intestinal changes that contribute to constipation also may cause you to feel full of gas. As your pregnancy advances, this bloated feeling intensifies, because your growing uterus and your ballooning intestines are competing for room. To alleviate gas:

- *Keep your bowels moving.* Avoid constipation, which contributes to bloating and gas. (See suggestions above.)

- *Eat slowly.* When you eat and drink fast, you gulp air. The more air you swallow, the more air your already sluggish intestines must deal with. Chew your food long and well. The better the upper end of your digestive tract does its food-processing job, the easier it will be on the lower end.

- *Eat nongassy foods.* Your intestines will tell you what they like and what they don't. Common gas-producing foods include cabbage, broccoli, cauliflower, brussels sprouts, beans, green peppers, and carbonated beverages.

- *Avoid fried and greasy foods.* High-fat foods can also contribute to your bloated feeling because they are very hard to digest and they stay in your intestines a long time.

- *Eat like a baby.* Eating small, frequent meals is more intestines-friendly than taking in three big meals daily. Most pregnant women feel more comfortable "grazing," eating five or six mini-meals at regular intervals each day.

I feel a little bloated, like how I feel before I get my period. I don't yet look pregnant, but I feel it's on my mind all the time and I wonder if people can see it in my eyes.

Prone to heartburn. Shortly after eating, and sometimes even between meals, many pregnant women belch and burp frequently and experience a burning, irritating sensation just below their breastbone. Once again, it's physiologically correct to blame heartburn on hormones. Pregnancy hormones (specifically, progesterone) cause an overall slowdown of the intestines, relax the stomach muscles, and delay the time it takes for food and gastric acids to be passed from the stomach. Thus, food and acids sit in your stomach longer than they do when you're not pregnant. Pregnancy hormones also relax the protective muscles at the entrance to the stomach, so it's easier for food and acids to travel back into the lower end of the esophagus when the stomach contracts. The medical name for this condition is "gastroesophageal reflux" (GER). (So, what you have is really "esophagus burn," not "heartburn.") GER also produces the uncomfortable sensation of "indigestion." Later on, as your uterus grows and begins pressing upward, the pressure on your intestines and stomach may make your "heartburn" even more irritating.

Here are ways to ease the discomfort of heartburn during pregnancy:

- *Eat small, frequent meals.* By taking in smaller amounts of food more frequently, you'll avoid overloading your stomach.

- *Use gravity to help keep the food down.* Avoid lying flat immediately after eating. Try to sit up for at least a half hour.

- *Lie on your right side.* This position allows gravity to empty the stomach. Later in pregnancy many women claim relief from heartburn when they assume the hands-and-knees position, which takes advantage of gravity to pull the uterus away from the stomach, allowing the stomach contents to move more easily into the intestines rather than refluxing up into the esophagus.

- *Keep a list of foods that aggravate your heartburn and avoid them* (e.g., spicy or greasy foods).

- *Avoid fatty foods.* Foods with a high fat content take a long time to digest, and therefore sit in your stomach longer.

- *Eat milk, cream, or low-fat ice cream right before a meal.* By coating your stomach, you may be able to relieve some of the acid burn.

- *Take a commercial calcium-containing, low-salt antacid just before meals.*

- *Avoid drinking large amounts of liquid with meals.*

Most women are delivered of all or most of their heartburn as soon as they deliver their baby, when their pregnancy hormones lessen and the uterus is no longer competing for space in the abdominal cavity.

Expanding waistline. Even though you don't yet show, you may begin to feel larger in the waist this month. It's normal to feel this way; while your uterus is only slightly bigger, your abdomen may be somewhat distended because of bloated bowels and a slight weight gain. As your waistband tightens, you will need to make adjustments in both your clothing and in your attitude toward your body. This is the first step in coming to terms with your pregnant body image. Some women look forward to showing and can't wait to declare their maternity by dressing the part. Others, for various reasons, may want to hide their pregnancy for a while and will dress accordingly.

HOW YOUR BABY IS GROWING (5–8 WEEKS)

Five weeks. By the end of the fifth week, baby is about the size of a green pea, 0.4 inches (1 centimeter) long. Pits that will become the eyes, ears, nose, and mouth begin to show. The arms and legs protrude from the body like tiny buds, and the paddlelike hands begin to show finger buds. The intestines are quite developed, and the pumping heart has already divided into right and left chambers. Breathing passages, called "bronchi," begin to appear. Imagine the miracle occurring in your body. More than a million new cells are added to your baby's growing body each minute.

Six weeks. Baby is ½ inch long. Special ultrasound pictures can now show a fluttering heartbeat of 140 to 150 beats per minute, about twice as fast as mother's. Arms lengthen, an elbow joint appears, fingers become distinct. Feet are distinct from the leg buds, and tiny toe notches appear. The humped-over head looks as large as the rest of the body. Eyelid folds begin to form, and tiny eyes the size of a period already contain a lens, iris, cornea, and pigmented retina. The tip of the nose begins to show.

Seven weeks. Baby is now about an inch long, about the size of a small olive. Elbow, wrist, and knee joints are obvious; toes have formed; the fingers have lengthened. Eyelids nearly cover the eyes, and external ear folds are evident. Ultrasound can now show the body and limbs moving. The head begins to be more erect. Nerve cells in the brain branch out, touch one another, forming primi-

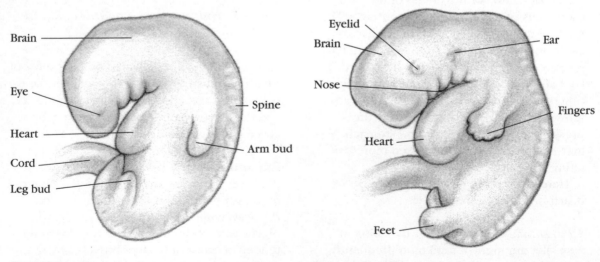

Fetus at 5 weeks.

Fetus at 6 weeks.

tive nerve pathways. The lobes of the cerebellum begin to be seen through the transparent skull. Researchers estimate that one hundred thousand new nerve cells are created every minute.

Eight weeks. Baby is around 1½ inches long, about the size of a large olive, and weighs around ½ ounce. The previously hunched-over head and curved body are now more erect. All the internal organs that will be present in the fully grown infant have already been formed. The heart is now divided into four chambers. Hands, feet, fingers, and toes are fully formed. Major joints, shoulder, elbow, wrist, knee, and ankle are evident. Mouth, nose, and nostrils are more formed, earlobes show, and all the structures of the eyes are found. External genitalia may begin to show, but whether baby is male or female cannot yet be determined by looking. Body and limb movements can be seen on ultrasound. The developing baby, previously called an "embryo," at eight weeks is now called a "fetus" (meaning "young one") and begins to look like a miniature human being.

CONCERNS YOU MAY HAVE

Difficulty Sleeping

The more pregnant you feel, the more trouble you may have sleeping, despite being very tired. Considering that your body is working day and night and that your hormones never rest, it's no wonder you have difficulty settling into a restful sleep. Even though you crave it, you may have trouble getting enough sleep, thanks to a developmental quirk that occurs in pregnant women. As your pregnancy progresses, your sleep patterns become similar to those of a newborn infant. The amount of deep sleep (also called "non-REM" sleep) you get lessens, and REM sleep increases. REM stands for "rapid eye movement," the state of sleep in which you are more aware of your environment and arouse

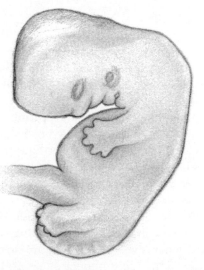

Fetus at 7 weeks.

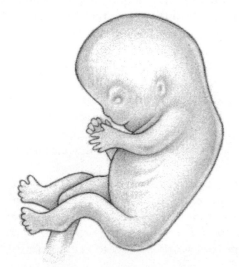

Fetus at 8 weeks.

from sleep more easily. Though it's hard to imagine a physiological purpose for this change, inconvenient as it is, it does prepare you for a realistic fact of parenting nightlife: motherhood is not a nine-to-five profession. The fact is, baby's metabolism doesn't slow down at night, so mother's metabolism can't slow down as much as it used to either.

While sleep loss is one of the inevitable side effects of motherhood, night feedings and diaper changes have yet to begin. Since the care and feeding of your preborn baby are now on autopilot, you'd like to convince your mind and body to enjoy a full night's sleep. While you must accept the fact that a sleep-through-the-night pregnant woman is as rare as a sleep-through-the-night newborn, there are a few ways to help your mind and body enjoy a better night's sleep.

Have a restful day. How you spend the day influences how you will rest at night. Increased exercise can convince a tired body it needs sleep, but don't rev up your body with strenuous exercise within an hour of bedtime; a racing heart and racing hormones do not help a body to sleep. Try also to keep stress to a minimum — a day filled with emotional ups and downs is likely to carry over into a fitful night. Learn ways to stay peaceful and relaxed. Read about methods for relaxing or try a relaxation tape. If you've been to an "early bird" childbirth class (see box), use the relaxation skills you learned there to relax into sleep. Work on managing your emotions.

Leave your work at the office. Mothers who successfully juggle two careers learn not to take their work, at least not their worries, with them from one to the other. Worrying about your work is likely to keep you awake.

An "Early Bird" Childbirth Class

Most parents-to-be begin taking their childbirth class in the sixth or seventh month of pregnancy so the information will be fresh in their mind by delivery day. However, by the time you take this childbirth class, you've already chosen a practitioner and birth place, and many of the important decisions about your birth have already been made. Try to take an "early bird" class in the first month or two. (If you have trouble finding one, check out Bradley instructors, who always have "early bird" classes.) The more you learn about birth options early on, the better your chance of choosing a birth attendant and birth place that will give you the kind of birth you want. An "early bird" class is also a good way to learn about the philosophy of the instructor and make certain that this is someone whose regular, late-pregnancy classes will be helpful to you.

Eat to sleep. Enjoy a light snack before bedtime. You're more likely to get restful sleep after eating foods that contain the natural sleep-inducing amino acid tryptophan; it is found in whole grains, dairy products, non-fatty meats (especially turkey), and fruit. Try intestines-friendly foods that lessen heartburn and are easily digested, such as fruit, yogurt, and whole grains. The complex carbohydrates found in grains have an added benefit: they release energy slowly, keeping your blood sugar levels up at night and lessening middle-of-the-night hunger pains. To lessen muscle cramps, try taking your calcium supplements at night. You might also try a cup of chamomile tea, which is known to have a soporific effect. Avoid caffeine-containing foods, at least after midday. Shun foods that you have learned, by trial and error, are unfriendly to your pregnant intestines. Unless prescribed by your doctor, avoid even over-the-counter sleeping pills, and don't drink alcohol, no matter how desperate you are to get to sleep. Alcohol is more of a drug than a sleep enhancer — it may get you off to sleep, but it is likely to disrupt your natural sleep patterns, causing you to wake up sooner and feel less rested the following day.

Eat to lessen midnight trips to the bathroom. If frequent treks to the bathroom disrupt your sleep, avoid diuretic foods (those that increase urination) after 3:00 P.M. Such foods include beverages containing caffeine (coffee, tea, colas), cranberry juice, and asparagus.

Also, use the triple-voiding technique (see pages 68 to 69) to empty your bladder before retiring. If you wake up in the middle of the night feeling like you need to urinate, get up and go. The sooner you do it, the sooner you'll get back to sleep.

Create a sleep-friendly bed. The sleep axiom that a firm mattress yields better posture doesn't always apply to the exaggerated contours of the pregnant body, so if you're shopping for a new mattress, get a soft one. To give yourself more space to stretch out during the final months, treat yourself to the luxury, if not the necessity, of a king-size bed. Still, your curves won't quite match the flatness of the mattress. Feather your nest with pillows or by using a pregnancy pillow: a body-size beanbag mat that conforms to the contours of your changing body.

My husband calls it "pillow addiction." It starts the first time you get pregnant and never goes away. Now, after three pregnancies, our bed contains piles of pillows — head pillows, body pillows, big ones, small ones — and half of them belong to my husband!

Many women tell us they sleep better with some fresh air. Open the window and see if you rest better. If it's too cold, at least humidify the room to avoid uncomfortable, dried-out breathing passages. A cool-mist humidifier is a healthy addition to a toasty bedroom with dry air from central heating.

Position yourself for sleep. Anticipate changing your sleep position as you grow. Just as you find a comfortable one, your body or your doctor will suggest another. (Front sleeping will, obviously, become increasingly uncomfortable.) In the first trimester, whatever sleeping position works is OK, though it is helpful to get used to sleeping on your side. If you're suffering from heartburn, it may help to sleep on your right side, which allows gravity to help empty the normal stomach acids. In the later trimesters, sleeping on the left side is best. A major vein in your body, the inferior vena cava, passes along the right side of your spinal column, so, theoretically, sleeping on your left side prevents your weighty uterus from compressing this vessel and slowing blood flow to your baby. Practically speaking, you need not worry about unsafe sleeping positions. Most mothers-to-be shift to many different positions throughout the night.

Relax your mind for sleep. Sleep is not a state you can force yourself into. Instead, set the conditions that will allow sleep to overtake you. Try the following sleep-inducing activities:

- Light reading (no mind-charging suspense thrillers, please).
- Light conversation. The before-bedtime hour is a time to wind the mind down, not up. Avoid arguments, debates, or any unsettling discussions that rev up your mind and send you to bed with overcharged emotions. Save the serious discussions with your spouse for daytime.
- Watch a movie, one that's easy on the nerves (comedy stimulates laughter; laughter settles the mind) and one that has a happy ending, of course.

Relax your body for sleep. Try a nice, long soak in the tub. Ask your mate for a head-to-toe rubdown. Maybe add some lovemaking for a finishing touch.

Listen to sounds that soothe. Create your own medley of songs that send you into dreamland. Ballads and classical pieces that have slowly rising crescendos and diminuendos work well, as do compositions containing multiple repetitions of somewhat monotonous themes. You can also try commercially available white-noise producers (they continually make sounds that are monotonous and repetitive, and lull the mind into oblivion) or compositions that play and replay environmental sounds, such as babbling brooks or ocean waves striking the beach.

Don't fight sleeplessness. You may find yourself getting angry at your mind for not cooperating with your tired body. Avoid falling into the cycle of desperately craving sleep, then feeling angry that you can't get to sleep, which makes you even more wide awake. Don't further complicate matters by worrying that you're not getting enough sleep; lack of sleep won't hurt your baby and you'll become even more tired from all the worry. If you find that you're not drifting into sleep, try sitting up to read, listening to soothing music (use headphones if your spouse is easily disturbed), or treating yourself to a glass of warm milk. When your mind is cleared, give sleep a second chance. Just lying in bed with your eyes closed and your mind resting has restorative value even though you're not asleep.

Bleeding or Spotting During the First Three Months

Vaginal bleeding during pregnancy is scary, but it does not necessarily mean something is wrong with your pregnancy. Many blood vessels are being formed as your placenta grows, so it's no wonder that an occasional tiny vessel breaks and you notice staining, spotting, or a little bleeding. Around 20 percent of all women who have healthy pregnancies experience slight bleeding or spotting during their early weeks of pregnancy. It's important for you to know when to worry, when not to, and what to do if you notice some bleeding.

Nonworrisome causes. Bleeding that you do not have to worry about (though every drop of blood is anxiety-producing and you should still consult your practitioner during his or her regular office hours) is painless, brief, slight, and not associated with any other symptoms. The blood is red or pinkish and does not contain fragments of tissue.

Three usual and nonworrisome causes of bleeding in the early months are:

- *Implantation "bleeding."* This occurs from two to four weeks after conception when the embryo burrows into the blood vessel–rich lining of your uterus. This may be mistaken for the beginning of your menstrual period, especially if your periods tend to be irregular.

- *Menstrual bleeding.* The developing placenta makes hormones that suppress menstruation, yet in the first few weeks the hormone level may not be high enough to completely prevent a period. So you may experience a slight and brief bleeding at the time when your menstrual period should occur in the first or second month of pregnancy.

- *Bleeding after intercourse.* Spotting after intercourse commonly occurs, but it is harmless (see page 122).

Worrisome causes. Of more concern is vaginal bleeding accompanied by pain or cramping, heavy and/or persistent bleeding, and dark-brownish or clotted blood, which may or may not contain tissue. Report these symptoms to your doctor immediately. Bleeding may signal a possible miscarriage (see page 79 for how to tell) or an ectopic pregnancy (see page 28).

What to do if you experience bleeding. If the bleeding consists of a small pink or reddish smear on your underwear once or twice and is neither painful nor persistent, you should consult your practitioner during regular office hours. This is not a middle-of-the-night emergency. If this type of bleeding occurs during exercise or intercourse, stop these activities until you consult your practitioner. If you pass any tissue (grayish-pink or brown) as opposed to blood, which is red or liver-colored, save the tissue in a clean container (a small plastic bag or clean jar will do)

and call your health-care provider for advice. The tissue can help determine whether a miscarriage or ectopic pregnancy occurred and can sometimes reveal the cause of a miscarriage.

If the bleeding is heavy enough to soak a sanitary pad, is painful, persistent, or accompanied by crampy abdominal pain or dizziness or faintness, seek medical attention immediately. Lie down and rest while you are waiting for the call back from your practitioner. Save the blood-soaked pad and any fetal tissue contents in a clean container.

When talking to your health-care provider, do your best to stay calm so that you can provide the information needed to decide whether this is nonworrisome bleeding or bleeding that needs medical attention. He or she will need to know how the bleeding began (sudden or gradual), how heavy the bleeding is, how long it has been going on, the nature of the bleeding (bright red, brown, pink, containing clots), if you notice any pieces of tissue, and especially whether or not the bleeding is accompanied by pain, cramping, or any other concerning symptoms.

Most of the time, occasional bleeding or spotting during early pregnancy does not mean a problem in pregnancy, and you probably will go on to deliver a healthy baby. If the doctor sees no need to worry when you call but you are still concerned, ask to be seen in the office in the next day or two just to relieve your anxiety. Your health-care provider may perform an ultrasound to determine whether or not the bleeding is threatening baby's health.

Fear of Miscarriage

It's normal to fear the loss of a treasured person, especially when that little person is growing inside you. You may find yourself checking for bleeding or spotting every time you go to the bathroom. This is a normal reaction, especially for women who have had previous miscarriages. Miscarriage — the medical term is "spontaneous abortion"— means the natural loss of the pregnancy before the fetus is developed enough to survive outside the womb.

Questions You May Have About Miscarriages

Why do miscarriages occur?

At least half of all early miscarriages (those occurring before twelve weeks) are due to chromosomal abnormalities in the fetus so severe that growth cannot continue. Other less common causes of early miscarriages include infections, hormonal deficiencies (especially progesterone), rare immune-system abnormalities (e.g., mother makes antibodies against the placental tissue), and exposure to environmental toxins, such as teratogens (see page 52), drugs, or cigarette smoke.

Late miscarriages (those occurring after twelve weeks) are more likely to be due to structural abnormalities of the uterus (for example, a uterus divided by a wall of tissue) rather than genetic abnormalities in the baby. Fortunately, these abnormalities affect less than 1 percent of women. Other causes of late miscarriages are abnormal attachment of placenta, uterine fibroids (benign tumors), an incompetent cervix, or infections.

For around a third of all miscarriages, the cause is unknown. Miscarriages are *not* caused by sexual intercourse (see page 126), safe exercises, heavy lifting, hanging pictures, doing your usual amount of work and play, a minor fall or accident, or stress or emotional upsets.

When are miscarriages most likely to occur?

Most miscarriages occur before the eighth week of pregnancy. As your pregnancy progresses, the chances of miscarrying decrease.

How common are miscarriages?

Most pregnancies begin with a healthy fetus, growing in a normal uterus, and result in a healthy baby. Studies have shown that around 10 percent of confirmed pregnancies end in miscarriage. Miscarriage very early in pregnancy, however, may be confused with an unusually heavy, late menstrual period. Therefore, the general figure for all miscarriages is thought to be around 20 percent.

Is there anything a mother can do to lessen her chances of miscarrying?

In most cases there is nothing you can do to prevent miscarriage, as most miscarriages are caused by factors outside your control. There are, however, a few things that might help: give your baby a healthy womb environment by following the guidelines on pages 44 to 60, refraining from smoking, harmful drugs, and excessive alcohol, and avoiding exposure to environmental toxins.

If you have had several miscarriages, your doctor will probably want to do special tests to see if a cause can be found. In many cases, he or she can help you achieve a pregnancy that goes to term. Structural abnormalities can be corrected by surgery. Hormone deficiency can often be compensated for by injections. Medical science has solutions for many of the common — and not so common — causes of repeated miscarriage.

How will I know if I had or am about to have a miscarriage?

These are the signs that a miscarriage has occurred or is under way:

• *Bleeding,* either bright red or dark brown, depending on how recently the miscarriage began. As many as 20 percent of women with healthy pregnancies may have one or two episodes of spotting or light vaginal bleeding early in pregnancy, so a bloody discharge from the vagina does not necessarily mean a miscarriage has occurred or will occur. Bleeding that is as heavy as a menstrual period or that continues for several days is more likely to be associated with a miscarriage.

• *Cramping abdominal pains,* similar to menstrual pains, and/or a low backache.

Later in pregnancy a miscarriage is more obvious. The bleeding is heavier and often includes the passage of clots. Uterine contractions can become very intense. Sometimes these signs and symptoms signal an impending miscarriage — called a "threatened miscarriage" — rather than a completed one. In general, the longer the bleeding occurs and the greater the accompanying symptoms of pain, the more likely the pregnancy will end in miscarriage. If you suspect a threatened miscarriage, your doctor will do a vaginal exam to see if there is fetal tissue protruding through the cervix. (This exam does not increase the chances of a miscarriage.) By using repeated ultrasound examinations and by monitoring the HCG hormone level in your blood, your doctor can tell you whether this pregnancy is likely to continue or end in a miscarriage. If serial ultrasound examinations

show baby is growing and the hormone levels stay high, chances are great that the pregnancy will continue.

Don't worry that every spot of blood or abdominal cramp signals miscarriage. Many women with healthy pregnancies show light bleeding (called "implantation bleeding") early in pregnancy as baby is implanting into the blood vessel–rich lining of the uterus.

What should I do if I suspect I'm having a miscarriage?

If you suspect you're having a miscarriage, call your health-care provider immediately, especially if you are passing clots or grayish-pink tissue. If your bleeding is heavy and persistent or your pelvic pains intensify, go to your nearest emergency room. (Try to collect some of the tissue in a jar. It can be examined to confirm the presence of fetal tissue and, if desired, to determine whether or not the genetic makeup of the tissue is normal.)

If you suspect you have miscarried, your practitioner will perform a vaginal examination or ultrasound to determine whether the miscarriage is complete (i.e., you have passed all the tissue) or incomplete (i.e., some of the fetal tissue still remains in your uterus). Miscarriages that occur prior to eight weeks are usually complete. The later in pregnancy a miscarriage occurs, the more likely it is to be incomplete. If your health-care provider determines that your miscarriage is incomplete, he or she will probably want you to have a D&C (dilatation and curettage). Since there are many other reasons for vaginal bleeding, your doctor may choose to do an ultrasound to confirm the diagnosis of miscarriage before doing a D&C. While you are under general or local anesthesia, your cervix will be dilated and any retained placental or fetal tissue will be removed from the uterus. During this procedure the doctor may attempt to determine the possible cause of the miscarriage by examining your uterus for any structural abnormalities. He or she may also send a sample of the fetal tissue to a laboratory for genetic analysis.

If you have not miscarried, your doctor may just send you home. Or, he or she may monitor you with ultrasound and blood tests.

If I have already had one miscarriage, does that mean I am more likely to have another?

Not necessarily. If this was your first known miscarriage, your risk of having a second one is only slightly higher than if you never had a miscarriage, especially if your first miscarriage showed a chromosomal abnormality or occurred early in pregnancy or you have previously given birth to a healthy baby. Even after experiencing two miscarriages, your chances of having a third one are not much higher than if you had never had one. For example, if you have had two miscarriages, you have a 65 percent chance of carrying your next baby to term; a woman who has never miscarried or who has had only one miscarriage has roughly an 80 percent chance of carrying to term. After three miscarriages, however, your chances of carrying your next baby to term go down to 50 percent. After three consecutive miscarriages, you would be wise to have a complete obstetrical evaluation to see if there are any underlying medical reasons that could cause you to have future miscarriages. If no reason can be found, you may reasonably assume that you still have an excellent chance of carrying a baby to term.

I'm so glad I had an ultrasound before I had a D&C because the ultrasound showed the problem was placenta previa and not a miscarriage. I think of this now as I hold my baby in my arms — what could have happened if they had acted on a misdiagnosis?

It's important to do all you can to work through your feelings and not let the visions of your previous miscarriage dampen the joy of your present pregnancy. Even so, some women with multiple miscarriages report not being able to fully overcome their fear until the moment they hold their healthy baby in their arms. It's also normal for a woman who has experienced previous miscarriages to want to keep the news of her next pregnancy private as long as possible (at least past the point when the previous miscarriage occurred), for fear of having to go through the trauma of "untelling." She may even subconsciously suppress the excitement of her pregnancy, delay choosing names, and even wait until the very last minute to decorate baby's nursery. It's important to bond with your baby in the womb even in the face of the risk of losing your baby. While it's normal to fear that this pregnancy may also end in a miscarriage, chances are greater than not that you will go on to deliver a healthy baby.

Because I had had two previous miscarriages, we decided not to tell anyone about our pregnancy for a while because it was previously so hard to "untell." We told only insiders and left the outsiders for later.

I'm afraid to get my hopes up for fear of losing you before you are born. I have been afraid to get to know you for fear I will lose you, because I have already lost one baby, but I know I'm only cheating both of us out of the joy of bonding.

Even though I knew all the stats were in my favor, because I had already had two mis-

carriages, *my fear of losing this baby didn't entirely disappear until after the final push, when I heard her first cry.*

Grieving after a miscarriage. People who have never had a miscarriage may not understand the sorrow women experience following the loss of a pregnancy. Their attitude may be "It's no big deal; you can have another baby." But for you it is a big deal, and it may take a long time to get over it. Everyone celebrates the news of a pregnancy, but few know how to acknowledge the end of one. You need to do whatever helps you come to terms with your grief and enables you to let go of your baby, and go on with having more children. You may need to name the baby you've lost or hold a private memorial service. Don't immediately try to "replace" this baby with another before you have finished your grieving process and have really let this baby go. Discuss with your practitioner when you can safely try to conceive again.

Our first pregnancy ended at eleven weeks, and we were devastated. The grief, pain of loss, and the excruciating crash of impending excitement cannot be shared by anyone except those who have been there. My husband suffered in silence (he did reveal his sadness to other men, but showed only support for me). Our second pregnancy ended at ten weeks. I had been fearful that the situation would repeat itself and felt as though it was a self-fulfilling prophecy. At that point I found myself asking, "Why are children born to unwed mothers?""Why are children born into abusive families?""Why do some women bear children without any problems?""Did I exercise and create the loss?""Is it something I did?" My friends, family, and acquaintances didn't know what to say, and that made it all the more

difficult to deal with. I could have joined a support group but chose to dig myself out of my private misery on my own. After surgeries for fibroids, I delivered a healthy baby, and then went on to deliver two more. Then I had two more miscarriages. I am now in my eleventh week with our next pregnancy, and it is very difficult keeping such an exciting secret from people I come into contact with every day. I know I would be saddened by another loss and would have to rise above it as I did before. But I'm happy to say there is life after miscarriage. It requires perseverance and a dose of the attitude that says if you want something badly enough, try, try again. I do not know if this eighth pregnancy will culminate in a fourth child, but for now the waiting game continues within a very busy life. (This mother went on to deliver a healthy baby boy.)

Having a Baby After Age Thirty-Five

I have just turned thirty-five and I've heard that older mothers have a higher risk of problem pregnancies. Is this true?

Yes and no. The worries you hear and read about do have some scientific basis. Statistically, women over thirty-five (along with teenagers) do have a slightly increased chance of having medical complications during pregnancy. Older women are slightly more prone than younger women to miscarry and to develop high blood pressure and gestational diabetes (the newer and more accurate term is "gestational glucose intolerance"; see page 209). You may also have heard that older women have more difficult deliveries. Researchers disagree about this, especially because the worries about older mothers are based on old statistics, when the older women who became pregnant may not have been as fit or as motivated to stay healthy as women are today. New studies have led obstetricians to conclude that except for an increased risk of chromosomal abnormalities, a healthy thirty-five-year-old woman should expect to carry and deliver as healthy a baby as would a younger woman. You are in good company. Over the past twenty years the number of women over age thirty-five having babies has more than doubled.

In our practices, we've noticed that women who have a baby when they are thirty-five or older have certain advantages. A more mature woman is likely to take better nutritional care of herself, make wiser choices in assembling her birth team and choosing a birth place, and ask more insightful questions during interviews to select an obstetrician or pediatrician. It's common for first-time senior parents coming to our medical office to open their interview with a statement like "This is a well-researched baby."

With today's advanced obstetrical care, which older women may utilize more wisely than younger women, women over thirty-five should no longer be frightened of having first babies. (For second babies after thirty-five, the risk of problems is even less, assuming earlier pregnancies were normal. You also have the benefit of hindsight. You know what to expect during pregnancy, how to position yourself for easier labor and delivery, and how to deal with a newborn and the stress postpartum entails.) If older mothers take advantage of all the advice in this book, we believe that the risks of being an "elderly primigravida" (the archaic term for first-time mothers over thirty-five) are insignificant.

Down Syndrome

Is it true that being over age thirty-five increases my chances of having a baby with Down Syndrome? Do I need to have all those tests?

Statistics on Down Syndrome can scare any "older" woman out of becoming pregnant. Age thirty-five is the usual age questions arise about genetic testing; this seemingly arbitrary dividing line has some statistical backing, which may or may not be meaningful for you. After researching these statistics, we believe the arbitrary age for concern over Down Syndrome should be at least forty years, although concerns over other chromosomal disorders may lower this age to thirty-five. Consider the figures yourself in deciding whether to get pregnant if you are over age thirty-five, and, if you are pregnant and over the age of thirty-five, whether or not to have prenatal testing.

The risk of having a baby with Down Syndrome (or any other chromosomal abnormality) increases as you get older, according to these statistics:

Mother's Age	Risk of Baby with Down Syndrome	Risk of Baby with Any Chromosomal Disorder
20	1:1667	1:526
30	1:952	1:385
35	1:378	1:192
40	1:106	1:66
45	1:30	1:21

But these statistics can be misleading. A 1 in 192 chance of having a baby with chromosomal abnormality at thirty-five is the same as a 99.5 percent chance of having a baby without a chromosomal abnormality. It's all in how you look at the numbers.

Discuss with your health-care provider the benefits and risks of prenatal screening tests. Don't feel you are being discriminated against just because of your age if your doctor pushes the tests. A medical doctor is legally obligated to inform a woman over thirty-five of the availability of prenatal screening tests for birth defects. Since the choice is up to you, consider these factors:

- Would the results of the test cause you to change the course of your pregnancy?

- Would knowing about a chromosomal defect beforehand help you adjust and prepare to parent a special-needs baby?

- Would not knowing such important information cause you to have a worry-filled or joyless pregnancy?

- Since the AFP test (see page 129) may not detect 30 to 40 percent of infants with Down Syndrome, having an amniocentesis (see page 131) is the only way for you to know absolutely if your baby has this chromosomal abnormality. Yet for mothers below age thirty-five, the risk of inducing a miscarriage from the amniocentesis may be similar to the risk of having a baby with a chromosomal defect. How do the risks compare with the benefits of the test in your particular obstetrical circumstances? Discuss the statistics with your doctor. Ask about the complication rate (especially the miscarriage rate) of amniocentesis in the hands of the doctor performing the procedure. The average risk of miscarriage following amniocentesis is one in two hundred (which at age thirty-five almost coincides with the risk of having a baby with

a chromosomal abnormality). This miscarriage risk in the hands of the doctor performing your amniocentesis may be more or less than this figure, so you need this valuable information in making your decision about whether or not to have amniocentesis.

Consider also that fears about having a baby with Down Syndrome may be based upon little knowledge of this condition or on outdated attitudes about special-needs children. On the one hand, you may know yourself and your family situation so well that you realistically conclude that you just could not handle parenting a special-needs baby. On the other hand, you may be surprised to learn of the special love and rewards that come from the experience. Our seventh child, Stephen, has Down Syndrome, something we did not know about beforehand (we elected not to have prenatal screening). Stephen has been a blessing to our family and has provided challenges that have made our lives richer. In some ways Down Syndrome children have fewer abilities than other children, but in many ways they have more. Stephen is perceptive, resourceful, lovable, and loving, and he has taught us a view of what's important in life that we never would have had without him. With the medical support, social services, and public education available for special-needs children today, they are no longer the burden they were once considered to be. Instead, they are a blessing to the family that cares for them — just as any child is a blessing.

Genetic Counseling

I have two friends who delivered babies with inherited diseases, but they didn't know it beforehand. Because I am so worried this may happen to me, my doctor recommends I have genetic counseling during my pregnancy. Is this advisable?

The availability of genetic counseling is a great boon to the relatively few parents who really need it (see below), but it can complicate life for low-risk parents. If counseling or technology can reassure you, should you take advantage of it? Will it change the decisions you make? Will it lower or raise your anxiety level? Or is it better to learn to deal with life's — and certainly parenting's — uncertainty? As with prenatal screening tests, the choice is yours, and it depends on your values and your life situation. Go through the decision-making steps (see page 83). What will you do with the figures the geneticist gives you? Have more children? Have fewer children? Worry more? Worry less?

Meeting with a genetic counselor to discuss your risks and options can provide many benefits, and, since this visit does not involve testing, it poses no risk to your baby. By meeting with a professional, you can get your facts straight (books you may have read may contain outdated statistics). The facts and figures you get from a genetic counselor enable you to make more informed choices about prenatal testing; many couples no longer agree to have a test done just because it is "routine." Genetic counseling can also help you to individualize your tests, ensuring that you consent to only those that you and your baby need — no more, no less. If you have no concrete reason to think you need genetic counseling, it may help to look at the chart on page 82 to remind yourself that for mothers under the age of forty-five, 98 to 99 percent of babies are born without any inherited diseases. If your worry is such that you cannot

enjoy your pregnancy, however, do see a geneticist, as he or she may be able to put your mind at ease.

My third pregnancy, at age thirty-eight, was a total surprise, and my husband and I were both reeling from the news. Our second child, only thirteen months old when I became pregnant again, has Down Syndrome. She was doing well, and we were coping, but the thought of having another baby with problems was adding greatly to the emotional turmoil we were experiencing. I looked into the various types of prenatal testing available to us and, after a session with a genetic counselor, decided to have an amnio. Waiting for the results was miserable — what would we do if there were problems? But when we found out I was carrying a normal, healthy boy, we were finally able to relax, enjoy the pregnancy, and look forward to our son's arrival.

Genetic counseling is usually recommended in the following circumstances:

- *You have previously given birth to or your spouse has fathered an infant with an inherited disorder.* A professional counselor can tell you how likely the disorder is to occur in subsequent children, and what prenatal testing, if any, is recommended.

- *You are particularly concerned about your baby having a certain disease.* Many parents, either because of a family history or personal experience with someone having a certain disease, are eager to rule out its presence. A geneticist can counsel them on the odds and recommend testing, if advisable. The presence of many diseases can be detected before birth, often by testing the blood of the parents.

- *You belong to an ethnic or geographic group at higher risk of carrying the genes of certain inherited disorders.* For example, Jews of eastern and central European ancestry may carry the gene for Tay-Sachs disease (a fatal enzyme deficiency). By testing the blood of the parents, doctors can tell whether one or the other is a carrier. The same procedure is used to rule out the possibility of sickle-cell anemia, a blood disease more prevalent in people of African ancestry. Genes for another type of inherited anemia, thalassemia, are carried by people of Mediterranean ancestry.

- *One parent has a congenital heart or kidney defect.* Some of these defects are inherited more easily than others; the counselor can inform you of the risks specific to your situation. Many inherited heart and kidney defects can be detected by prenatal ultrasound.

- *You and your mate are closely related.* Since genetic diseases do run in families, the closer you are related, the greater are your chances of passing on a genetic disorder to your child.

Genetic counseling is best done before a couple gets pregnant, especially in situations where a known, inherited disorder has occurred on either side of the family. Nevertheless, if you are already pregnant and are concerned about genetic abnormality in your baby, talk to your health-care practitioner. He or she may be able to dispel your worries or recommend a good genetic counselor.

Single Mothers

I'm glad about being pregnant, but I'm finding it's harder than I thought it would be to go through pregnancy without a mate.

Having a baby on the way means big changes in your life, and change is stressful even if it's positive. It's natural to wish you had a partner in this endeavor. Whether you are alone as a mother-to-be by choice or by circumstance, you will need significant others with whom to share your pregnancy. Once they've digested the news, most friends and families will be delighted to listen to your joys and worries, accompany you to prenatal classes (and some prenatal checkups), help you prepare a nest for your baby, and assist you in getting ready for life as a single parent. You may even want one of these special people to act as a labor support person. As the months go by, you will be able to identify the most supportive people in your life, those who are willing and able to help during your pregnancy, labor, delivery, and beyond.

If you don't already know other mateless moms, try to meet some. You'll be able to learn a lot from these women about what to do and what not to do. Sometimes the best advice comes from someone who has already walked the same path and has made wise decisions for herself and her baby. Your main source of support and love, however, will probably be your family, assuming they are able to have a healthy, accepting attitude toward you and the pregnancy. If you find that your family is not supportive, consider seeing a counselor. He or she can help you sort through some tough issues. Keep in mind that your family's heritage is the only one your child will be able to experience. If lasting tensions prevent you from having the kind of family environment you want for your child, don't just give up. Do all you can reasonably do to see that your child has a community of loving friends of all ages in which he or she can thrive. Don't worry if pregnancy is not what you'd hoped; all your child can expect of you is that you do the best you can in this less-than-ideal situation.

I got pregnant by artificial insemination, and when I told my mother over the phone I was pregnant, she was struck speechless. She now thinks her four-year-old granddaughter walks on water.

Making a Move

We live in a small apartment and we know we'll run out of space shortly after the baby comes. Would it be smarter to move now rather than later?

Questions like this one underscore how much your life is changing: you now have another person to consider in major family decisions. In this case, the new person is the impetus for the decision. Before you pack your bags, however, think about why you need to move. Is it because you always envisioned yourself decorating a large nursery? Because you want a yard for baby to play in? Because you associate having a baby with having a house? Will moving mean a long commute for one of you? Will a new mortgage mean you both have to work?

For the first year of his or her life, baby can live happily in the smallest of places. He doesn't care if he has his own room or not (he'd prefer to be with you, anyway); she won't miss pink polka-dot wallpaper. After the baby can walk, he needs a place to stretch his legs — but that can be done on a sidewalk, in a department store, or at grandpa's house. If you're worried about a place to put the baby toys, you'd be surprised how much can fit under a bed or a crib. A few built-in cabinets are a lot cheaper than a move.

If you do decide to move, the best time to do it is mid-pregnancy. In the first trimester, you're likely to be too sick and too tired, and the reality of how much your life will be changed may not have yet sunk in. In the final months, you are just too pregnant to leave your nest, let alone change it. In the last month of pregnancy, especially when that nesting instinct kicks in, it's nice to be settled in. Moving is very stressful and not at all conducive to the emotional well-being of a woman about to give birth. The first few months of parenthood, too, are stressful enough without coping with house-hunting, mortgages, and movers.

In the middle trimester, you're more likely to feel like shopping for a home. In deciding where to move, think first about what you can afford, then consider what you most want life with your new baby to be like. What is most important to your family? A ground-floor apartment? Proximity to a park? A safe street? A fenced-in yard? A location near work? Try to anticipate what life will be like with a baby in tow. If you're moving to a new neighborhood, spend some time there to get a real feel for what it's like — not the Realtor's-eye view.

Sharing in the decision about where you live doesn't mean you should share the heavy work of moving. While you can still be the brains (or co-brain) of the expedition, you shouldn't be the brawn. Let your movers, mate, and friends lug boxes while you direct traffic or pack china.

Hold off making a move if it will complicate rather than improve your life with your baby. Consider whether the move will bring new stress about money, commuting, or making new friends. A baby will change your lives enough without adding other major changes.

The Necessity of Prenatal Checkups

How necessary are prenatal visits to my doctor? I eat well, exercise daily, get enough sleep, and I've read all the pregnancy books. I've got a time-consuming job and a lot to get done before the baby comes. These monthly weigh-ins seem like a waste of time.

Even though you may know all the right things to do to grow a healthy baby, everyone profits by being held accountable to another person. For many people, knowing they have to check in regularly helps keep them on the straight and narrow. And no matter how well informed and confident you are about your pregnancy, you must remember that whereas pregnancy books and classes generalize, your pregnancy is unique. Furthermore, prenatal visits include more than just checking your weight and blood pressure, measuring your baby, and testing your urine. They afford an opportunity to discuss the emotional and lifestyle changes most women experience during their pregnancy, and they provide a sounding board for the many worries (minor and major) that nearly all pregnant women have. Prenatal checkups give a mother-to-be a chance to work through her birthing decisions and, perhaps most important, a chance to become comfortable with the people who will be with her when she delivers her baby.

The usual schedule of prenatal visits to your practitioner is monthly for the first twenty-eight weeks, every two weeks from twenty-eight to thirty-six weeks, and weekly thereafter until delivery. The frequency and complexity of these visits may vary according to your practitioner's philosophy, your previous obstetrical history, and any special needs you and your baby may have. (What is likely to happen at each visit and how to get the most out of your visits is discussed at the beginning of each chapter.) Your obstetrician or midwife will use office visits to monitor the changes you and your baby are experiencing. Most of these changes will be normal, indicating that mother and baby are growing and developing normally. Other changes signal an actual or potential complication that may not be obvious to untrained eyes and hands and that, if detected early and monitored vigilantly, can be corrected or curtailed. In other words, these visits increase your chances of delivering a healthy baby.

In raising a child, there are no guarantees of the adult person that child will later become, yet there are things parents can do to increase the chances that that child will turn out well. Likewise in pregnancy, there are things parents can do to increase their chances of delivering a healthy baby. Regular prenatal checkups rank at the top of this list. In growing a baby and raising a child, new moms soon learn a valuable lesson — to take good care of themselves so that they can take good care of their babies.

EATING RIGHT FOR TWO

During pregnancy you need to consider a very little person's needs as well as your own in planning your menu. While you're pregnant, digesting all the worries about eating right may be more difficult than digesting all the food. While you should give some thought to what you eat, it's not realistic to scrutinize every morsel that passes your lips.

Food lists, menus, and recipes often create unrealistic expectations for the busy pregnant woman who has neither the time nor the energy to count every calorie and measure every mouthful. Better to think in terms of general principles rather than prescribed diets. Eating right during pregnancy means following the same nutritional guidelines for health and well-being that you should when you're not pregnant, plus considering the nutritional needs of the additional person inside your body. By understanding basic nutritional principles you can choose the healthiest foods and the healthiest amounts that fit with your eating habits and your lifestyle.

Your body, pregnant or not, needs the six basic nutrients: proteins, carbohydrates, fats, vitamins, minerals (mainly calcium and iron), and water. "Balancing" your nutrition during pregnancy means trying to get the right mix of these nutrients: 15 to 20 percent of your calories from proteins, 50 to 60 percent from carbohydrates, and 20 to 30 percent from fats, plus the recommended daily allowance (RDA) of vitamins and minerals. Here's how much you need of these basic nutrients and why:

Figure in some fats. The pregnant body needs fats. Besides being a valuable source of energy, certain fats (called "essential fatty acids") are necessary building blocks of vital tissues, especially the brain and nervous system. While pregnant, you may not have to eat less fat, but you do need to eat healthier fats. The best nutrition is found in the fats of fish, nuts, avocados, and most vegetable and seed oils (olive, canola, and flax oils). Less healthy but still necessary fats are found in dairy products. Less healthy still and the least necessary fats are those that come from meat. The only "bad fats" are artificial ones made by processing natural fats. Omit from your diet any food with the word "hydrogenated" on the label. This is a nutritionally unhealthy fat used to give packaged foods an oily taste.

Martha notes: I make butter more nutritious by making "better butter." I mix a stick of melted butter with one-half cup of canola oil and let it harden in the refrigerator.

What about cholesterol, that nutritional "bad word" that marketing managers have used to their advantage in food labeling? The good news about cholesterol is there are two stages in life when you don't have to worry about it: during infancy and during pregnancy. Your pregnant body and your developing baby need extra cholesterol. Growing little brains need cholesterol. Cholesterol is also a building block for pregnancy hormones. Pregnancy hormones make and metabolize cholesterol anyway, so it's natural for cholesterol levels to increase during pregnancy.

Being pregnant doesn't mean that you can now slather butter on everything guilt-free. Calories from fat can make up about 20 to 30 percent of your total daily calories. This is the same proportion of fat recommended for nonpregnant people.

Proteins are powerful. Proteins provide the structural elements for your body and the body of your growing baby. Your baby's tissues and organs grow by piling up millions of proteins on top of each other until each organ has reached full growth. Proteins are composed of tiny building blocks called "amino acids," and a protein is essentially a pile of amino-acid boxes. Most of the amino acids necessary to build proteins are homemade, that is, manufactured in your body. Some amino acids, however, cannot be manufactured in your body and must be taken in with food. These are called "essential amino acids." Without these essential amino acids, a body will not grow properly. Foods that contain all of the essential amino acids are called "complete proteins": meat, fish, poultry, eggs, and dairy products. Complete proteins come from animal sources. Vegetables, whole grains, and legumes (e.g., soybeans, lentils, dried beans, and peanuts) are also good protein sources. However, unlike animal sources of food that are complete proteins, with the exception of soy, foods grown in the soil are incomplete proteins, meaning they contain some, but not all, of the essential amino acids. So in order to get all the essential amino acids, it is necessary to combine different sources of protein. Grains combined with legumes provide complete protein needs, as does any plant source of protein combined with an animal source (e.g., vegetable and dairy, grain and dairy, grain and meat). Try these food combinations to get complete proteins:

- bread and cheese (whole grain and dairy)
- cereal and milk (grain and dairy)
- whole wheat pasta and cheese (whole grain and dairy)
- bread and peanut butter (whole grain and legume)
- granola and yogurt (grain and dairy)
- bean or lentil soup with whole-wheat or rice crackers (legume and whole grain)
- rice pudding (grain and dairy)
- beans and rice (legume and grain)
- pasta with meat sauce (grain and meat)
- broccoli in cheese sauce (dairy with some veggie protein mixed in)

Pregnant women need to eat 100 grams of protein a day. If you normally eat three or four servings of the big five (meat, fish, poultry, dairy, and eggs) each day, you can probably get enough protein by just adding an extra helping. This extra protein is primarily needed during the second and third trimesters, so don't worry if the nausea prevents you from eating more protein during the first three months. Some women who normally avoid red meat say they crave steak when pregnant. If you don't eat meat, are sensitive to dairy products, or are vegetarian, you will have to do some counting of protein grams to be sure you get enough, as well as some planned mixing and matching. (See the discussions of vegetarian eating while pregnant, page 98, and some alternatives to dairy, page 92.) A common nutritional myth is that most people eat more protein than they need. The fact is that most people, especially pregnant women, eat more carbohydrates but less protein than they need.

Carbohydrates should be complex. Sugar has gotten an undeservedly bad reputation among nutrition–conscious eaters. Even when you're pregnant, 50 to 60 percent of your daily calories should come from sugars — the body's main source of energy. Yet all sugars are not nutritionally equal. Least nutritional are the simple sugars, so-called because their molecules are so small that they are easily digested and quickly pass through the intestinal lining into the bloodstream. This causes your blood-sugar level to rise, which triggers insulin release, which then causes the blood sugar to rapidly fall. Some persons experience "sugar blues," the mood swings that accompany this roller-coaster effect of blood-sugar swings. Simple sugars come in a variety of forms: sucrose, dextrose, and glucose; they are the granular sugar in the sugar bowl and the sugar found in candy, icings, syrup, and most commercial foods. Because the hormones of pregnancy change sugar metabolism, some women who were not previously sensitive to the ups and downs of blood-sugar levels find themselves exquisitely sensitive to "junk sugars" during their pregnancy.

Healthier sugars are the fructose sugars, which come primarily from fruits, and the lactose sugars, which come from dairy products. These sugars provide quick energy, yet, unlike the simpler sugars, do not excite insulin release and therefore do not cause the roller-coaster mood swings that the simple sugars do.

The best sugars, especially for pregnant mothers, are complex sugars, so-called because their molecules are larger and thus are absorbed more slowly into the bloodstream, giving a more steady blood-sugar level, which lasts longer. These are also called "complex carbohydrates" or "starches." Best sources of complex carbohydrates are pasta, potatoes, grains, legumes, nut butters, and seeds. Unlike simple sugars, starches, fructose, and lactose provide slow, steady energy and give the feeling of fullness longer, resulting in steadier blood-sugar levels and a greater overall feeling of well-being.

You need extra iron. Iron is necessary to make the extra blood you need to nourish your baby and to make the billions of red blood cells your baby needs. Insufficient iron (anemia) or "tired blood" makes for a tired mom. Toward the end of the first trimester (coinciding with the time when morning sickness usually subsides), your health-care provider will advise increasing the amount of iron in your diet and taking iron supplements. Most women need to double the amount of iron in their diet when they're pregnant, taking in at least 60 milligrams of elemental iron each day, more if anemic or carrying multiples. Do you need iron supplements during your pregnancy? Usually *yes!* Even though mother nature gives your iron levels a boost by increasing the absorption of

iron from foods when you are pregnant, it is nearly impossible to consume enough dietary iron while pregnant without eating excess calories. It's best to begin taking iron supplements early in pregnancy (or even before), in order to store extra iron. Some women find that iron tablets upset their stomachs and aggravate constipation. If iron upsets your already upset stomach, ask your doctor if you can safely delay taking iron supplements until after your morning sickness subsides, since the greatest demand for iron is in the second half of your pregnancy. If iron supplements still upset your intestines, try taking them in small doses throughout the day. Try these tips for eating iron-rich foods and maximizing iron absorption from the foods you eat:

- How much of the dietary iron you absorb depends in part upon what you eat along with the iron-containing food. Some foods help iron absorption, others hinder it. Foods high in vitamin C (e.g., citrus fruits, strawberries, green pepper, kiwi), when eaten along with iron-containing foods, increase iron absorption. Milk, tea, coffee, and antacids inhibit the absorption of iron. So, to get the most benefit from the iron in your foods, drink orange or grapefruit juice with meals, and save the milk for between meals.

- Consider the myths about iron. Remember when your mother made you eat your spinach? Yes, spinach is rich in iron, but most of it cannot be absorbed through the intestines. And there are other foods like spinach, ones that contain a lot of iron that is not absorbable. The figures look good on paper, but that's all it is — "paper iron." The iron found in vegetables and egg yolk, for example, is not well absorbed. Read the label on iron supplements. The amount of

Best Iron Foods

Food	Milligrams of Iron*
liver (4 oz.)	8.5
oysters (½ cup)	8
beans (1 cup)	5
chick peas (1 cup)	5
soy beans (1 cup)	5
blackstrap molasses (1 tbsp.)	5
artichoke (1 cup)	5
cereals, iron-fortified (1 oz.)	4–8
barley (1 cup)	4
lentils (1 cup)	4
beef (4 oz.)	3.5
sardines (4 oz.)	3.5
sauerkraut (1 cup)	3.5
pumpkin (1 cup)	3.4
clams (4 oz.)	3
apricots, dried (½ cup)	3
peaches, dried (½ cup)	3
beets (1 cup)	3
peas (1 cup)	2–3
potato, with skin	2.7
tuna (4 oz.)	2
shrimp (4 oz.)	2
figs (5)	2
pasta (1 cup)	2
sunflower seeds (1 oz.)	2
broccoli (1 spear)	2
bagel (1)	1.8
cherries (½ cup)	1.6
raisins (½ cup)	1.5
brewer's yeast (1 tbsp.)	1.4
prunes (5 large)	1.2
chicken, turkey (4 oz.)	1
bread (1 slice)	1
nuts (1 oz.)	1
tofu, extra firm (3 oz.)	1

* *The RDA of iron for pregnant women is 60 mg.*

iron listed on a bottle label may be misleading. More nutritionally important is "elemental iron," which means the amount of iron that is available for absorption. For example, a 300-milligram ferrous sulfate tablet contains 60 milligrams of elemental iron. If the iron supplement you are using doesn't reveal the amount of elemental iron, ask your doctor or pharmacist how much it contains. For a list of the most iron-rich foods, see the box "Best Iron Foods."

You may have difficulty telling if you are anemic, since the symptoms of iron deficiency — fatigue, irritability, poor concentration, tired muscles — may occur simply by being pregnant. The blood count (hemoglobin and hematocrit) your doctor routinely checks reflects the late stage of anemia. You still could be iron-deficient even though your blood count is normal. If you suspect you are anemic, ask your doctor to check the ferritin level in your blood. This is a more accurate measure of the iron stores in your tissues. A low ferritin level (less than 20) is a sign that your tissue stores of iron are being depleted. Not only is iron deficiency tiring for mother, it's unhealthy for baby. Anemic mothers are more likely to deliver low-birthweight or premature infants. Alternatively, the hemoglobin and hematocrit that your doctor measures may reflect that you are anemic when you aren't. Because fluid volume in your blood normally increases during your pregnancy, a process called "hemodilution," your hemoglobin and hematocrit may reflect lower values than before you were pregnant. This is called the "physiological anemia of pregnancy."

Care about your calcium. Your calcium needs double during pregnancy so that your body can build healthy baby bones and maintain mommy's healthy frame. Baby's teeth and bones begin to form in the second month and double their growth by the sixth. If the calcium in your diet is insufficient, baby's needs will pull calcium from your bones, making them more brittle — a condition called "osteoporosis." You and your baby together need an average of 1600 milligrams of calcium daily, 800 milligrams more than before you were pregnant. New studies show that pregnant women who take 1500 to 2000 milligrams of daily calcium supplements can reduce their chances of developing high blood pressure and preeclampsia by 60 to 70 percent. Be sure your calcium reserves are adequate when your baby begins to need large amounts, which is primarily during the third trimester. Unless you must avoid dairy products, it's not too difficult to ingest this

amount. One quart of milk contains your total daily calcium requirement. The calcium champion, the food that packs a lot of calcium into the fewest number of calories and agrees with most women, is yogurt. If you dislike milk, yogurt is an excellent choice for you; an equivalent amount of yogurt is higher in calcium and more nutritious than milk anyway. Treat yourself to a daily yogurt shake. Three 8-ounce cups of yogurt will meet the total daily calcium needs of most pregnant women. Cheese is also a concentrated source of calcium that can be an alternative to milk. If you have trouble digesting regular milk, try acidophilus milk. If you have a lactose intolerance, try calcium-enriched soy or rice milk or a lactose-reduced milk, or take the enzyme lactase (Lactaid), available in tablet form, along with your milk. If it's the fat or the calories in dairy products that you're not fond of, try low-fat or nonfat dairy products, which may contain slightly higher amounts of calcium.

Best Calcium Foods

Food	Milligrams of Calcium
yogurt (8 oz.)	400–450
milk (8 oz.)	300
Fish: salmon, with bones; tuna; sardines (4 oz.)	250
cheese (1 oz.)	200
tofu, firm (8 oz.)	200
rhubarb (½ cup)	174
cottage cheese (8 oz.)	150
blackstrap molasses (1 tbsp.)	137
figs (3)	80
almonds (1 oz.)	75
collards (½ cup)	74
refried beans (½ cup)	70
soy beans (½ cup)	66
broccoli (½ cup)	50
kale (½ cup)	47

Get a Head Start on Nutrition

If you are planning or trying to get pregnant, plan ahead for good nutrition for yourself and your baby, before the ravages of nausea make it difficult to keep vitamin supplements down and make drastic changes in your previous eating habits. It's easier to change unhealthy eating habits before you're pregnant. Begin taking iron supplements (see page 90) and folic acid (see page 94) at least a couple months before conception. Studies have shown that women who take folic-acid supplements prior to becoming pregnant lower their baby's risk of spinal defects.

Understanding the Food Pyramid

In attempting to reshape the high-fat American diet, in 1992 the U.S. Department of Agriculture published a food pyramid, which illustrates the basic nutritional guidelines for a healthy, balanced diet. Unlike the old four basic food groups, which gave all foods equal rating, the pyramid shows consumers that foods that are of plant origin, not from animals, should be the foundation of a healthy diet. You will notice that grains, vegetables, and fruits occupy first, second, and third positions in the pyramid; the animal-source foods (dairy, fish, poultry, and meat) occupy the fourth and fifth positions. Also, the human body needs a bit of "oiling" with healthy fats. Besides being nutritious, food can taste good with a bit of vegetable oil or seed sprinkled on top.

1. **Grains: bread, cereal, rice, and pasta.** 6–11 servings (1 serving = 1 slice of bread, ½ cup of rice, pasta, or cooked cereal, ½ cup of potatoes or beans, or 1 ounce of ready-to-eat cereal). Use whole grains whenever possible.

2. **Vegetables.** 3–5 servings (1 serving = 1 cup of raw, ½ cup of cooked, or ¾ cup of vegetable juice). Use fresh whenever possible; organic is best.

3. **Fruits.** 2–4 servings (1 serving = 1 medium-size orange, apple, or banana, ½ cup of canned fruit, or ¾ cup of juice). Use fresh whenever possible; organic is best.

4. **Dairy products: milk, yogurt, and cheese.** 2–3 servings (1 serving = 1 cup of milk or yogurt, ½ cup of cottage cheese, 1½ ounces of cheese, or ½ cup of ice cream).

5. **Meat, poultry, fish, eggs, legumes (beans and seeds), and nuts.** 2–3 servings (1 serving = 3 ounces of meat, fish, or poultry, 2 eggs, 2 tablespoons of nut butter, or 1 cup of cooked legumes).

Note: The above pyramid food groups and recommended servings apply to all healthy eaters, whether pregnant or not. The range of servings accounts for levels of activity. Very active persons would consume the higher number of servings. Pregnant women would also consume the higher number of servings, add an extra serving to groups four and five, and eat lean meat and low- or nonfat dairy products.

Satisfy with salt. There once was a time when swelling in hands and feet during pregnancy was blamed on too much salt. Nearly all women experience some degree of swelling; excess salt is not to blame. Unless advised by your health-care provider, you should not restrict your salt intake while pregnant. The craving for salt that many women experience during pregnancy is another of nature's necessary nutritional messages. Salt causes your body to retain fluid, of which you need more during pregnancy. Your fluid requirements while pregnant will nearly double to support the 40 percent increase in your blood volume and the constant replenishing of the amniotic fluid surrounding your baby. Farmers recognized the need for extra salt long ago. Travel past any dairy farm and you'll see pregnant cows licking salt blocks. Be sure to use iodized salt (not sea salt), since your body needs the extra iodine to prevent thyroid deficiency while pregnant. Salt your food to taste.

Value your vitamins. While the body's needs for protein, calcium, and iron increase greatly during pregnancy, the need for most vitamins increases only slightly. In most women eating a healthy diet, these needs will be met by the extra food they eat. Vitamins are found in nearly all foods, so as long as you are eating a reasonably healthy and balanced diet, it is unlikely that you or your baby will suffer vitamin deficiency. For this reason, as long as a woman's diet is good, many health-care providers no longer recommend the routine use of multivitamin supplements during pregnancy.

Take extra folic acid. An exception to this no-supplements suggestion is the vitamin folic acid, also known as "folacin," a B vitamin essential for a healthy, growing baby. Folic acid is plentiful in such common foods as raw, leafy vegetables, legumes, kidneys, nuts, liver, dark yellow fruits and vegetables, and broccoli. Your need for folic acid at least doubles while you are pregnant. Since your body does not store this vitamin, and as the kidneys excrete much more of this vitamin during pregnancy, you need a daily source of 400 to 800 micrograms. Deficiency in folic acid has been linked to congenital malformations of the baby's central nervous system, primarily spina bifida. In recent studies, pregnant women who took between 100 and 4000 micrograms of folic acid during the first six to twelve weeks of pregnancy had a much lower risk of delivering babies with spinal column defects. Recent research suggests that people with different genes require different amounts of folic acid. Perhaps some women come genetically predisposed to

folic-acid deficiency and are more likely to need supplements of this vitamin while pregnant. Since there is no way to tell if you are one of these women, all women should take a folic-acid supplement as early in pregnancy as possible, since these malformations occur in the first few weeks. Even better is to take a folic-acid supplement a few months before conception. The Food and Drug Administration (FDA) recommends that beginning in 1998 all enriched foods, including flour, cornmeal, pasta, and rice, be fortified with folic acid. This addition will not meet a pregnant woman's daily requirements, though; supplements will still be necessary. Even though the risk of spinal abnormalities from folic-acid deficiency is greatest in the early months of pregnancy, it is necessary to continue supplementing with this vitamin throughout the pregnancy. New studies show that deficiency of folic acid throughout pregnancy increases the chance of giving birth to a premature baby.

Don't megadose on vitamins while pregnant. While much is known about the average daily requirements for vitamins during pregnancy and the effects of vitamin deficiency, little is known about overdoses, and more may not be healthier for a preborn baby. Excesses of vitamins A, D, and E have been linked to birth defects or health problems in the mother. For example, a 1995 study showed that pregnant women who took more than 10,000 IU of vitamin A supplements daily were nearly five times more likely to give birth to babies with defects such as cleft lip and cleft palate or heart defects. Even though the body usually protects against overdosing on most nutrients (especially water-soluble vitamins), excess vitamins A, D, and E are not automatically eliminated from the body because they are fat-soluble and therefore stored in body fat. Large doses of vitamins C and B complex used to be considered harmless because these vitamins are water-soluble and therefore the excess is easily excreted through the urine. Newer studies cast doubt on the safety of large doses of these vitamins too. Newborns of mothers who take megadoses of vitamin C can enter the world dependent on these high doses and actually develop signs of vitamin deficiency after birth. Some infants of mothers who took large doses of vitamin B_6 during pregnancy may be more likely to develop seizures. The bottom line on this new research is that it's safest to stick with what we know: the dosage of vitamins recommended by your health-care provider — no more, no less.

I couldn't tolerate citrus because it gave me heartburn. I realized my body might be low on vitamin C when I walked into the supermarket and began craving strawberries and kiwis, foods high in vitamin C. It's amazing how the body tells you what it needs when you're pregnant.

Don't forget your fluids. Extra fluids are necessary not only to increase your blood volume by 40 percent and to keep refilling the pool of amniotic fluid but also to maintain your overall well-being during pregnancy. Drinking lots of water and other fluids helps keep your skin soft and smooth. More fluids in your diet put more fluids in your bowels, lessening constipation. Keeping your body primed with extra fluids helps move along and dilute the body's waste products and causes you to urinate more frequently, lessening the risk of urinary tract infections. You will need eight 8-ounce glasses of fluid a day to keep your body and your baby well hydrated. Avoid alcohol and caffeine, since, be-

Pregnancy Nutrition in a Nutshell

When reading all the stuff about the importance of proper nutrition during pregnancy, it's easy to lose your appetite. So much information can overwhelm you with its complexity, leaving you fearful that there's no way you can eat right for yourself and your baby. Eating right while pregnant is really quite simple. If you already know the basic principles of good nutrition and were eating healthy before you became pregnant, simply add an extra:

- 300–500 calories per day of nutritious food
- 25 grams of protein
- 800 milligrams of calcium
- 0.4 milligrams of folic acid
- 40 milligrams of iron

The extra daily calories, calcium, and protein can be obtained by eating an extra cup of yogurt and six ounces of fish (or the nutritional equivalent). The extra folic acid can be obtained by taking one tablet of supplement (0.4–0.8 milligrams), the calcium by taking a 500-milligram calcium supplement, and the extra iron by taking one 30-milligram tablet of ferrous sulfate (or the 60-milligram elemental-real-food equivalent, if you want to eat liver every day for nine months).

So, don't be intimated by the volumes written about proper nutrition while pregnant. You simply eat like you should anyway, plus an extra helping for your inside guest.

sides the problems discussed on pages 48 and 50, these substances have a diuretic effect, robbing your body of fluids. Make it a habit to use extra-large cups and glasses, and make a large water bottle your constant companion. While most of your fluid requirement should be satisfied in the form of plain water, it's okay to treat yourself to more flavorful fluids, such as juices and soups. Have juice as an alternative to drinking a glass of milk with meals (vitamin C enhances the absorption of iron from your food), but be careful not to overdose on juice, since it is not a nutrient-dense food; ounce for ounce it contains nearly as many calories as milk, with much less nutrition. Instead, try diluted juice or flavored seltzer water, or flavor your water with just a teaspoon of frozen juice concentrate. It's best to space your fluid intake evenly throughout the day. As you're eating smaller, more frequent meals, you should be consuming larger, more frequent drinks.

Questions You May Have About Nutrition

Here are some questions you may have about eating right while pregnant:

Why is it so important to eat right during pregnancy? Don't I simply need extra calories so that my baby and I can grow?

Studies show that the better a pregnant woman's nutrition, the more likely she is to deliver a healthy baby. Eating too little (or too little of the needed foods) increases the risk of giving birth to a baby who may be born too soon or too small, have birth defects, or have breathing and blood chemistry problems at birth. Poor prenatal nutrition increases the risk of problems ranging from

stillbirth to developmental delay. Poor prenatal nutrition increases your risk of having an uncomfortable pregnancy with more morning sickness, constipation, fatigue, heartburn, and muscle cramps; and obstetrical complications, such as anemia, toxemia, a more difficult delivery, and a greater chance of needing a cesarean section. Also, an undernourished mother is more likely to deliver a premature or low-birthweight baby.

Think of your pregnancy as a baby-building process. You yourself need energy — calories to do the building. This energy comes from fats and carbohydrates. Then you need the right mix of materials for a solid structure — proteins, vitamins, iron, other minerals, and water. If, in building your baby, you don't have enough energy, the work doesn't get done. If you don't use the right mix of materials, the building isn't constructed well. Fortunately, you don't need the skills of an architect or engineer to build a baby. The growing infant self-engineers his or her construction. All you have to do is provide enough energy and make the right materials available.

What changes in my eating habits am I likely to experience while I'm pregnant?

Your eating habits will change because both nutritional needs and your intestinal function change. Sometimes your body will be wise, causing you to crave the extra nutrients you need, for example, extra salt. Other times the "wisdom of the body" is not so wise. You may crave what you don't need, say, a hot fudge sundae (sometimes good for the soul, but seldom a legitimate nutritional need). That's why before giving in to your cravings, rationalizing that your body knows best, double-check your urges with your knowledge of good nutrition.

You are likely to want to eat lighter, smaller portions more slowly and more frequently. There will be days when you graze like a toddler, snacking all day long. Sometimes you'll satisfy the "always hungry" feeling by eating all the time. You don't have to make a conscious effort to eat like this — your body is likely to compel you to do this. The usual sluggish digestion that accompanies pregnancy will voice its preferences. After a while you will know what foods are most friendly to your digestive system and how much and how often to eat them.

What does having a "balanced" diet while I'm pregnant really mean?

While there are principles in nutrition that apply to all pregnant women, each pregnant woman must customize her diet to what's digestible for her. In a nutritional nutshell, "balanced" means eating the right amount of food and the right mix.

Yet you need not be obsessed with balancing every meal every day. The combination of food cravings, fluctuating appetite, lifestyle choices, the other facets of pregnant life, and just plain human nature, means that you won't eat the right amount and the right mix at every meal, and you don't have to. The body has a marvelous way of parceling out the food it gets. One day you may undereat an important nutrient, another day you may eat more of it to compensate. The body recognizes this erratic pattern, stores the excess (except for a few vital nutrients), and releases it when you and your baby need it. Rather than worry about balanced meals, shoot for a balanced week.

Which foods are best to eat while I'm pregnant, and how much?

Depending on how much you exercise and whether or not you started your pregnancy over- or underweight, you will need to eat an extra 300 to 500 calories per day to ensure adequate nutrition for both of you. A sit-a-lot mother may need only 300 extra calories; an active mom chasing small children all day will need around 500 extra. You may be surprised how little extra food this is (300 calories equals two glasses of low-fat milk and a slice of buttered bread; 500 calories equals three glasses of low-fat milk and two slices of buttered bread).

Even though your caloric needs increase only around 20 percent while you're pregnant, your nutritional needs for some nutrients increase by 50 to 100 percent. So, you have to eat a little more food but be a lot wiser in your choice of food. In other words, while pregnant you need only a small increase in the *quantity* of food you eat, but you do need to give a lot of attention to the *quality* of food you eat. This means eating foods that are more nutrient-dense, foods that pack more nutrition into each calorie. In applying the concept of nutrient-dense eating to your diet during pregnancy, choose foods that are highest in protein, calcium, and iron for the least number of calories. Examples of favorite nutrient-dense foods for most pregnant women include the following:

- nonfat cottage cheese
- nonfat yogurt
- tofu
- fish: tuna, salmon
- beans: kidney, garbanzo (chick peas)
- eggs
- turkey

Here is one of Martha's favorite nutrient-dense recipes:

The Pregnancy Salad

8 oz. nonfat cottage cheese
4 oz. water-packed tuna
4 oz. kidney beans
4 oz. garbanzo beans (chick peas)
3 cups dark green leaf lettuce

Mix together with a generous squirt of lemon juice.

This salad contains around 600 calories and provides about 75 grams of protein (three-quarters of your daily requirement), 350 milligrams of calcium (approximately 20 percent of your daily requirement), and 8 or 9 milligrams of iron (about 20 percent of your daily requirement). For extra flavor (and 125 extra calories), add a tablespoon of cold-pressed olive oil. For an extra touch (and 80 extra calories), add a tablespoon of raw sunflower seeds. Besides being nutritious, this type of salad is extremely filling. Some women may find it too much for one meal and may prefer to cut the recipe in half or to make the full portion and graze on it throughout the afternoon.

I'm a vegetarian and I feel great, but I'm worried I may not be getting adequate nutrition for my baby and myself later in pregnancy. Do I have to change my diet?

Much of the world's population is vegetarian, and healthy vegetarian mothers birth healthy babies. Yet during pregnancy you do have to be more savvy about nutrition — and perhaps sometimes compromise a bit — to ensure enough nutrition for a growing mommy and baby. The nutrients that are marginal in vegetarian diets are iron (more plentiful and better absorbed from animal sources), vitamin B_{12} (found mostly in animal sources),

and, unless you get plenty of sunlight, vitamin D (added to dairy products). Even though folic acid (see page 94) is present in green, leafy vegetables, as is the case with iron, you would have to eat a huge amount of vegetables, almost like a foraging animal, to get enough folic acid. So, vegetarian pregnant women need iron and folic-acid supplements just as nonvegetarians do.

If you are an ovo-lacto vegetarian (eggs and dairy, but no meat or fish), you can get adequate vitamin D and additional protein from these sources, but iron and B_{12} may still be insufficient, and you may need to take supplements of both. If you are unwilling to take commercial supplements but are willing to compromise, eating 4 ounces of fish (e.g., fish liver oils, salmon, sardines, tuna) daily will provide enough of the otherwise missing nutrients for you to safely continue being "almost" a vegetarian while pregnant.

If you're a strict vegetarian (a vegan — no eggs, dairy, meat, or fish), you will need to monitor your diet most carefully. To increase your and your baby's chances of getting enough nutrients, consult a nutritionist to work out alternative sources of marginal nutrients. Follow these tips to be sure you get enough nutrients:

• Maximize your iron absorption by combining plant sources of iron with foods high in vitamin C (e.g., citrus fruits, strawberries, kiwi, green pepper).

• Be sure to tell your health-care provider you're a vegan, and have your hemoglobin checked at least every other month. Because you can still feel anemic with a normal hemoglobin level, your health-care provider may want to do an iron profile, which is a more accurate measure of iron-sufficiency in your blood (see page 91).

- If your practitioner recommends that you take an iron supplement, protect yourself from discomfort by taking smaller doses and with meals — for example, 100 milligrams of ferrous sulfate tablets three times a day rather than 300 milligrams once a day. To increase the amount of iron absorbed from these pills, take a 100-milligram vitamin C tablet at the same time.

- Sunlight is a valuable source of vitamin D. Cloudy days, cold climates, varying layers of clothing, and the growing realization that sun-browned skin is cancer-prone make the sun an unpredictable and suspect source of vitamin D. Since the body does not store vitamin D, you will need to take a supplement daily. Excess vitamin D is not readily excreted, so be sure you take only the required amount, which is 400 IU per day.

- You will need a vitamin B_{12} supplement, since animal foods are the primary source of this vitamin. Consult your health-care provider. Some vitamin B_{12} is also found in yeast, wheat germ, and whole grains.

I don't eat red meat, but I eat everything else, including poultry and fish. Will my baby and I get enough nutrition?

Yes. There are no nutrients in red meat that you or your baby needs that are not found in poultry or fish. In fact, ounce for ounce, you may be happy to know that fish is more nutritious than all the meats. You don't have the extra fat that laces most meats or the worry of additives (hormones and antibiotics), which are present in beef and poultry. Ocean fish tend to be safer than fresh-water fish, which could be contaminated with mercury and PCBs; try to check the safety of the water before you eat fresh-water fish. You will find wild fish more tasty and less fatty than farm-grown fish (which are grown in water tanks).

I'm a busy person. I grab breakfast on the run, eat a quick lunch, and often order a take-out dinner for my husband and myself. Now that I'm pregnant, I worry I'm not eating right. How can I still eat fast yet healthy?

The four basic food groups does not mean McDonald's, Taco Bell, Pizza Hut, and KFC. One of the valuable lessons learned by a busy woman in the life of growing a baby is that it's important to slow down and smell the roses. It's unlikely that you'll have to make a conscious effort to slow down — your body, if it hasn't whispered it already, will soon give you the clear message to relax your pace of living and eating. Before you were pregnant, you could get away with erratic and less nutritionally sound eating habits. Your body was more likely to forgive your hit-or-miss nutrition, and you may even have been able to jog off your indulgences. Now that you have another mouth to feed and a body that prompts you to be more nutritionally correct, you will need to slow down and read labels, read menus, and even change where and what you order.

Fast foods can still be healthy foods, but not unless you become a savvy consumer. If it isn't posted, ask to see information on the nutritional content of the fast food you like. (See "Learning to Read Labels," page 101.) Many fast-food establishments offer pre-made salads or create-your-own salad bars. Today's supermarkets, too, often have salad bars, deli counters, and other good food "to go." For healthy salad dressing, bring your own or use oil and vinegar. You can enjoy an occasional burger binge, but you might want to try veggie burgers as a substitute, if you haven't already. How you dress your food can determine its healthiness. Frequent the establishments that let you have it your way. Ask for a whole-wheat bun for your burger, hold the mayo, double the lettuce and tomatoes, and ask the cook to blot the excess grease out of your burger with a paper towel before it's put between the buns. Drink juice (at home, drink nectar, which is even more nutritious and a natural laxative) instead of soda, have fruit instead of fries, and skip the shake (as a healthier choice, treat yourself to a custom-made shake from a frozen-yogurt shop). Instead of high-fat dressing, try a little oil and vinegar with a sprinkle of fresh cheese and nuts; instead of sour cream and butter on your baked potato, bring your own low-fat yogurt. All-fruit spread is a healthy alternative to syrup on pancakes. Skip the fat-laden desserts and pick up an apple or an orange at the convenience store. Instead of grabbing a doughnut for a snack at work, bring a supply of fruit or yogurt, trail mix of raisins, nuts, and dried fruit, and a bottle of mineral water.

My husband and I are careful to watch how much cholesterol we eat. We eat very lean meat, skinless poultry, and low-fat everything. Now that I am pregnant, should I continue to limit my cholesterol, or do I and my baby need more?

Growing persons need more cholesterol. There are two groups of people who can and should indulge in cholesterol-containing foods: infants and young children; and growing, pregnant women. Cholesterol is a vital nutrient for infant brain development, and your pregnant body automatically responds to baby's increased need by increasing its internal cholesterol production by at least 25 percent. You don't have to purposely increase the cholesterol in your diet, as your

body will automatically provide this, but you can permit yourself an occasional cholesterol-rich treat without worry.

Yet pregnancy is not a license to indulge in cholesterol-rich foods. Most high-cholesterol foods are also high in unwanted calories and unneeded fats. Besides, serving your cholesterol-watching spouse low-fat pasta as you indulge in a juicy steak is not likely to promote mealtime goodwill in your marriage. Continue setting a healthy-heart eating example for the rest of your family. (If you must take advantage of your temporary license to cheat on cholesterol, do it on the sly, so you're not rubbing it in.) Don't let yourself slip back into high-cholesterol eating habits that may be difficult to change after birth. Don't let your taste buds get used to fat-flavored foods.

Now that I'm pregnant I'm afraid to eat any kind of processed food. Could all those chemicals and additives hurt my baby?

While you certainly don't have to farm or fish for your food because you're pregnant, neither can you afford to become lax about labels. The body, at least the nonpregnant one, has a remarkable way of ridding itself of unnecessary and oftentimes unsafe chemicals. Yet it is unwise to apply this cavalier modern attitude to the diet of the preborn baby. Chemicals added to our foods have received a "generally regarded as safe" (GRAS) designation from federal agencies. But "generally regarded as safe" can be interpreted as meaning "not 100 percent certain." GRAS designations come from the offices of number-crunching statisticians or the laboratories of researchers who have fed unrealistically high levels of the suspect chemicals to unsuspecting rats; little is known about how these chemicals work in humans. Two concerns should make you

Learning to Read Labels

For the sake of yourself and your baby, learn the language of labels. Ingredients are listed in order; the main ingredient is listed first, then the next most prevalent one, and so on, and the least one last. Also useful is the amount of protein, carbohydrate, fat, and calories in the food. These facts are helpful in counting calories and protein grams and in keeping your fat intake under control.

Watch out for all of sugar's different names. You may see it listed as sugar, but sucrose and dextrose may also be mentioned, and though they sound healthier, they are still sugars. Corn syrup and high-fructose corn syrup are other common sweeteners that masquerade as natural, yet yield little more nutrition than plain old sugar. Some foods may have two or three different sweeteners in the ingredient list; if you add them together,

sugar might turn out to be the main ingredient in the food.

The term "natural" on a label is nutritionally deceptive. It conjures up thoughts of "homemade," "home-grown," and "fresh," when all it really means is derived from natural, as opposed to artificial, sources. Beware of the labels "fortified" and "enriched." This means that extra vitamins and minerals have been added to the food — usually because the natural nutrients have been processed right out. If you are allergic to milk, watch for the milk derivatives casein, sodium caseinate, and whey.

As a general rule, if you can't pronounce it, don't eat it! While it's no longer practical or necessary to grow, hunt, or catch everything you eat, it is up to you to forage through the supermarket to find the best foods for yourself and your baby.

more careful, but not paranoid, about what you eat during your pregnancy. The first is that much of our knowledge about pesticides and chemical additives is incomplete; ditto for pregnancy. We know only that major problems are caused by consuming huge amounts of these chemicals, but we have little or no knowledge of what minor effects can be caused by eating small amounts. Of even greater concern is the fact that the immature waste-disposing system of the pre-born baby is unlikely to be as tolerant of toxic chemicals as that of an adult. Conceivably, toxic substances could remain in the baby's system (e.g., liver) for a longer time and in higher concentrations than in the

mother's, and therefore there is greater potential for trouble.

I'm expecting twins. How much extra nutrition do I need?

While it's unlikely that you need to eat twice as much because you're carrying two babies, you will need to consume more calories, more protein, more vitamins, more calcium, and more iron. Each day you will probably need an additional 250 calories, 25 grams of protein, 20 milligrams of an iron supplement, and a higher dose of folic acid, as determined by your health-care provider.

Nutritional Nuggets for Mothers-to-Be

1. **All calories are not created equal.** All foods contain nutrients, but some are more nutritious than others. "Empty-calorie" food (better known as "junk food") contains calories, but very little else needed by your body. Appreciate the concept of "nutrient-dense foods," foods that provide a lot of nutrition in a small volume and for a reasonable number of calories. Foods that provide little nutrition in a large amount of food and a lot of calories have low-nutrient density (i.e., empty calories). The key to healthy eating while pregnant is to eat efficiently, consuming nutrient-dense foods that ounce for ounce contain both the nutrients and the calories you need. (To make every calorie count, see the "Best Foods" lists, pages 91 and 92.)

2. **Crossover corrects for different tastes.** Food likes and dislikes are part of human nature, and when pregnant you will be as human as ever. Don't worry if you develop an aversion to broccoli during your pregnancy, because you will find the same nutrients in many foods you do like, a nutritional quality called "crossover." There is a wonderful variety of choices on the "should haves" of the daily menu during pregnancy.

3. **Excess calories turn into excess fat.** Eating too many calories, regardless of the food source, will deposit excess weight on your baby in the form of excess fat. In fact, in practical terms, excess weight means excess fat. (Excess weight can be due to increased muscle, but that kind of weight is gained by body builders, not pregnant women.) Every person has a basic caloric need, meaning the minimum number of calories the body needs to grow and function. Eat less than this, and your body must burn stored fat; eat more, and your fat deposits grow.

4. **Every bite adds up.** You may be surprised that even a little nibble can show up on

Figuring Out a Healthy Weight Gain

Pregnancy may be the only time in your adult life when you can watch the numbers on the scale climb steadily upward and be pleased. For many scale-gazers, being happy about weight gain is not what they are used to. You may have to change your mind-set and learn to smile at your monthly weigh-ins. After all, this weight gain is not you getting fat. It's your body performing an amazing and wonderful feat.

Even though you may know that weight gain goes with the package of pregnancy, nevertheless, you are bound to wonder about how much is too much, how little is too little, and whether the weight you are gaining is the right amount for you. Too little weight gain is not healthy for baby; too much is not healthy for you. Mothers-to-be who are undernourished are more likely to deliver premature babies; those who gain excessive weight are more likely to have problem pregnancies and difficult deliveries.

Common Questions About Weight Gain During Pregnancy

How much weight gain is healthy for me and my baby?

your body. An extra chocolate chip cookie each day (over your basic caloric need) adds up to an extra pound of body fat each month or an extra 9 pounds of excess fat you will need to shed after giving birth. Unfortunately, for most people it is easier to put fat on than to take it off. Consider what you have to do to work off the extra 9 pounds gained in nine months of chocolate chip cookie nibbling. It takes at least one hour of vigorous exercise to burn off 500 calories, and one week of one-hour-a-day vigorous exercise to burn off the 3500 calories in one pound of fat.

5. **Control weight by exercise, in addition to healthy eating.** An hour walk every day, besides being healthy for your mind, is good for the body. Exercise burns calories from unneeded fat stores, a much healthier method of weight control than risking undernourishment from dieting. Also, by stimulating your body to produce endorphin hormones, exercise improves your sense of well-being.

6. **Too much fat in the food yields too much fat on the body.** One gram of fat contains 9 calories, more than twice as many as 1 gram of protein or carbohydrate. That's what makes fat a more efficient fuel. Yet, it's also the nutrient that contributes most to unneeded weight. Body fat is the body's fuel storage system. Everyone needs a certain amount of it, and the pregnant body needs more. But excess fat in the diet is all too readily stored on the body as fuel you may never use.

7. **Value the fiber factor.** Pregnant women need extra fiber to speed up the passage of food waste through their slowed-down intestines. (See page 69 for an explanation of how pregnancy affects digestion.) Best fiber foods are raw fruits and vegetables, whole grains, beans, and the *P* foods: prunes, pears, plums, peas, and psyllium (a branlike laxative product found at nutrition stores).

The currently recommended healthy weight gain is 25 to 35 pounds. Where you fit into this range depends on two factors: your body type and whether you start your pregnancy under, over, or close to your ideal weight. Tall and lean women (ectomorphs) tend to gain less, short and pear-shaped women (endomorphs) tend to gain the most, and women of average build (mesomorphs) gain somewhere in the middle of the 25- to 35-pound range.

If you are underweight at the beginning of your pregnancy, you may need to gain more to pay your debt to your body. If you bring excess weight into your pregnancy, you may need to gain less. Every pregnant woman needs a fat reserve — consider it "baby fat"— to ensure there will always be a steady supply of calories available to her baby in case she undereats for a day or two. This fat reserve also supplies energy for milk-making after the baby is born. If you start pregnancy with this reserve already in place, you don't have to increase your investment by much. If you start your pregnancy too lean, a few pounds of extra fat is metabolically necessary.

Weight charts for growing mothers, like those for growing babies, present ranges and averages. It doesn't necessarily mean you're unhealthy if you don't weigh in just right according to the chart through every month of your pregnancy. Here are some guidelines to help you evaluate your weight gain:

- If you begin your pregnancy close to your ideal weight, a healthy weight gain would be 25 to 35 pounds.
- If you begin your pregnancy slightly above your ideal weight, a healthy weight gain for you would be 20 to 25 pounds; if you are obese, less than 20 pounds.
- If you begin your pregnancy below your ideal weight, a healthy weight gain for you would be 30 to 40 pounds.

More important than what the scale shows is what you show. If you are feeling healthy, looking healthy, and your baby is growing, you are likely to be gaining the *right weight for you.* If you are eating the right foods (see page 87), you really don't need to think about your weight. The only reason to check the numbers is to help warn of abnormal conditions that would cause a sudden sharp increase in weight gain (e.g., toxemia). Wise practitioners know that weight gained in pregnancy is extremely individual, and that it depends on individual body chemistry. A woman eating appropriate amounts of healthy food could gain quite a bit more than the "allowed" 35 pounds and lose it all quite quickly postpartum. Another woman, eating less wisely, may gain less but lose it much more slowly.

How fast should I put on the weight?

As a rule of thumb, a healthy rate of weight gain for a woman of medium build, starting pregnancy at her ideal weight would be:

- 4 pounds during the first trimester. Add 1 pound if underweight, subtract 1 pound if overweight;

- 1 pound per week thereafter. Add ¼ pound if underweight, subtract ¼ pound if overweight;
- During the last month it's normal for mother to gain less, even though baby is growing quickly. Some mothers normally gain 1 or 2 pounds; some stay the same; and a few may even lose a bit. All are normal.

Most women gain most of their weight during the second trimester, which coincides with the period of most rapid weight gain for baby (from 1 ounce to 2 pounds, or a thirty-two-fold increase). Most women normally bounce up 5 to 10 pounds quickly between fifteen and twenty weeks due to the rapidly expanding blood volume necessary to nourish the growing uterus and its resident. Once again, individual chemistry is at work (or perhaps mother splurged during the holidays or on a vacation). It usually happens only once and then things settle down. Most babies gain 90 percent of their weight after the fifth month, and 50 percent of their weight in the last two months.

Some women gain 8 to 10 pounds during the early weeks of pregnancy due to fluid retention; other women actually lose weight due to nausea and diminished appetite. Most women of normal weight do not have to worry what their weight does the first three months. Underweight women, however, need to avoid weight loss during their first three months.

I'm in my fourth month now, and finally I feel like eating. I was so sick during the first few months I could barely keep any food down, and I didn't gain any weight. Could I have harmed my baby because I didn't eat right?

No. You need not worry. It's the rare mother who eats by the balanced book during the nausea-prone first trimester. Besides, from conception to three months, baby gains only 1 ounce anyway. Nearly all women enter pregnancy with enough nutritional reserves to provide for mother and baby, even if mother eats barely anything during those early food-aversion months. Research shows that most women gain the most weight during the second trimester, and that mother's second-trimester eating habits have the most influence on baby's eventual birthweight. So it isn't until the middle trimester that your baby's needs require you to eat extra well.

My pregnant friend is dieting because she heard it's easier to deliver a smaller baby. Is she right?

No. She's doubly wrong. First, it's a dangerous medical myth that smaller babies are usually easier to deliver. There are many factors that influence the "ease" of delivery. Second, being smaller because of being nutritionally deprived is not a fate any mother would wish for her baby. Nutritionally deprived babies (also called "low-birthweight infants" or "intrauterine-growth-retarded infants") have a higher risk of newborn complications and delayed growth and development. New studies show that a mother who is undernourished is more likely to deliver a baby that is undernourished.

The warning on tobacco packaging that smoking can lead to low birthweight in infants does not mention the risks attached to having a small baby. As a result, some women may purposely continue to smoke during pregnancy, not realizing that a smaller baby does not mean an easier delivery. A nutritionally deprived baby isn't only going to have

narrower shoulders; all the baby's organs will be deprived.

Quite honestly, I want to get back my prepregnant figure as soon as possible after birth. What can I do during pregnancy to make this happen?

How quickly you get your figure back depends not only on how well you care for this body during pregnancy, but also on the body habits you brought into your pregnancy. If you exercise regularly and eat wisely before and during your pregnancy, you are likely to reclaim the figure you want more quickly than if you brought a poorly toned and undernourished body to the birth.

If you gain more fat than you and your baby need, it will naturally take you longer after birth to lose the excess. You will lose

How Your Weight Adds Up

Less than one-third to one-quarter of your weight gain is actually baby, even though he or she is the star of the show. The rest is an all-important supporting cast, without whom there would be no production.

baby	7½ pounds
enlargement of uterus	2 pounds
placenta	1½ pounds
amniotic fluid	2 pounds
breast enlargement	2 pounds
extra blood and fluid volume	8 pounds
extra fat stores	7 pounds
	30 pounds

around half the weight you gained when you deliver your baby (baby, amniotic fluid, and placenta). During the first few weeks postpartum, you will lose a few pounds of excess fluid. You will continue to shed pounds if you continue to eat carefully and exercise regularly. Breastfeeding may help take off some of those pounds between three to six months postpartum, when milk production is at its highest. During the first nine months postpartum, anticipate having around 5 to 10 extra pounds to "work" off. And, realistically, expect to take a full nine months to take off what it took you nine months to put on. Even women with ideal eating habits and a regular exercise regimen during and after their pregnancy will usually remain a few pounds heavier and a bit more full-figured after becoming a mother.

I'm carrying twins. How much weight is healthy for me to gain?

Oftentimes, a greater-than-average weight gain is the first clue that you are nourishing more than one baby. To all the before-mentioned guidelines for ideal weight gain, add approximately another 10 pounds for twins, more for additional multiples.

Why must I gain so much weight during my pregnancy, and where does that extra weight go?

That excess weight may be unwanted, but it is certainly needed. It goes to three vital areas. Naturally, most of the weight gain is lavished on the star of this drama, your baby. Next, is the supporting cast, all those structures and behind-the-scene players that the actor depends on: extra blood volume, amniotic fluid, uterus, placenta, and breast tissue. Then a few pounds are deposited as cash re-

serves to keep the show going in the event of hard times. (See "How Your Weight Adds Up," page 105.)

I'm not a health-food nut, an exercise freak, or a calorie counter. Do I have to be all of these just to be a good mother?

To be a healthy mother, most women will have to become amateur nutritionists. The good news is there is little you need to do differently during pregnancy than you should do anyway for your health and well-being. In pregnancy you just do a little more (or less); and now you have an added incentive. All the advice we offer for healthy eating and healthy living we would offer to everyone. It's just more important when you're pregnant. Pregnancy convinces many women to improve their style of eating and living and to get their whole family on a healthier track. Becoming a wise nutritionist during pregnancy prepares you to feed your growing family well after birth.

I began my pregnancy 20 pounds overweight, and I'm worried that I'll be even more overweight after the baby. Can I safely diet during pregnancy without harming my baby?

Yes and no. You can "diet" in the sense of changing your eating habits for the better, learning to eat healthy, but you shouldn't diet to lose weight. An undernourished baby has a higher risk of complications at birth and of delayed growth and development. There are safe ways to take off excess body fat and still give yourself and your baby the extra nourishment you both need. Remember, it is the fat you are trying to lose. You don't want to deprive your baby or yourself of important nutrients.

First, establish your basic caloric need, which is how many calories you need each day to maintain your health (see below). This figure depends partly on your body type (see page 103). Some body types naturally burn more calories than others. In addition to knowing your body type, assess your past history of weight control. Do you gain weight easily, such as during the normal binge of vacation eating? Are you envious of friends who eat twice as much as you do yet don't gain weight, while all you have to do is look at a banana split and you feel fatter? Each of us came genetically programmed to burn off food calories differently. If you've always had to watch your weight, you will need to become even more weight-conscious while pregnant. Yet "the leaner the body, the less the worry" principle of nutrition doesn't hold true for all women during pregnancy. Even some ectomorphs, if nutritionally careless, can enter the ranks of the obese.

The average pregnant woman needs about 2500 calories per day (2200 to nourish herself, 300 for baby). Women with a high metabolism and/or high levels of activity need an additional 300 calories; women with low metabolism and/or low levels of activity need around 300 calories less, so, depending on your individual metabolism and level of activity, you will need to consume an average of 2200 to 2800 calories a day. For the best advice, consult a nutritionist to figure out your particular basic caloric needs. Eat what you need and no more.

Another thing you can do to control your weight is increase your exercise. *It is safest while pregnant to control or shed excess fat by exercise, not by diet.* Exercise burns off excess fat and, when coupled with healthy eating, doesn't rob your body or your baby of needed nutrition. One hour of sustained, low-impact exercise each day (swimming, walk-

ing briskly, cycling) can burn off 300 to 400 calories a day, which translates to losing or not gaining a pound of fat every nine to twelve days. And since exercise is a natural mood elevator and anxiety reducer, it also lessens the food-for-pleasure temptation.

The combination of eating healthy within your basic caloric requirements plus exercising for one hour daily will increase your chances of completing your pregnancy either with less excess fat than you had when you started or at least with no more.

To take off excess fat while putting in enough nutrition for your growing self and baby, try these fat-trimming tips:

• Avoid using food as a reward or as a pick-me-up when you're down. Eat only when hungry (unless depression suppresses your appetite and you need to force yourself to eat). Gratify your food-for-pleasure need with a healthier alternative that won't add unneeded pounds: go shopping, call a friend, read a good book, take in a movie. Pregnancy is a good time to enjoy a hobby or other activity you've been putting off. Becoming a mom may be just the added push you need to discover and do the things you truly like to do.

• Since you will and you should graze while you're pregnant, keep a bag or tray of nutritious snacks readily available. Make your less nutritious cravings harder to reach. Put them in the farthest room in the house, or, better still, don't even have them in the house. Not only is out of sight out of stomach, but if you do indulge, you'll burn off some of the penalty if you have to walk to the store to find the temptation.

• Trim off excess fat from foods before you eat them — it's easier than trimming it off yourself months later. Peel the fatty skin off poultry, trim the fat off meat. After cooking meat, use a paper towel to blot off the remaining fatty juice.

- Choose foods with lower fat content. (See "Learning to Read Labels," page 101.) Hold the mayo on sandwiches and in dressings. Substitute strained low-fat yogurt (removing some liquid through a yogurt strainer gives it a creamier consistency) for butter and sour cream on your baked potato. Just about every food worth its weight in sales is now packaged with a "reduced-fat" or "low-fat" alternative. Befriend these less fatty choices, but read the labels carefully: many reduced-fat foods still have more fat than is good for you.

Trying to lose excess weight while growing a baby is always a bit risky, but it can be safely done. Review your nutrition and your weight gain monthly with both your practitioner and a nutritionist. You may have to make periodic adjustments in your exercise regimen and your eating habits. Don't long

for a fat-free figure while pregnant. An overall increase in body fat is a normal part of the process of pregnancy. Just try to keep it under control. As long as you practice a healthy lifestyle and develop healthy eating habits while pregnant, your weight gain is likely to be right for you.

Maybe one day I'll get back into my old clothes. As for now, they just hang in my closet with a weepy look like, "Please put me back on."

Fitting into my jeans would be nice, but not necessary for a happy life.

I tend to get obsessed with not gaining more weight than I need to, and I was getting depressed after every monthly weigh-in. Eventually I just didn't look at the scale and asked my doctor not to tell me what it said. If my doctor didn't comment on the weight, I assumed it was just right.

THE SECOND MONTH

❖ ❖ ❖

Emotionally I feel: _____
_____
_____
_____

Physically I feel: _____
_____
_____
_____

My thoughts about you: _____
_____
_____
_____

What I'm eating: _____
_____

Most stomach-friendly foods (remember this list for labor day): _____
_____
_____

Food cravings: _____
_____

My top concerns: _____
_____
_____
_____

My best joys: _____
_____
_____

My worst problems: _____
_____
_____
_____

VISIT TO MY HEALTH-CARE PROVIDER

Questions I had; answers I got: _____

_____

_____

_____

_____

_____

_____

_____

Tests and results; my reaction: _____

_____

_____

_____

_____

_____

My weight: _____

My blood pressure: _____

What I imagine you look like: _____

_____

_____

_____

_____

What I would say if you could hear me: _____

_____

_____

_____

_____

photo at two months

Comments: _____
_____
_____
_____
_____
_____
_____
_____
_____
_____
_____
_____
_____
_____
_____
_____

Third-Month Visit to Your Health-Care Provider (9–12 weeks)

During this month's visit you may have:

- examination of your abdomen to feel the top of the uterus
- examination of the size and height of the uterus
- blood tests: hemoglobin and hematocrit
- urinalysis to test for infection, sugar, and protein
- weight and blood-pressure check
- an opportunity to hear baby's heartbeat with a Doppler ultrasound device
- discussion of tests if advised: ultrasound, chorionic villus sampling, amniocentesis, AFP, and prenatal screening for genetic problems
- examination for swelling of hands and legs or fluid retention
- an opportunity to discuss your feelings and concerns

The Third Month —
Almost Showing

MANY WOMEN FIND that the unpleasant physical reminders of pregnancy (the constant tiredness and ravages of morning sickness) begin to lessen this month, and although they haven't begun to "show," their jeans are feeling a little snug. (Women with second or third babies often begin to show earlier than first-timers.) By the third month you're also likely to be tiring of the sort of limbo you've been in when it comes to receiving sympathy and help. During the first trimester you feel pregnant — tired, nauseated, grouchy, short-tempered, and generally on an emotional roller coaster — even if your body has not yet revealed to others what's going on inside. Accordingly, friends, relatives, and especially your spouse may not be offering you either the sympathy you want or the help you need.

HOW YOU MAY FEEL EMOTIONALLY

The emotional ups and downs of the first two months often continue into the third month. The good news is that the level of pregnancy hormones in your blood will prob-ably peak during this month, meaning that at least their side effects won't get any worse. For most women, the almost constant PMS feeling will begin to diminish by the end of twelve weeks.

During the first two months I cried all the time. Now my husband wonders, "What's going on? You haven't cried for a while."

Confident. The fear of miscarriage, so prevalent in the first two months, now lessens a lot, since miscarriages most often occur within the first eight weeks. If you've had a previous miscarriage, you may enter the third month with a sigh of relief and allow yourself to feel the surge of maternal love and hopefulness that you have been holding back in case this baby didn't make it. It is in this month that most women begin to feel confident that they really are going to go on to deliver a healthy baby.

Craving solitude. Throughout much of the first trimester, but especially at its end, many women report that they just want to be alone. Perhaps this is another one of nature's messages to slow down, retreat, and consider yourself first. It's also a sign that you are ready to become acquainted with the little life that's growing inside you.

I've been so tired and meditative lately. Baby must be growing some important parts.

Worried about weight gain. In the first two months you may have worried less about weight gain than you do now. Chances are you were just happy you could keep any food down at all. (Women who experience more than their fair share of nausea and food aversions during the first two months may not begin to gain weight until the third month.) Now that you are craving food more and able to keep most of it down, it's normal to become conscious of the weight this extra food is going to put on. Some mothers-to-be, however, are just so happy not to feel sick that a little weight gain is easy to accept.

Please try to relax about the prospect of

Don't Worry

Some women find their worry list growing as their pregnancy does. If you tended to be a worrier before pregnancy, you are likely to find this tendency escalating. You probably worried ahead of time — that you wouldn't get pregnant. Then once you were pregnant, you worried about miscarriage. Now that the pregnancy is well established, you worry about the delivery, and whether your baby will be healthy. (Even after you are delivered of all of your pregnancy worries, you will probably worry about how you are adjusting to motherhood and whether or not you are a good parent.) Because the stakes are so high, you may fret about everything you eat, drink, breathe, or feel. To make matters more worrisome, you worry that you are worrying too much.

While it is true that there is a lot you can fret about during pregnancy, all worry does is aggravate the tension-related discomforts you are already experiencing. Worry releases stress hormones, and the last thing you need are unnecessary hormone challenges on top of those you already have to deal with. It may help you to remember that each year millions of women go through healthy pregnancies and have healthy babies. Most choose to do it a second or third time (or more!).

As soon as you find yourself worrying, change your thoughts. Think about the joys of pregnancy rather than the problems. Focus on the miracle that is going on inside you rather than all the lifestyle changes that are going on outside. If you are labeled "high risk," think about positive ways you can reduce your risk instead of worrying about circumstances you can't change. In addition, don't sweat the small stuff. Why waste nervous energy on trivial worries when you can concentrate on more important matters that are within your control, such as how to get more calcium in your diet?

If you feel yourself getting worried to a frazzle during a rough week of pregnancy, treat yourself to a change of environment. Go shopping. Eat out. Take a mini-vacation. Finally, rely on the old standby that is bound to change your worry to wonder: think, "I am doing the most valuable job in the world — growing a human being."

Discovering Your Personal Bests

Here's a word of advice we give to all new parents: *What your baby needs most is a happy mother.* The truism holds for pregnancy, too; what's good for mother is good for baby. Pregnancy presents a wonderful opportunity for personal discovery. Your thoughts naturally turn inward.

Early on in your pregnancy, think about what you need for your overall well-being. Discover what works best for *you;* your preferences may well differ from those of your pregnant friends. Discover your best foods, your best exercise, your best forms of relaxation, your best home remedies for the pains and discomforts of pregnancy. Post your "I need . . ." list strategically in your home and constantly update it as your pregnancy changes. Include what you need from other family members, and be sure your mate pays attention to this list. To help you figure out your personal bests during your pregnancy, list the following:

- Best foods: _____
- Best exercise: _____
- Best relaxation: _____
- Best conversation: _____
- Best sleep schedule: _____
- Best work schedule: _____
- Best activities: _____
- Best romantic dates: _____
- Best clothing styles: _____
- Best hairstyle: _____
- Best sex: _____
- Best comforting measures: _____
- Best things mate can do: _____
- Best reading material: _____

Certainly, neither life nor pregnancy is happy all the time, but unless you know what makes you happy, you're unlikely to work toward those things that satisfy you. If you can keep on top of your list most of the time, you are likely to have a pregnancy that is a personal best for you.

getting heavy — you are supposed to be heavy when you are pregnant. Ironically, now that health-care providers have relaxed about weight gain, women seem more disturbed by it. Nearly thirty years ago, when Martha was expecting our second child, her O.B. laid this "heavy trip" on her:

I weighed 9 pounds more than at the beginning of my first pregnancy (134 versus 125 — at 5 feet 6 inches, this was not a problem). I still remember my doctor's remark when he looked at my chart: "If you don't watch your weight, you'll turn into a blimp." Times change: with my third (six years later) and subsequent pregnancies, weight gain was never an issue. I gained more and enjoyed the pregnancies a lot more (license to eat!).

(See pages 102 to 108 for weight-gain guidelines and nutrition.)

Worried about coping. If you are one of the few women whose morning sickness does not begin to diminish by the end of this month, you may wonder how you are ever going to get through the next six. Even the sickest women usually experience some relief by the end of four months, so hang in there. Some women now begin to feel so much better they worry how little pregnant they feel. Don't worry — as your pregnancy progresses, you'll feel more pregnant.

Antsy. It's common at this stage of pregnancy to feel eager to get into "real" pregnancy, where you look pregnant and feel the baby moving. Waiting is especially hard if you're feeling out of sorts.

By the end of my first trimester, I had had it with pregnancy. This wasn't a baby, it was a long-term illness. I wasn't beautifully rounded, I was bloated and fat. Even though I knew intellectually that I'd soon be able to feel my baby move (and maybe enjoy some of the much ballyhooed solicitude you're supposed to receive when you're pregnant), at twelve weeks I just felt blah.

HOW YOU MAY FEEL PHYSICALLY

Your still-rising hormones and your growing baby continue to make their presence felt. Nausea, vomiting, heartburn, and constipation often continue during the third month but typically begin to subside by the end of this month. In addition to these familiar discomforts, you may feel differently physically.

Pelvic discomforts. Even though you don't yet show, you will begin to feel that something important is going on in your pelvis. You may feel a fullness in your lower abdomen. You may also notice mild stabbing pains when you suddenly change positions, going from lying to sitting, or from sitting to standing. As your uterus grows, it stretches its supporting ligaments, causing these twitches of pain on both sides of your waist. Gradually easing into changes of position lessens the sudden stretching of these ligaments and the accompanying pains. During the first trimester, uterine ligament discomfort tends to be sporadic, mild, and more of a nuisance or discomfort than truly painful. To relieve pelvic-ligament pain, try the standing leg lift. Stand barefoot. Steady your body with your hand against a countertop or chair and lift the foot on the side of the pain around 2 inches off the floor. Hold for 10 seconds. Repeat ten times; then reverse legs.

Between clothing sizes. From the third to the fifth month you may find nothing fits. Your regular clothing and underwear feel too tight but you feel silly in maternity clothes. Buy some comfortable nonmaternity pants and skirts one size larger and with elastic waistbands. You'll wear them again after the baby is born.

Martha notes: When I was just beginning my third month of pregnancy, I was not yet ready to part with my previously slim figure. One morning while getting dressed I decided to wear my sleek slacks — as long as I still had my waistline. I cinched the belt in with a vengeance and immediately felt a wave of nausea hit, and came close to vomiting. I realized I had to make a sudden adjustment in my clothing as well as in my attitude toward my body. I had been holding on to my prized waistline, but I now had to surrender to this slowly expanding middle that was declaring my maternity.

Hearing life. By the twelfth week, you and your doctor may be able to hear your baby's heartbeat using a Doppler ultrasound device (called a Doptone). Baby's heartbeat is about twice as fast as yours and sounds like rapid-fire "swoosh-swoosh." You may have expected to hear a faint twittering and not the loud

Feeling Your Uterus Grow

Empty your bladder, lie on your back, relax your abdominal muscles, then feel the area just above the middle of your pelvic bone (see illustration). The height of the growing uterus varies from woman to woman, but the illustration shows the uterine growth pattern for most pregnant women. Around the twelfth week, you might begin to feel the tip of your uterus protruding from just beneath the pubic bone. (You can feel your uterus earlier in subsequent pregnancies because you know what it feels like and because the abdominal muscles are looser.) You may find yourself constantly feeling this hard ball in anticipation of feeling your baby move and even imagine you do. By sixteen weeks, it feels like a melon midway between the top of your pubic bone and your naval. By twenty weeks you will feel your uterus around the level of your navel. At each visit your health-care provider will measure the size of your uterus as a rough guide to how well your baby is growing and to determine whether you are growing more than one baby. (If you are having trouble identifying the location of your uterus, ask your health-care provider to show you where to put your hands.) If you haven't yet had an ultrasound, feeling your uterus may be the most convincing sign that there really is a baby in there. (You

won't feel the first kicks for another month or two.) Feeling your uterus may prompt you to begin those stereotypical abdominal embraces; it's almost impossible not to place your hands affectionately above your pelvis as a prelude to the next few months when there really will be a bulge to embrace.

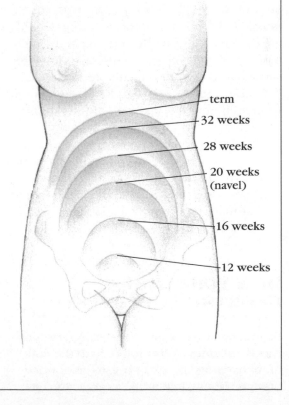

booming sounds that the ultrasound will reveal. You will be amazed how strong your baby's heart sounds. Remember, the Doptone magnifies the sound many times.

I was unprepared for how deeply I would be affected by the sound of my baby's heartbeat. The first time I heard that boom, boom, boom, it took my breath away. Much later in pregnancy I took my mother-in-law to an appointment with me. I had forgotten that this technology wasn't available when she was pregnant, and I neglected to prepare her. When she heard the heartbeat, her eyes got very wide and she burst into tears. It was a great moment.

Noticing more breast changes. Your breasts are continuing to gear up to feed your baby after birth. By the end of this month your nipples will probably have enlarged considerably and the areolae, the pigmented area around your nipples, may seem to take up a lot of your breast. According to folklore, this darkening makes the nipple an easier "target" for the newborn to find. Getting used to the different feel and look of your breasts and realizing the importance of these changes will prepare you for the more pregnant look that is soon to come to the rest of you. If you are anxious about adjusting to your new body image and don't look forward to that fuller look, now is a good time to work through those feelings.

HOW YOUR BABY IS GROWING (9–12 WEEKS)

Beginning at week nine, your baby, previously called an "embryo," is promoted to the rank of "fetus"; now all baby's organs are formed, though they will continue to grow and de-

velop during the rest of the time in the womb. Baby's liver, spleen, and bone marrow start making blood cells this month. The yolk sac, which previously supplied these cells, is no longer needed, and begins to disappear. Baby's teeth begin to form; by the end of this month baby will have twenty little tooth buds beneath his gums. Fingernails, toenails, and rudimentary hair appear, and baby's very thin skin, which is still transparent (allowing many of the blood vessels to show through), now responds to touch. Baby's intestines, previously part of the umbilical cord, now move into the abdominal cavity and become covered with skin. The tongue and vocal cords form this month. The circulatory system is operating, and heart valves are now develop-

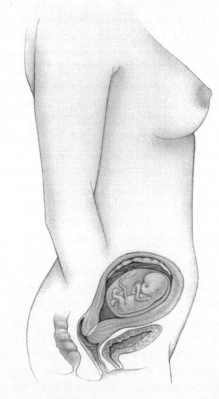

Baby at 9–12 weeks.

ing, meaning a heartbeat can be detected by a Doppler ultrasound. The liver secretes bile. The pancreas begins to produce insulin. The urinary system discharges urine into the amniotic fluid. Until this month, the external genitalia of both sexes looked very similar, making it difficult to tell a proportionately large clitoris from a penis. During the third month, these external genitalia differentiate clearly into male and female, so that by the end of the month ultrasound pictures can often reveal whether baby is a boy or a girl.

In the previous month baby's head was about half the size of his entire body, but now the body catches up, so that by twelve weeks the head is around a third of the size of the body. During this month baby grows rapidly, more than doubling his length and weight. He'll go from 1½ inches at the end of the second month to 2½ to 3 inches long by the end of the third and weigh from ½ to 1 ounce. As baby's neck and body grow, his previously hunched-over head and curved body will become more erect. Toward the end of this month eyelids grow and begin to fuse. The baby can open his mouth, move his tongue, swallow amniotic fluid, open and close his fists, move his limbs, even hiccup. His tiny feet can now kick, but you are unlikely to be able to feel it yet. He also shows other purposeful movement, such as swallowing. Not only does baby begin to look like a little person, he begins to act like one too.

CONCERNS YOU MAY HAVE

Vivid Dreams

The hormones that play with your emotions while you are awake also make their presence felt while you are asleep. By understanding why you dream differently during

pregnancy you can make these sometimes disturbing nighttime thoughts and fantasies work for you.

How pregnancy dreams are different. Pregnancy dreams tend to be more intense, vivid, disturbing, and bizarre than your nonpregnant dreams, and sometimes even funny. Women we have interviewed report that pregnancy dreams seem more real than regular dreams and that the usual life worries seem more grossly exaggerated. Pregnancy dreams, besides being more exotic, occur more frequently and are more likely to be remembered than nonpregnancy dreams. Dreams are recalled more easily because a pregnant woman wakes up so frequently, often during or at the end of a dream, when it's fresh in her mind.

I dream a lot anyway, but my pregnancy dreams were so realistic! I dreamt that I told my husband he could date his ex-girlfriend, and the dream went downhill from there. I dreamt he took her out to dinner on my birthday, and eventually ran off with her. I woke up drenched with sweat, shook my husband, and screamed, "How could you do that to me?"

Why pregnancy dreams are different. You dream differently while pregnant because you sleep differently. During pregnancy, especially during the last trimester, you will spend a larger percentage of your nap and nighttime sleep in REM sleep, the stage that encourages dreaming and easy awakening. During REM sleep the body rests, but the mind doesn't. However, pregnancy dreams cannot be blamed entirely on hormones, since many expectant fathers also report having more vivid, even scary, dreams. A baby on the way means big life changes for everyone in the household. Because of these changes, a pregnant woman's mind is ready for thought and introspection day and night.

I dreamt we left our two-year-old with my parents and forgot to pick her up. I think this dream means I'm scared I will neglect our older child when the new baby comes.

Dreams grow as your pregnancy does.

Pregnancy dream content often reflects a woman's pressing concerns, which change with the stages of pregnancy. Early in pregnancy, dreams seem to focus on fertility symbols: potted plants, fruit, seeds, water, ocean waves. Toward the middle of pregnancy, dream babies appear in your fantasies, and your dream life may be filled with images of "your" baby, babies in general, and even tiny animals, such as puppies or kittens. Some women dream that they aren't pregnant at all and wake up confused and horrified. Many women find the "builder" theme repeated in their dreams, perhaps reflecting their roles as creators. Toward the end of pregnancy, the dreams may become nightmares; your baby is not healthy, you have a problem delivery, someone is stealing your baby. While it's also normal toward the end of pregnancy for dreams on other topics to become more anxious — you might dream about career upsets or problems with your spouse — most women report their fearful dreams are baby-related incidents, such as having empty breasts when baby wants to nurse, or doing something terrible as a mother. Dreams of dropping the baby are common.

I kept dreaming about deformed babies. My therapist says this is a common dream for pregnant women and perhaps is symbolic of the real threat the baby poses to an established lifestyle and body image.

Making your dreams therapeutic.

It is best not to overinterpret your dreams and become anxious about their content. Sleep, especially pregnancy sleep, distorts and exaggerates realities anyway. While dreams do not foretell the future, pregnancy dreams, especially those that have a recurring theme, can reveal hidden anxieties and bring your attention to issues that need to be dealt with. While you don't need to attach a great deal of meaning or importance to your dreams, some pregnant women find reflecting on their content can actually alleviate a lot of their anxiety. Many women find it helpful to write down a negative dream and then rewrite a happier ending. If you dream you deliver a deformed baby, it just means you have the normal, healthy fears a good mother has for her child.

It's helpful to write down the recurring story line of your dream to see if a pattern emerges that might reflect some hidden issue that needs to be addressed. Encourage your husband to talk about his dreams as well. He's making a big adjustment, too.

I kept dreaming that I discovered extra rooms in my house. We have enough room here, but, nevertheless, it felt so good to find these hidden surprises! My friend told me that new rooms in a dream represent new capabilities in oneself. I hope this means I'll rise to the occasion in my new role as a mother.

Enjoying Sex While Pregnant

Pregnancy can change your appetite for many of life's simple pleasures, from making dinner to making love. How you will feel about sex while pregnant depends on your individual feelings about sex, your partner's feelings, and the physical and emotional changes from this particular pregnancy. We can give you one guarantee: while pregnant you will feel different about sex. For many women and their partners, this difference is exciting. Some women become aroused more easily and climax more quickly, pleasurably, and frequently, and many men find their pregnant wives sexier than ever. Yet while some couples experience pregnancy as a peak erotic time in their married life, others experience a downturn in desire or satisfaction. Most couples report both ups and downs. Fortunately, all of these feelings are normal. And the good news is, a little knowledge helps most couples increase their sexual pleasure during these pregnancy months. Once you and your mate realize why sex is different during the nine months of pregnancy (and for that matter, the nine months after birth), you'll find it easier to adjust to this biological fact of life. It is just one more season of your marriage, one that needs sensitive understanding.

In the early months, fatigue along with nausea and fear of miscarriage turns sex into an uncomfortable obligation for many women. During the second trimester — called "pregnancy's honeymoon" — hormonal surges level off. Fatigue and morning sickness usually lessen, the fear of miscarriage subsides as the statistical risk decreases, and many women feel a surge in sexual desire. It is not uncommon for men, enjoying the new erotic feelings of their mates, to feel that the sex they didn't get earlier was worth waiting for. The heightened sensitivity of the erogenous zones is so thrilling to many women that they experience more enthusiasm for sex during the middle months of pregnancy than at any time in their lives.

Do not be surprised if in the final months you are too large, too awkward, or too preoccupied with the coming birth to enjoy sex. In the third trimester, as a ballooning abdomen literally comes between a woman and her partner, most women report that they focus more on becoming maternal than on being sexual. Even if the body is willing, it is clumsy.

Expect change. For most women sexual desire parallels their energy levels: down in the first trimester, up in the middle, and declining again in the third.

Sexual organs change. The changes in the sexual organs that accompany pregnancy can lead to one woman's pleasure and another woman's pain. The same hormones that prepare your body to birth and nourish your baby also change the way your body experiences sex. During pregnancy, your breasts become increasingly full and your nipples become larger and more sensitive; during lovemaking, blood flow to your breasts increases even more. While your more voluptuous look may be a turn-on for your mate, heightened breast sensitivity can be either irritating or stimulating for you, depending on where you are in your pregnancy.

The changes in your vaginal canal that get it ready for baby's passage also make it feel different during lovemaking. The increased blood flow to the muscles and lining of your vagina cause a feeling of fullness. For some women — and their partners — this change can accentuate sexual joy; for other women it's uncomfortable. Vaginal secretions increase and the odor changes. The naturally increased lubrication of the pregnant vagina may seem a perk to women who previously experienced dryness during intercourse. For other women, this is just another nuisance that will soon pass. The increased snugness and lubrication of the pregnant vagina may accentuate sexual enjoyment for some couples. Other couples may feel the venous congestion makes the vagina feel too snug, leaving less room for the penis. Changes in sexual organs during pregnancy tend to be more pronounced in subsequent pregnancies than for first-timers.

Due to the increased blood supply to the cervix, you may experience occasional bleeding or spotting after intercourse, caused by the breaking of tiny blood vessels at the tip of the cervix. This harmless but scary sight can be lessened by avoiding deep penetration during intercourse. If bleeding occurs during intercourse and it worries you, your practitioner can examine you to determine whether the bleeding is coming from your uterus (which is of concern) or is harmless bleeding from the congested vessels lining your vagina or cervix. For suggestions on positions for intercourse, see page 273.

Communication changes, too. You will find that the language of lovemaking changes during pregnancy. You will need to show and tell your mate what produces pleasure and what produces pain or irritation. There may be days or nights when the increased sensitivity of your breasts and vagina gives you immense pleasure during foreplay; at other times, the ultrasensitivity in the sexual organs makes breast- and clitoral-fondling off-limits. To increase your pleasure and help you avoid discomfort, tell your partner what feels good and what doesn't. When your breasts or sexual organs enjoy touch, welcome it; if they don't, nudge those caressing hands toward less sensitive areas.

Your attitude makes a difference. While some of pregnancy's side effects dampen sexual pleasure, others soup up the fun. How

you approach sex during these months can tip the scale either way.

The workings of nature that can make you feel and act more sexy while pregnant can also serve to cool your passion. During the first three months you may be barely surviving nausea and fatigue caused by pregnancy hormones, and sex may be the farthest thing from your mind. Physical discomforts are not the only feelings that separate a pregnant woman from her man. Myths and misunderstandings add mental anxieties to the already tired and queasy body. Fear of endangering the life that is just getting started may hinder the desire for and frequency of sex. Both you and your mate may need periodic reassurance that baby is well protected from the goings-on outside.

Sex during pregnancy is safe for most women. There is seldom a reason to fear causing a miscarriage or harming the baby (see "When to Abstain," page 127). Sex during pregnancy can be more relaxed than "regular" sex. This may be the first time in your life you will have sex without the fear of getting pregnant or the pressure to get pregnant. Sex while pregnant can thus be less planned, more spontaneous. There are no ovulation dates or messy menstrual periods to plan around, no birth control to worry about. You can enjoy a spontaneity rare for couples of childbearing age. For many couples, especially those who treasure a long-awaited pregnancy, each instance of lovemaking is a replay of the moment they conceived this precious baby.

The pregnant body is marvelous. Feeling sexy and being pregnant need not be mutually exclusive. During pregnancy many women need to redefine their sexuality. In fact, how you handle your sexuality during pregnancy sets the tone for how you will later blend sexuality and motherhood. Prior to marriage, you may have subconsciously defined your sexuality in terms of your ability to flirt, how you dressed, or how much you looked like a magazine model in her size 6 dress. After marriage you probably found the need to look and act sexy less compelling as you settled down into connubial bliss. Ironically, you became better and better at being sexy; in the security of a committed relationship, we are freer to accept — and be — ourselves. Then one day you found yourself pregnant, and now you face the same kind of sexual self-invention you did at another point of dramatic physical change: adolescence. Now that you're pregnant, you may start wondering, "What will it take to make me feel and act sexy?"

Your biological destiny is on the threshold of the ultimate expression of female sexuality — birth and nurturing. Being pregnant is, after all, the incontrovertible proof of your sex appeal. In anthropological terms, you are the very symbol of sexuality, the fertility goddess incarnate. When, however, you start off pregnancy feeling sick, you'll probably also feel asexual for a while. And once that hurdle is past, if you are a victim of the somewhat unnatural culture we live in, you face another challenge — that Barbie-doll body you worked toward for so many years literally goes to pot in a few months, causing your sexual self-image to take a dive. You may worry that you'll never get your body back, a normal reaction that research shows is second only to physical discomforts on the "pregnancy concerns" list. It's time for Demi Moore to come to the rescue. Pregnant was never so beautiful! Actually, men and women have known this for ages. What has happened is that our culture, via Hollywood and *Playboy* (and Mattel) has betrayed twentieth-century women.

It is a rare woman who can completely ignore our society's values and revel in nature's magic, but do your best. Relax and enjoy your body for how it is changing; don't be obsessed with controlling your waistline. You are growing a whole new person! If you have been culturally programmed to believe that slim is beautiful, remind yourself that being fuller and rounder is even more beautiful when you're carrying a baby. Parting with that girlish figure may be easier if you admit that you are no longer a girl. And, even though the cliché "baby makes it all worthwhile" may not yet be totally convincing, you will soon find that it is true. If you long to keep your prepregnant figure as much as you long to be a mother, do yourself the favor of easing up on your expectations of the former — you have only a slim chance of emerging from maternity with the same body you had before. You may have to work very hard, particularly after a second or third pregnancy, to look the same as you did before you became a mother. Your goals and expectations for your body may change.

If you find yourself not yet ready for a more mature look, try these image-enhancing suggestions:

- *Go ahead and mourn the "old you."* You may find it hard to give up your previous self-image, especially if, somewhere deep inside, a part of you wasn't ready to be a mommy. It's hard to retain a virginal appeal with a baby in tow. Take time to say goodbye to the image you had of yourself (or showed others) that doesn't fit this new life experience. Assure yourself that the "new" you will be just as sexy — just different. If you have real trouble giving up an old role, or feel you need help with your evolving self-image, talk to a professional.

For the Pregnant Father

Men, while you may read or hear that a woman's desire for sex (translation: intercourse) lessens during pregnancy, the real fact of pregnant life is that a woman's need for sex (translation: affection) increases while pregnant. It's important to meet your mate's need for cuddling and caring during her pregnancy.

Show affection for your mate and the body she has now. If she senses you appreciate and even get excited about her changing shape and sexuality, you are likely to be rewarded with a livelier-than-ever sex life — at least during mid-pregnancy. If, however, she perceives that her ballooning belly is not appealing to you, you are in for a sexually flat pregnancy. In one study, researchers interviewed 260 pregnant women, asking them to cite the reasons they felt less sexual while pregnant. The most common reasons were physical discomfort (46 percent); fear of injuring baby (27 percent); feeling awkward during lovemaking (17 percent); sex discouraged by practitioner (8 percent). It's comforting to know only 4 percent felt less sexual because they perceived their mate found them less attractive.

Some men lose interest in sex during their mate's pregnancy for reasons not directly related to how their partner looks or acts. A man may fear that penetration will harm the baby, though in most situations this is nothing to worry about. Adding to this fear, normal pregnant-father feelings can click into overdrive — some men just feel more paternal than sexual during their wives' pregnancies. For them, it takes a while to integrate the roles of father and lover. They may also need some time to adjust to thinking of their partner as both mother and lover.

Then there is the uneasy feeling that the baby is an intruder. Sometimes feeling movement from the life a couple has created can turn a man on, but it can also be a turn-off when he realizes that little thumper is just an inch or two away from his penis. More than a few men have lost

• *Think positive.* Think round, think big. Consider what you're getting, and not what you're losing. Your new roundness provides more surface area for your lover to see and touch. Whenever you feel yourself falling back into your old mind-set, call a friend who's been there and ask her to talk you out of it. Stand in front of a mirror and embrace the new version of yourself. Take pride in your "new" body — give it the respect it deserves.

• *Give yourself a sexy look.* Just because your body is getting bigger doesn't mean you shouldn't look your best. Treat yourself to a new hairstyle, change your makeup, buy a new nightgown that reveals what's appealing. This is likely to spark your mate and push your sexual image up a notch.

• *Act sexier than you feel.* Social scientists have shown that acting can affect feeling. Smiling, for example, causes your brain to release the same chemicals it would if you their erections when they (or their wives) suddenly felt baby kick.

This real-life scene is a preview of what's to come, when your baby awakens crying in the midst of your longed-for lovemaking. Maintaining a sex life as new parents will mean working around your wife's still recovering body, her exhaustion (and yours), her dripping breasts and vaginal dryness, and the new picture each of you has of yourselves as both parents and sexual beings. Sex is bound to be different for a year or more after the baby is born. It may never be the same. But it *can* be even better.

Don't be surprised if your pregnant partner turns tiger, even if she was previously passive. Some women experience new sex cravings while pregnant, stunning their mates with their sudden and unexpected sexual voracity. Some men feel overwhelmed when a woman demands more intimacy than they think they can supply; feeling pressured for sex can weaken your performance, but don't retreat! Typically, in the first trimester, she can't meet your sexual needs; in the second, you can't satisfy hers. Don't be alarmed if you don't always rise to the occasion, especially as you try new positions. It may take you a while to adjust to her changing body. Engorgement of her vagina and greater lubrication (see page 121), especially, may cause you to lose your erection until you get used to a different feel and fit. And don't feel cheated if your wife does not experience second trimester hypersexuality, which we may have set you up to expect. She may be too sick, too shy, or just too tired.

Your sexual enjoyment will probably wane as her sexual interest dwindles in the last trimester. And it's normal to feel guilty that you are enjoying sex and she isn't. Such is the sex life of the pregnant couple. Talk to each other about your desires and try to find a way to satisfy both of you. Understanding and enjoying each other's sexual needs during pregnancy is a season of the marriage. Approaching this time with compassion and affection can have an enriching effect on your whole relationship.

were actually happy — thereby making you happier. If you act unsexy, you may cause your partner to feel unsexy, making him retreat. (This cycle reinforces your belief that you really are unattractive to your partner.) If you act sexy, you may soon surprise yourself with feeling sexy!

• *Believe in your attractiveness to your mate.* If you convince yourself that your blossoming belly is no longer attractive to your husband, you are setting yourself up for a sexual slowdown. Besides, this probably isn't true. It's the rounder shape that attracts males. And certainly during pregnancy you will look rounder than at any other time in your life. Research doesn't support your assumption that you are not attractive to your mate; most men find their wives' newly rounded bodies appealing. Your mate is likely to love the fleshy feel and curvy look of your pregnant body. Add to these features the possibility that once you are past the yucky early months of pregnancy, you are initiating lovemaking, and your mate is likely to feel excited about your sexuality while pregnant.

• *Have a sex talk.* Tell your mate about the way pregnancy is affecting your sexuality; and ask him to tell you how he feels about your new look. Each partner should explain his or her feelings. Be sure that he does not interpret your lack of interest in sex as lack of interest in him, for example, and don't you assume his confusion over how to touch you now means he's not interested. By the same token, avoid projecting your sexual uneasiness onto your mate. He will probably find you more attractive than ever.

• *Share your body.* Be sure to include your husband in the pregnancy by being proud of — rather than hiding — your body's milestones: your darkened nipples, the first tummy bulge. Focus on what is new and exciting that you will both enjoy only during pregnancy. For example, your new breasts will be "all his" for the rest of the pregnancy — what a turn-on, without resorting to silicone! Lie nude together watching and feeling the baby move. Your mate will enjoy side views that he has never before seen. One fun project can be taking "as you grow" photos, month-by-month photos showing, from all angles, your changing pregnant image. Your mate will enjoy his "pinup wall."

• *Have a fling.* Have periodic weekend "dates" before baby arrives; after he or she comes, you will have less energy for each other. The best time for ambitious sexual retreats is during the middle months of pregnancy, but make an effort to spend ro-

mantic time enjoying each other throughout the pregnancy.

• *Avoid the "sex as a service" feeling.* While for most women a certain amount of "obligatory" sex is usual during pregnancy, don't let your mate feel you are always "servicing" him, even though you sometimes may be.

My husband took a video of me in the nude every month so we could document the exciting and beautiful changes my body went through. Now that I have my old body back and can hardly remember what being pregnant felt like, it's a wonderful reminder of a very special time in our lives.

(Also see "Enjoying Late-Pregnancy Sex," page 272.)

Questions You May Have About Sex While Pregnant

I've had two miscarriages already and I'm newly pregnant. Could having sex cause me to lose another baby?

There is no scientifically proven link between sexual intercourse, orgasm, and miscarriage, yet the fact that uterine contractions are a part of orgasm compels some practitioners to advise women who have a history of miscarriages to avoid orgasm during the first trimester. Even though science is on your side, and it is unlikely that having sex could cause you to lose another baby, it is best to discuss your individual obstetrical circumstance with your practitioner. Fortunately, at the time when your chance of miscarriage is highest, in the first trimester, your interest in sex is likely to be at its lowest. Your libido naturally increases after the first few months, when your chances of miscarrying are far less.

When to Abstain

Most healthy women and their partners can have intercourse right up to the day of birth. Yet there are some conditions in which sex during pregnancy can put the health of the mother and baby at risk:

- If you or your partner has a sexually transmitted disease (STD) that has not completely cleared up after treatment, intercourse could transmit the disease up into your uterus.
- If you experience spotting or bleeding, check with your health-care provider. Blood can be a sign that you might miscarry, so your practitioner may ask you to avoid intercourse for a while.
- If your practitioner has found you to be in preterm labor, orgasm could further stimulate contractions and increase your risk of delivering a baby prematurely.
- If you had an ultrasound that diagnosed placenta previa, intercourse could cause the placenta to further separate from the uterus.
- If you have a history of previous miscarriages, your health-care provider may advise you to abstain from orgasm-inducing sexual activity during the early months, until your pregnancy becomes securely rooted. (Even though most research suggests there is no link between orgasm and inducing

miscarriage, every woman with a high-risk pregnancy should consult her own practitioner regarding the advisability of orgasm.)

- If you are in the last trimester of a high-risk pregnancy (if, for example, you have an incompetent cervix or are experiencing an impending premature birth), your practitioner may feel that intercourse or orgasm increases the risk and advise you to avoid sex.
- If your membranes (the protective sac surrounding baby) have broken, intercourse increases the risk of bacteria from the vagina and cervix infecting your baby, and therefore is not advisable.

When asking your practitioner about sex during pregnancy, be sure you get a clear answer on *what* you may do *when,* and *why* or *why not.* The two main concerns are orgasm and penetration. For some couples, medical circumstances may limit sex to cuddling and caressing; for them, even breast touching is discouraged since nipple stimulation can induce contractions after twenty weeks. If because of your particular medical circumstance, you are advised to limit sexual activity while pregnant, explore other satisfying ways of being together.

I'm at risk for having a premature birth because of an incompetent cervix. My doctor prescribed bed rest and no sex, but I'm feeling like I need some intimacy and certainly my husband does.

The warning of "no sex" need not mean "no pleasure." What your doctor means by "no

sex" is no orgasm and no penetration. These restrictions compel you to invent ways of pleasuring each other without intercourse. Enjoying sex without intercourse now forces you to a new level of intimacy. Communication is the key. Show and tell each other what pleases you the most.

If orgasm is to be avoided for medical reasons, be aware that masturbation for the woman is not an option. The uterus contracts even more intensely in response to an orgasm through masturbation than to an intercourse-induced orgasm. In fact, the hyperresponsiveness of the pregnant uterus to orgasm is sometimes used to the pregnant woman's advantage — once the practitioner has determined that the cervix is ripe and the baby is ready to be born — sex can be a way of inducing labor.

Sometimes when we have sex, the baby starts to move and our passion fizzles. Is this normal?

You will find that there is very little that is "normal" or "abnormal" about sexuality during pregnancy. It's what feels right to you that counts. Both your baby's movements and your feelings are normal. You're not used to having another person in the bedroom while you're making love, even if that person is behind a closed womb. Approach this interruption with humor, and take it as training for the real sex life that is to come; this is your preparation for learning to enjoy sex despite the possibility of ill-timed intrusions from a baby needing to nurse or (someday) a teenager coming home early from a date.

My doctor advises no sex in the last three months for fear of inducing a premature delivery. Should I get a second opinion?

You could get a second, and a third, and a fourth, and they may all differ. The possible cause-and-effect association between orgasm and preterm delivery is primarily a theoretical one (studies are conflicting), yet many advisers stick to the theory. Many women experience strong uterine contractions dur-

ing and following orgasm, and some doctors worry that these contractions may stimulate preterm labor. Based on new research finding no link between orgasm and preterm birth, more and more practitioners are telling couples that they can safely enjoy lovemaking throughout pregnancy. Still, you may have a particular circumstance, such as an incompetent cervix, in which lovemaking would not be in the best interest of your baby. In most cases, though, orgasm-induced labor is unlikely unless your cervix is "ripe" for delivery, something your doctor can determine.

Obstetricians do agree that there is no correlation between sex without orgasm and premature labor. Also, researchers used to worry that hormones in semen, called prostaglandins, might trigger labor; new research shows this worry is not warranted. (For more on when it is advisable to avoid sex, see page 127.)

I'm carrying twins. Should I worry about having sex?

Unless advised by your doctor, you don't have to double your worry about enjoying sex just because you are carrying twins. Because women carrying multiples have an increased risk of delivering prematurely and because orgasm can stimulate uterine contractions, in the past, conventional wisdom advised these women to abstain from orgasm during the third trimester. Recent studies, however, have shown no relationship between intercourse and the premature delivery of twins.

Screening Tests for Birth Defects

The fact of nature that some infants will be born less than perfect is difficult to deal with while you're waiting for the birth of your own child. Modern prenatal testing attempts to identify babies with serious problems even before they are born, but these tests are, as the name implies, only "screening" tests for birth defects and not absolutely diagnostic. Although prenatal tests can answer a lot of questions about what's going on in the womb, they can also both falsely reassure and needlessly worry expectant parents, causing them, for example, to become unnecessarily anxious over ambiguous results. One of the truisms we teach medical students is "The problem with tests is that you are forced to do something with the results." Herein lies the problem with some of these tests too. Some of these tests pose no risk to mother and baby, but the results are notoriously inaccurate. Other tests are highly accurate in predicting a problem prenatally but carry a higher risk to mother or baby. In this section we discuss the most commonly available prenatal screening tests and offer some ways to help confused parents choose the tests they feel are right for themselves and their baby.

AFP (Alpha-Feto Protein) Screen

Why is it done? The most commonly available prenatal screening test for birth defects is the AFP screen. AFP, a natural substance produced by baby's liver, normally enters the mother's bloodstream during pregnancy. Maternal levels of AFP are elevated if the mother is carrying a baby with a neural-tube defect (NTD) — the vertebrae that normally enclose the spinal cord fail to develop — because AFP leaks out of an open spinal column. These defects include spina bifida (in which the spinal cord is not enclosed in the spinal column, often causing paralysis from the waist down) and anencephaly (in which the baby's brain is either severely underdeveloped or doesn't develop at all).

Maternal AFP levels are lower than normal if the baby has Down Syndrome or another chromosomal defect. A new test, called the "triple screen" (also known as the "prenatal risk profile" or "expanded AFP"), measures maternal levels of AFP, HCG (human chorionic gonadotropin, which is elevated if mother is carrying a baby with some chromosomal abnormalities), and estriol (a byproduct of the hormone estrogen, which is lower if mother is carrying a baby with some chromosomal abnormalities). The triple screen raises the accuracy from 25 percent with the AFP alone to 60 percent. The triple screen may detect 70 percent of Down Syndrome babies in women over age thirty-five, and 60 percent in women under age thirty-five.

When is it done? The AFP screen is done between the sixteenth and eighteenth week of pregnancy. The results are available within one week. Some parents may feel put off when the doctor mentions this test, usually at the first or second prenatal visit, feeling that it dampens the otherwise joyful experience of being pregnant. Early in the pregnancy, many parents are not yet ready for the "what ifs" of pregnancy and may feel their doctor is being an unnecessary alarmist. Yet, realize that your doctor is professionally obliged to offer this test to you. Some states even have laws that require doctors to offer the AFP screen.

How is it done? The AFP screen is performed on a small amount of blood taken from the mother's arm.

Is it safe? The blood test itself is as safe as any maternal blood test for mother and baby. But there is disagreement on the usefulness and wisdom of this test. Some parents and professionals feel that prenatal screening programs are the product of the kind of thinking that makes decisions based on the overall cost and convenience to society, not on the risk or the benefit to the individual parent or infant. Others feel reassured by prenatal screening tests, especially parents who have a higher risk of delivering a baby with a birth defect. They feel that they would, of course, be reassured by negative results and that even if the test revealed problems, they would want to be able to prepare themselves for the challenges ahead.

While this test is physically safe, it can be psychologically traumatic. One of the risks of AFP screening is that it can lead to unnecessary worries. If the first AFP test is positive, a second one is recommended because of the possibility that the first test was wrong. This means another week of anxious worry, waiting for the results, which may well be negative. A confirmed positive test will be followed by other tests, which carry greater risks and cause more anxiety, and usually you find out there was nothing to worry about in the first place (or nothing you want to do about it anyway).

In deciding whether or not to have a prenatal screening test for birth defects, consider these points:

• Would the results matter to you? Would you change the course of your pregnancy? Are the results of the test going to create or alleviate anxiety? Would having the test or not having the test worry you more or less? Would knowing about a birth defect beforehand dampen the joy of your pregnancy, or do you feel it would be better for you to have the time to prepare yourselves to handle a special-needs baby? Do you need the results from the test to alleviate overwhelming worries, or do you feel that you could handle the sudden adjustments

necessary if you were surprised? In our own experience, giving birth to a baby with Down Syndrome was not nearly so horrendous as we had always imagined it to be. We were able to focus on Stephen, the baby we were holding in our arms, and to us this seems less traumatic than spending five or six months thinking about Down Syndrome. (Of course, parents who have had the experience of being able to prepare for the birth of their special-needs baby may feel that their choice was the better one for them.)

• If you've already decided not to act on the results (i.e., termination of the pregnancy is not an option), then you may feel it's unnecessary to have the test.

• What is the accuracy and meaningfulness of the expanded AFP test? This test is designed to detect some of the most rare defects that may occur: the incidence of neural-tube defects is one to two per thousand births; the incidence of anencephaly is one in seven thousand births; and the incidence of defects in the abdominal wall muscles (also detected by this test) is a minuscule one in thirty thousand babies. Also, the incidence of a mother having the chromosomal abnormalities that are detected by this test is less than 1 percent (see page 82 for how the incidence varies with maternal age).

• Also, consider that this test can detect only 80 to 90 percent of infants with neural-tube defects and 60 to 65 percent of babies with chromosomal abnormalities, such as Down Syndrome. Moreover, meaningful AFP results depend upon accurate dating of your pregnancy. If your dates are off, if you are carrying more than one baby, or if you are diabetic, your AFP levels won't match the norms. An "abnormal" AFP puts you on a track toward needing more expensive and risky tests. Ninety-five to 98 percent of "positive high" or "positive low" AFPs turn out to be false (i.e., the baby has neither a chromosomal abnormality nor a neural-tube defect).

- Are you at genetically higher or lower risk for having a baby with one of the problems the test is designed to detect? Have you delivered a baby with a previous such defect? Does your maternal age or family history put you at a higher genetic risk? On the other hand, if you are a mother in her twenties with a normal genetic and previous birth history, you already have a 99.9 percent chance of not having a baby with Down Syndrome or a neural-tube defect. Do you feel it is necessary to have a test to exclude most of the remaining one-tenth of 1 percent risk?

What do the results mean? Suppose the results come back "negative" or "low" AFP. This can be reassuring, but not absolutely. It simply takes more of the worry out of having a baby with these problems. If the result is "positive," this will obviously increase your worry. If your AFP test is abnormally high or abnormally low, your health-care provider may recommend that you have further tests, such as an ultrasound and/or amniocentesis. Yet realize, as we said above, 95 to 98 percent of suspicious findings go on to be disproven by further tests.

Amniocentesis

Amniocentesis falls into what we call the "high-yield–high-responsibility" category of prenatal testing. While amniocentesis provides a lot of valuable genetic information, it is not without risk to mother and baby.

Therefore, parents and practitioners must exercise a high level of responsibility in deciding whether or not to have this prenatal test.

Why is it done? The material obtained in amniocentesis reveals the gender of the baby, his or her chromosomal makeup, the maturity of the baby (especially the lungs), and whether or not he or she may have certain inherited diseases. Amniocentesis is considered if:

- Parents have had a previous child with a genetic abnormality, such as Down Syndrome.

- Parents already have a child with a metabolic disease. (Amniocentesis can identify only about 10 percent of all the various genetic and biochemical abnormalities that a baby can be born with.) Since each special test, such as a Tay-Sachs or cystic fibrosis screen, costs several hundred dollars, these tests are run only if the doctor specifically requests them.

- Mothers who are carriers of inherited genetic disorders. If mother carries a sex-linked genetic disease, such as hemophilia, she has a 50-50 chance of passing this trait on to her son; generally, however, amniocentesis can identify only the sex of the baby, not whether the gene has been inherited. If genetic mapping studies on the family have identified the chromosome involved, amniocentesis may be able to determine if the fetus inherited this abnormal chromosome.

- Parents already have a child with a spinal defect.

- Mother's AFP levels are high for no apparent reason.

- Triple-screen test indicates the fetus is at high risk for Down Syndrome.

- Both parents are carriers of an inherited genetic disorder, such as Tay-Sachs disease or sickle-cell anemia. The baby has a one-in-four chance of inheriting the disorder.

- Ultrasound has identified a fetal abnormality that suggests a serious or even lethal genetic defect.

- A preterm induced delivery is being considered for the best interest of mother or baby. Amniocentesis is used to assess the maturity of baby's lungs in order to weigh the risk of allowing the baby to mature further in the womb against the risk of being born too soon.

- A mother is over age thirty-five.

When is it done? This test is usually performed between the twelfth and the sixteenth week after conception, when there is enough fluid surrounding the baby that a sample is possible. Amniocentesis may also be performed in the last eight weeks of pregnancy when a preterm delivery is being considered. It takes a week or two to get the results on chromosomal abnormalities and the baby's sex. Results on conditions such as spinal defects, metabolic disorders, such as Hunter's syndrome, and Tay-Sachs disease are available the next day.

How is it done? Mother lies on the examining table and her abdomen is washed with antiseptic solution. As the doctor numbs the skin with a local anesthetic you may feel a little sting. Using ultrasound to locate an area where baby and placenta are not in the way, the doctor inserts a long needle through the skin on your abdomen into the uterus and withdraws some amniotic fluid. This sample is then sent to genetic and biochemical laboratories for analysis. The whole procedure takes around thirty minutes. The procedure is usually painless, yet some women may experience temporary discomfort at the puncture site.

Is it safe? It is safe, though not without a slight risk of damage to the organs of the baby, placenta, and umbilical cord (though ul-

---

Giving Your Doctor a Prenatal Test

If your doctor recommends or you wish a certain prenatal test, be sure you ask your doctor the following questions:

- What are the risks and benefits of the particular test? Could it harm me or my baby or increase the risk of complications during my pregnancy or birth?
- Is it necessary in my particular pregnancy? Will information about the genetic well-being of my baby increase my well-being in managing my pregnancy or making medical decisions?
- What is your particular experience and complication rate with the procedure? Should I be referred to a fetal-medicine specialist?
- How much will it cost? Will it be covered by my insurance?
- What information does the test give? When will I hear the results? How reliable are the results?
- Are there alternative procedures that are safer and yield nearly as much information? Will the procedure hurt? What complications might I expect? Can my husband and I watch the procedure on the ultrasound screen?

trasound guidance reduces this risk considerably). The main concern about amniocentesis is the one in two hundred chance that it will induce a miscarriage. Risk levels may be higher or lower depending on the experience of the professional performing the procedure, so be sure to ask the doctor about his or her own complication rate, especially the rate of postamniocentesis miscarriage. Unless your practitioner has a lot of experience performing this procedure, he or she may refer you to a fetal medicine specialist. Amniocentesis also carries a tiny risk of infection. Waiting one to three weeks for the results may also take an emotional toll on parents.

Weigh the risks and benefits of amniocentesis together with the advice from your health-care provider to make the decision that's best for you.

(See the related discussion "Having a Baby After Age Thirty-Five," page 81.)

Chorionic Villus Sampling (CVS)

CVS provides more genetic and biochemical information than amniocentesis and can be performed earlier in pregnancy and with quicker results. Yet CVS carries a much higher risk of miscarriage than amniocentesis does. So, this higher-yield–higher-risk procedure demands even greater responsibility in making the decision about whether to have the test.

Why is it done? Like amniocentesis, CVS yields a lot of information about the genetic makeup of the baby, but with CVS the results are available up to four weeks sooner.

When is it done? CVS is usually performed between the eighth and twelfth week after the last menstrual period in situations where an earlier diagnosis is needed or wanted than could be obtained a few weeks later by amniocentesis.

How is it done? There are two methods of performing CVS — transabdominal and transcervical. Which approach your doctor chooses depends on which is safest in your particular pregnancy. The transabdominal approach is similar to an amniocentesis (see page 131). A needle is inserted through the abdomen into the uterus to obtain a small amount of tissue from the chorionic villi, which are fingerlike projections of tissue that surround the baby in the early weeks and ultimately form the placenta. In the more common transcervical approach, a catheter is inserted through the vagina and cervix and into the uterus near where the placenta is forming. Both approaches rely on ultrasound for guidance. Preliminary genetic results may be available within forty-eight hours with confirmatory results available within a week.

Is it safe? Even though CVS provides information earlier in pregnancy than amniocentesis does, it carries a risk of miscarriage that is two to four times higher, depending on the expertise of the physician. Temporary vaginal bleeding and cramping may occur following CVS. Physical and emotional recovery may take a day or so, unlike the immediate recovery following amniocentesis. Recent studies also suggest a possible increased risk of limb deformities in the fetus.

Because the cells in the chorionic villi may not always contain the same genetic material as those in the baby, false positives (suggesting the baby is not normal when in fact he or she is) may occur in 1 percent of procedures. This is not a problem with amniocentesis. Because of the increased risk of miscarriage and misinterpretation, CVS is losing favor among most obstetricians and parents. It stands to reason that cutting off and removing a tiny piece of tissue near the baby carries a higher risk than taking an ounce of amniotic fluid that surrounds the baby. Waiting a few weeks to have an amniocentesis makes a lot of sense to most parents.

WORKING WHILE PREGNANT

Many women find themselves juggling the inside "job" of growing a baby and the outside job of working for pay. For some, especially those who do not suffer from morning sickness and whose jobs are important to them, work is a welcome way to wait out the nine months. These mothers want to work right up until the first contraction. Other women may need a month or more before the birth to prepare their nest and focus on the life inside; they may plan to leave their jobs at a particular time, often in the last trimester. Some mothers, due to pregnancy complications, need to leave in the early months. Whatever your pregnancy situation and your job, here's how to work out the best maternity-leave package for you, your family, and your company.

Informing Your Employer

As soon as you learn you are pregnant, start planning when and how you will tell your boss. How you handle yourself in the next four months or so may well determine how he or she treats you for the rest of your pregnancy and beyond.

If you intend to stop working after your baby comes, you need to give your employer plenty of time to find a replacement, and yourself enough time to finish up important projects. Tell him or her when you plan to quit and ask how you can help make the transition a smooth one.

If you want to return to your job after the baby is born, you must be careful. You want to keep your options open for a satisfactory maternity leave and at the same time protect your position. While it is illegal to discriminate against someone who is pregnant, the corporate world is often confused when a worker becomes a mother. A promotion for which you are in line may be jeopardized by the fact of your pregnancy. You may be given less challenging assignments because of your "condition." You may be uncertain about how your co-workers will handle the news. Some may be sympathetic to your occasional memory lapses and your first-trimester miseries. Others, you fear, will be worried about having to "cover" for you on days when you aren't at your best.

When to tell. The best time to tell your employer and co-workers is just after people begin to suspect you might be pregnant and before they are sure. Although you are excited about your news, most women recommend against revealing a pregnancy in the early months. Here are a few women's experiences:

I'd had an especially good year the year I got pregnant, and several other companies were showing interest in me. No way was I going to take a new job while pregnant, but they didn't need to know that. Of course, these things have a way of getting around, and in my third month my boss walked into my office with the "we don't want to lose you" speech and a fat raise! I was so surprised. I intended to work part-time after the baby came, and this boost of confidence was a real help in my negotiations.

I told everyone right away and, unfortunately, had a miscarriage at ten weeks. People were very nice, of course, but they were all waiting for me to get pregnant again.

After I announced I was pregnant, I got "promoted" to a less visible job within the company. If I'd been showing at the time, they wouldn't have dared, because it would have looked like the discrimination it was.

I told several people before I had thought out my postpregnancy plan and was called to my boss's office to discuss the matter. Ill prepared, I did not negotiate a good maternity leave.

Be careful not to wait too long to tell, either. You don't want to give your employer any reason to think you are untrustworthy; any suggestion that you concealed your pregnancy for your own gain may make you look as though you are not a team player.

Don't be afraid of revealing your pregnancy earlier than planned if you are finding yourself unable to do a good job. You don't want your boss to get it into her head that you're not a good worker, especially at a time when you need her support.

In the first months I did not want my colleagues to know I was pregnant, so I tried to look and behave as usual, but it was not easy. I tried to hide my pale face with makeup and wore clothes that concealed my bulge until they got so tight they left a rim around my waist that took all night to disappear. I tried to concentrate, but I lost interest in what I was doing at work. I had previously regarded my work as challenging, but now it seemed to be a monotonous routine without any serious sense and purpose. It was unusual for me not to enjoy my work, but I couldn't get over the feeling that

now I was working only to earn money and provide a good future for our baby.

Don't expect to function every day on your job at the same level as you did before you were pregnant. If you want to stay employed but find your current position too strenuous, ask for a temporary transfer to a less demanding job. Better to be honest with your supervisor than be disgruntled and inefficient. If you don't want to change jobs, ask if you could work part-time, do some of your work at home, or have flexible hours, so that you can work harder or longer on more comfortable days to make up for the less productive days.

Negotiating Your Maternity Leave

Do your homework before you negotiate, and you're likely to be happier with the maternity-leave package you end up with.

Negotiate with yourself. Interview yourself. If you truly know what you want, you are more likely to get it. Determine what you ideally want; what you can afford; what's best for your pregnancy and your family. Can you grow a baby and do your job? Do you want to? Bear in mind that complications or situations during your pregnancy or after delivery may make some of these decisions for you. Explore your options. Unless your doctor or your baby determines otherwise, could you work through most of your pregnancy? Would you rather start maternity leave early? Do you want to continue your job on a part-time basis from home? After the baby is born, do you want to come back to your present job or to one that is more compatible with family life? Do you want full-time or part-time work?

Working while pregnant should not mean being torn between protecting your job and mothering your baby. You can do both. Whether you want to take off as early as possible and return as soon as possible or work as long as possible and return as late as possible, you should be able to work out the best plan for you, your baby, and your family. That plan may be very specific or quite general. One mother we know was certain that she was more committed to her baby than to her job, so she had nothing to lose by asking for everything she wanted. Not knowing how she'd feel about working after the baby came, she asked her employer if they could negotiate after the baby came. During her pregnancy leave, she offered to keep up with projects from home on an hourly-pay basis. After the baby was born, she worked a few hours a week from home, went in for meetings at four and six weeks (with the baby), and at eight weeks knew enough to negotiate a continuation of work from home for an hourly wage — that way she felt neither party would be short-changed. She worked ten to twenty hours a week from home for the company for four years.

Admittedly, most employers are not that flexible. But if you do a unique job in the company or can afford to quit, you may be able to call your own shots. If not, try to anticipate as best you can your feelings toward motherhood, your financial needs, and your parenting philosophy. And relax. No career decision lasts forever. You can always change your hours, quit, or get a new job.

Know your rights. Know what your company's maternity-leave policies are (you should have been given a copy of them when you were hired) and what the laws allow (see page 140). If you know and trust a co-worker who previously negotiated a leave package with your company, ask what she did, what she got, and what she'd advise you to do. If you do not have a copy of the maternity-leave policy, you can get one from your Human Resources director. (Be aware, however, that he or she may inform your boss.) If your company does not already have a maternity-leave policy and is small enough not to be legally required to have one, you may have to be a pioneer, negotiating the policy for the benefit of your future pregnant co-workers. If you can, check out the maternity-leave policies of other companies before you talk to your supervisor.

When reviewing your company's policy, be sure you understand the following:

- Is your maternity leave paid, unpaid, or partially paid?
- Are you eligible for disability-insurance benefits (complete or partial)?
- Does your company have a medical disability-insurance policy that pays a portion of your salary while you're on leave? Pregnancy is legally considered a medical disability. Find out which forms you have to complete and where to send them, and follow up: Has the appropriate office received, processed, and finalized your application? Be sure your doctor has signed and completed the appropriate forms stating when you will be able to return to work.
- Does your company's policy guarantee that you can return to your same job or one that is equivalent in pay and advancement possibilities?
- How much time off are you allowed?
- May you use your present benefit days (sick leave, personal leave, vacation time) to extend your paid maternity leave?

- What are the company's provisions for extended maternity leave (paid, unpaid, partially paid, working from home)?
- What is the possibility of your continuing your present job part-time at home during and after your pregnancy, and of being tied in to the office by phone, fax, or modem?
- What options are available should medical complications or maternal desire necessitate a change in plans?
- Is your health plan still in effect while you are on extended leave, and does it provide partial or full coverage? How long will your company keep you on its medical insurance policy at full or partial benefits? Do you have to share the cost?

Whom to tell. Officially, you should tell your immediate supervisor first, before she or he hears about your pregnancy from the company grapevine. Or, you may want to talk to the Human Resources department, if it typically handles such matters or if you have real reason to fear discrimination from your boss. (You may need to visit Human Resources for information on your company's maternity-leave policy, anyway.) If you want to tell close co-workers a bit earlier, be sure they have your best interests at heart.

If you have a choice of supervisors to tell, select the one who is most likely to be sympathetic. The supervisor's own parenting experience and philosophy matter more than his or her gender. Find out ahead of time if your supervisor has previously had to juggle working and parenting. If your supervisor is female, find out if she is a parent, the ages of her children, and if anyone knows about her maternity-leave history. If your supervisor is male and has children, find out what kind of package his wife had. The more you know about your supervisor's parenting situation,

the better insight you have into how he or she will approach your situation.

How to tell. After selecting the time and person to tell (and preferably when that person is having a good day), present your case. How to tell depends upon your pregnancy, your job, your wishes, and the reception you imagine you will get from your supervisor and co-workers. As in any negotiation, consider where the other person is coming from. Your supervisor wants to know when you are leaving, when you are coming back, and how best to fill the gap while you're gone. Be ready with those answers. Realistically, your supervisor is more concerned about the company's operations than about your personal needs. Your employer must consider the possibility that you may later decide not to return to work. (Incidentally, studies show that attractive maternity-leave policies and a family-friendly workplace make it more likely that women will return.)

While listening to you, your supervisor will be trying to sense your current level of commitment to your job, though he or she is probably wise enough to know that the company often can't fight the pull of motherhood. In presenting your case, first convey that you are committed to your job (if you really are) and that you are committed to working out a maternity-leave package that considers both the needs of your family and the needs of the company. Opening with "The law allows me . . ." is likely to put your employer on the defensive and get you only what the law allows — which in some states and some companies is precious little. If a special situation later arises and you need to ask for more than the law allows, you will need your boss's continued goodwill and some leftover negotiating power. It is better to open your dialogue by reviewing the company's maternity-leave policy (if there is one) and presenting your plans in the spirit of co-operation. To show your commitment to your job and your respect for the needs of the company, include in your plan specific ideas on selecting and training your replacement. Depending on your familiarity with your supervisor, you may even interject comments such as, "I know you've been faced with these decisions before yourself, and I'd appreciate your help," or "Did your wife take a maternity leave? What worked for her and her company?" Remember that the company is more likely to extend your maternity leave beyond what its policy or the law allows if you show your willingness to extend yourself as well.

Working Out the Right Maternity-Leave Package for You

Only you can guess how much maternity-leave time you will need; only your company can guess how much time it can afford to be

---

A Safe Workplace for Pregnant Women

There are bodily changes that occur during pregnancy that not only change your capacity for work but necessitate your being more safety-conscious at work. Your body is working to increase the blood supply to your growing uterus (and its resident), which may mean you have less energy for your work. As pregnancy hormones increase, your joints and muscles relax, making them less stable and you more prone to losing your balance in certain work-related tasks. You are also more prone to strains and sprains during heavy lifting. All of these changes may mean changes in your work.

Unfortunately, protecting your baby and your job isn't always easy. While you and your preborn baby have a right to a safe workplace, don't rely on federal laws to protect these rights; it is often difficult to determine whether a company has made a decision with the intent of protecting the baby or discriminating against the pregnant mother. You may have to identify unsafe work for yourself, then fight for your right to transfer to a safer job temporarily without being permanently assigned to that position. If your job requires you to stand for long periods of time, for example (studies show that pregnant women who stand for long periods of time are more likely than sedentary women to experience preterm deliveries), and you ask for a position that allows more sitting, you may have to work hard to get your old job back after you deliver. (If you are required to sit too long, periodically stand, walk, or at least use the foot and leg exercises suggested on pages 182 and 195.) It helps to know your legal rights (see "What the Laws Allow," page 140).

If you work with dangerous materials, see "Workplace Hazards," page 59. If your job requires any physical strain (e.g., lifting, standing for long periods, sitting without a chance to stretch), talk to your health-care provider, but be thinking about ways to adapt your work to your new bodily needs. You may have to take a different job temporarily, or quit until you have delivered.

THE THIRD MONTH — ALMOST SHOWING ~ 139

without you. Remember, your bargaining power depends not only on how you present your case but also on your value to the company. If you have a unique skill required for a special job, you'll have more clout than if there are many others within the company who can do your job just as well. Be realistic about your needs, your negotiating power, and the needs of your company, but remember, too, that companies want to be seen as family-friendly in their maternity-leave policies. Try these negotiating specifics:

Offer to stay connected while on leave. If you are in the middle of a project or have specific knowledge or skills that the company relies on, show your commitment to the company and strengthen your negotiations by offering to be available by phone, fax, or E-mail. Fax or E-mail allows you more choice about when to respond to what's needed. Leaving your employer with a message of "Feel free to contact me whenever you need me" is more likely to leave your supervisor feeling that he or she does need you.

Offer to help with the transition. Leave right. Offer to help select and train your temporary or permanent replacement, if any. Remind your supervisor of your availability by phone, fax, or E-mail in case your replacement runs into a snag that requires your special knowledge.

Display your willingness to work hard to the end. When leaving your present job, either temporarily or permanently, show your desire to tie up loose ends. Finish the jobs that need finishing or be sure you have appropriately delegated them.

Develop a contingency plan. Be sure to address the many what-ifs of pregnancy and

Pregnancy Etiquette in the Workplace

You can be pregnant and professional at the same time. You should be. Don't use your pregnancy "disability" to your work advantage, as co-workers and supervisors may resent your flaunting your pregnancy to get special treatment. While snacks in the desk drawer and crumbs on the boardroom table are part of the pregnancy package, respect your co-workers by cleaning up your own messes. You may need a rest after lunch, but be sure your work is done on time.

Choose those to whom you complain. Women who worked while they were pregnant are likely to be more sympathetic than childless co-workers. Carefully select which colleagues you ask to cover for you when you need to use the bathroom, and show you appreciate their help by leaving them "thanks for understanding and helping" notes or small tokens. Find ways to return the help on days when you are feeling better. Use humor to defuse a particularly unsympathetic co-worker: "Your mother probably had days like this when she carried you." Who could argue with that?

If you are having serious trouble getting your job done, talk to your health-care provider first, then to your supervisor. Remember that while you are changing dramatically, your job responsibilities have not. Respect your prior commitment, and if you find you cannot honor it, negotiate in good faith.

What the Laws Allow

Astonishingly, current federal laws do not guarantee the right to maternity leave for all women in all companies. State laws vary.

In 1978, Congress passed the Federal Pregnancy Discrimination Act, which applies only to federal workers and companies with fifteen or more employees. This act states that "women affected by pregnancy, childbirth, or related medical conditions shall be treated the same for all employment-related purposes, including receipt of benefits under fringe benefits programs, as other persons not so affected but similar in their ability or inability to work." This act does not entitle you to special treatment because you are pregnant, but it does entitle you to the same disability rights as any other employee in your company. Pregnancy is treated as a medical disability under the law to ensure that women are not denied medical or other workplace benefits. These are the practical applications of this act.

A company cannot:

- deny you a job because you are pregnant.
- fire you because you are pregnant. Your employer may change or terminate your job only for business-related reasons (such as downsizing or failure to perform), not just because you are pregnant.
- force you to take maternity leave if you are still able to do your job.
- terminate your employment on the grounds that your job will harm your preborn child. You have a legal right to stay on the job even if your employer maintains (correctly or not) that it is unsafe for you or your baby.
- deny pregnancy-related benefits that are offered to married women if you are not married.
- treat your pregnancy disability differently from any other employee disability or medical condition. You are entitled to the same disability rights and benefits as any other employee in your company. For

parenthood. What if a medical complication during your pregnancy or after delivery requires a doctor-mandated period of bed rest or extended maternity leave? What if you have a special-needs baby who, for medical reasons, requires a full-time mother? And what if you should get hooked on motherhood and can't bear to leave your baby after those magical six weeks are over? (Maternity leaves of six weeks reflect the needs of commerce rather than the needs of the family; there's nothing in maternal biology or infant development that marks six weeks as a good

time for mothers to return to work.) Many a career train has been derailed by the lure of a beautiful baby.

Dr. Bill notes: Many doctors are willing to write notes for mothers to extend their maternity leave. Oftentimes, mothers come in with a six-week-old infant, pleading for help for just two more weeks at home . . . and then two more weeks . . . and so on. For a mother who works for a less family-friendly company and who lives in a country whose maternity-leave example, if employees unable to perform a job because of disability are transferred to other jobs, you have the right to likewise be transferred. If their jobs are held for them, your job must be held for you.

Depending on company policy, you may not be eligible for benefits if it is determined you were pregnant prior to being employed by your company.

The Family and Medical Leave Act (FMLA) of 1993 permits you to take unpaid, job-secured leave to meet the health needs of your family. This law requires that:

- companies with more than fifteen employees provide their employees with twelve weeks of unpaid leave in the case of the birth or adoption of a child or the care of a foster child; or in the case of the need to care for a child, spouse, or parent (or yourself) with a serious health condition. (The company may choose to offer some or all of the twelve weeks as paid leave, but this act does not

require any paid leave.) Eligible employees include regular full-time employees with at least one year's service, and part-time employees with at least 1250 hours of service during the twelve months before the beginning of the leave. The employer may require that you first use your paid vacation or personal time for any part of the twelve-week period.

- the employee must be returned to the same job or a job equivalent in pay, benefits, and other terms and conditions of employment.

- the employer must maintain your preexisting health benefits for the period of the leave.

An important exception to this act is that if you are among the highest-paid 10 percent of employees and if the employer can prove "substantial and grievous economic injury" to the company by your absence, he or she can deny you the same job when you return. (For more about what the law allows, see "Resources for Women's Working Rights," page 142.)

policies undervalue motherhood as one of its greatest natural resources, many doctors are happy to oblige by offering a variety of reasons to extend her "disability" leave.

Put it in writing. Outline your desired maternity-leave package on paper and present it to your supervisor during your negotiation. Include specific dates and desired compensation. If your supervisor sees exactly what you want, you are more likely to get it. Of course, a prudent negotiator always asks

for a little more than she needs as a built-in hedge toward getting less.

Get it in writing. After you have worked out a maternity-leave plan acceptable to both you and your supervisor, ask for the plan in writing (you may have to offer to do the writing), and be sure that all specifics, such as the questions listed on pages 136 to 137, are addressed. Include the specific dates of your leave and return, if possible, and offer suggestions on how to fill the gap while you're gone. To be sure there are no misunderstandings, it is

Resources for Women's Working Rights

To learn more about your rights to a safe workplace and job protection while pregnant, consult the following resources:

- The Women's Bureau, U.S. Department of Labor, PO Box PM, Washington, DC 20210. Ask for information on the Family and Medical Leave Act and for the publication "A Working Woman's Guide to Her Job Rights," available free from the Department of Labor.
- Your regional office of the U.S. Department of Labor. The telephone number should be available in the government listings (blue pages) of your phone book.
- The Federal Equal Employment Opportunity Commission (EEOC), for information about the Federal Pregnancy Discrimination Act.
- The National Association of Working Women (800-245-9865).

- *The Working Woman's Lamaze Handbook: The Essential Guide to Pregnancy, Lamaze, and Childbirth* (New York: Hyperion, 1992), by O. Robin Sweet and Patty Bryan.
- 9-to-5, National Association of Working Women, 614 Superior Avenue NW, Suite 852, Cleveland, OH 44113 (800-522-0925).
- Coalition of Labor Union Women, Reproductive Rights Project, 15 Union Square, New York, NY 10003 (212-242-0700).
- "Sex Discrimination in the Workplace: A Legal Handbook," a booklet available from the Women's Legal Defense Fund, 2000 P Street NW, Suite 400, Washington, DC 20036.
- "Guidelines on Pregnancy and Work," available from the American College of Obstetricians and Gynecologists, 409 12th Street SW, Washington, DC (202-638-5577).

wise to run the written plan by a knowledgeable friend or attorney before signing it.

Besides being fair to your employer, be fair to yourself. If you do not plan to return to your present job, save as much money as you can during your pregnancy and get used to living on one income. Be sure you collect all of the benefits that you are owed, such as pay for unused sick days. Talk to Human Resources about extending your medical insurance through the completion of your pregnancy and beyond, as far as you can.

No matter how carefully you map out the rest of your maternity-leave plan for after the delivery, *pencil in* the date when your leave ends. Maternal instincts and baby protests may change your plans. When the reality of motherhood hits and you feel a baby at your

breasts, you may push back for weeks, months, or years the date you return to work.

Wardrobe Wise: Dressing for the Job

By the beginning of the third month of pregnancy (and perhaps before), you'll notice yourself gravitating to your loosest, most comfortable clothes. Soon you may notice these outfits begin to feel a bit uncomfortable; even formerly loose jeans are harder to zip, buttons strain on a previously roomy blouse. With the help of a few strategically placed button extenders, rubber bands, or safety pins and the wearing of oversized tops, you can probably wear most of your regular clothes for a few more weeks. But near the end of the third month many women feel larger even if they don't look larger, and by the fourth month most women need to ease into expandable clothing.

Today's pregnant woman has more choices in maternity wear than ever, and a fashion-conscious shopper will find a variety of maternity selections. Of course, you will have to sacrifice some style. Consider your physical comfort as well as how you look. Try these practical tips for choosing maternity wear:

Borrow before you buy. You will find your friends quite eager to shed their maternity clothing after their babies are born. Most women have limited maternity wardrobes and are pretty sick of even their nicest outfits by the time they give birth. Discarding the old wardrobe (or at least lending it out) is a deserved rite of passage for the no-longer-pregnant woman. Yet remember, just because it looked good on your friend doesn't mean it will on you. Also, if you live where the seasons change every three months, many of your friends' clothes may be too warm or too cool for your pregnancy. Last, many pregnancy staples, such as leggings, get very hard wear or often see the mother through the first few months postpartum as well, so there will be no way for you to avoid buying some maternity pieces yourself. Nevertheless, borrow whatever you can that suits you, and be sure to share your own maternity clothes with your friends when they become pregnant. Also, check resale shops in your area. Many stores that sell secondhand children's clothes also sell gently used maternity items.

When I got pregnant, I dreaded the day when I would have to shell out money for maternity dresses. I'd rather spend money on the baby! So I began to notice what my pregnant friends were wearing. If I liked what a soon-to-deliver friend was wearing, I would ask her if I could borrow it after her delivery. All my friends were extremely flattered, and most said yes unless the clothes were borrowed to begin with or already promised. I put in my reservation for some nifty-looking clothes, and no one seemed to mind. Everyone knows how expensive it is to buy a whole wardrobe you can wear for only six months. I can't wait until I can return the favor!

Make your own. Even if you don't make whole outfits, you may want to find some fabric you really like and whip up some simple tops, jumpers, or skirts. Inspect the racks of maternity shops and copy the manufacturers' ideas, such as using wide elastic bands and expandable elastic inserts. Also, notice that the seams on quality maternity wear are extra strong. This option may be especially attractive to you if you want to wear cotton, since much ready-to-wear clothing is made from synthetic fabrics.

Know the fashion tricks. Fortunately, the days of cutesy, bow-under-the-chin maternity clothes are long gone. Maternity clothing does not have to be childish, drab, or matronly. Maternity shop clerks and your fashion-conscious pregnant friends can offer suggestions to help you get the look you want. For example, most pregnant women wish to appear slimmer, and thin, vertical lines are more slimming than wide, horizontal ones. Tapered pants and the right arrangement of prints, stripes, and shoulder pads can make you appear taller and thinner. Balance bulky tops with sleek, tapered bottoms. Note that the length of a dress or overblouse is crucial — it can hit wrong and accentuate a fuller thigh or just right and conceal it.

Dress for comfort. Choose comfort over fit. While you don't have to look and feel like you're wearing drapery, think "loose," rather than "tight"; "flowing" rather than "clingy." Forget the perfect fit. If it fits exactly this week, it's likely to be too tight the next. Buying maternity clothing to "grow into," however, may leave you feeling like you're wearing a tent — another incentive for borrowing. If you can't borrow, plan to buy as you grow.

In assessing comfort and fit, pay attention to areas of your body that you may never before have considered, such as your waist, thighs, crotch, breasts, and belly. These are the areas where clothing will become tighter as you grow. Remember that wide elastic bands are more comfortable than narrow ones. If you see deep band marks around your waist, your clothing is probably too tight. Time to move up a size. Clothes that are too tight and are uncomfortable can contribute to indigestion. But resist the temptation to go too big. Clothes that are too large and baggy are unappealing and often awkward.

Choose cotton garments that breathe and that don't irritate your already sensitive skin. Loose knits are friendly to the ever-changing contour of the pregnant woman's body. Don't worry too much about buying really warm outfits for cold weather unless you live where it is unusually cold. Your increased metabolism and the extra insulation of normal body fat will make you feel warmer anyway. Try the layered look, and gradually remove outer clothing as the temperature of the day or your environment changes.

Choose loose, stretchy clothing that will grow with you. Select designs that have tie-backs, drawstrings, alligator clips, elastic waist, side-button adjustments, and a maternity panel — a stretchy section that expands as your abdomen does. To help your baggy clothing have a more shapely fit, use alligator clips to cinch in the sides of the dress.

Accessorize. If you wish to draw attention to other parts of your body rather than your belly, give more attention to your head, neckline, arms, and shoulders. Try snazzy scarves, earrings, necklaces, hats, watches, collars, and shoulder pads. Accessories are wonderful for dressing up your plain, but comfortable, favorites.

By the time I got pregnant with my second child, most of my maternity wear was out-of-date. Luckily, I no longer had to dress for the office, but I did have church and social functions to attend. I found a wonderful, slimming, name-brand dress in navy blue at a consignment shop and wore it everywhere. I changed my hair, added scarves, wore dramatic earrings, necklaces, and bracelets, and always felt attractive.

Sport your spouse's clothes. As the top half of your body begins growing out of proportion to the bottom, you may find yourself rummaging through your mate's closet for oversized shirts and sweaters. If he wears large or extra-large clothes, you may also find his T-shirts, worn loose or knotted at your hips, practical cover-ups for around the house.

It's what's underneath that counts. Choose loose-fitting, cotton underwear. Cotton breathes and won't irritate your ultrasensitive skin. Cotton underwear is also durable and can stand many washings. Some women prefer bikini underwear, which rides under their belly, while others like maternity briefs, which come up and over their abdomen. This latter type can get very stretched out by the end of pregnancy, so don't count on wearing it next time around!

When it comes to hosiery, stockings rather than panty hose may be the most comfortable, though many women find putting them on awkward, especially in pregnancy. Most opt for maternity panty hose, which are more expandable and have a larger and extra-absorbent crotch. You can even buy maternity panty hose with special support in the legs. Very tall women often find maternity panty hose too short, however, and report that standard queen sizes work well.

Choosing the Right Bra

As your belly grows, so will your breasts. By the fourth month of pregnancy, most women feel more comfortable wearing a maternity bra. Here's what to look for in choosing the right bra:

- **Fit.** Think comfort above all. Be sure the cup size and closure system are adjustable to accommodate your expanding breast size. The cup should fit smoothly without puckering and the center of the bra should lie against your chest without any gaps. Even though most women find their cup size peaks by the sixth month of pregnancy, continued expansion of your rib cage may require easing the band. When you purchase the bra, be sure it fits comfortably at the tightest hook closure. This will allow room for expansion.
- **Construction.** Choose a cotton fabric that is comfortable and that breathes. Look for cups that are cotton rather than scratchy lace. An underwire bra is a no-no for many moms during pregnancy and nursing, because it can compress expanding, sensitive breast tissue. If you do buy an underwire maternity bra, be sure that it's not too tight. If it pinches as you grow, put it away until two to three months postpartum, when your breasts are no longer swollen with extra fluid.

- **Band.** Feel how the band rests on your rib cage. In the back, it should be comfortably below your shoulder blades. It should fit loosely enough not to bind your breasts, yet be snug enough not to ride up when you raise your arms or shrug your shoulders.
- **Straps.** They should be wide and padded, so they don't dig into your shoulders as the weight of your breasts increases.
- **Nightwear.** Some women find that wearing a lightweight maternity bra at night gives extra support and eases discomfort.
- **Nursing bras.** You may want to buy nursing bras during the last few months of pregnancy. (These have cups that open for baby's easy access.) If you plan to use bras bought during pregnancy for nursing, buy them on the roomy side to allow for the rapid expansion of your breasts when your milk comes in. (Breast size may increase by two full cup sizes in the days after birth.) Buy only two of these nursing bras; you may even want to reevaluate the fit later. Many mothers stick to maternity bras throughout their pregnancy and switch to nursing bras after their milk comes in. You will find a full range of maternity and nursing bras in maternity shops and maternity catalogs.

Beginning in the second or third month you will notice the need for a larger bra. Some women just buy progressively larger bras. Others opt for maternity bras, which can be found at maternity shops, in the maternity-wear section of department stores, and in maternity-wear catalogs. Many women save money by buying nursing bras, which they can wear after the baby comes, too. This is often not a bad idea, but it is not uncommon to find yourself going up still another size in the first months of lactation. Note that you can lessen the chances of postpartum sagging by wearing a supportive bra throughout your pregnancy, even at night if you need to. (See "Choosing the Right Bra," page 145.)

Be sure your shoes fit. As you grow and your center of balance changes, so must your shoes. Because of the extra fluid throughout the pregnant body, your feet may swell, perhaps even going up a size as your pregnancy progresses. Buy new shoes if you need to instead of suffering. Many women also find that wearing high heels in the second half of pregnancy throws them off balance and contributes to backache. As your pregnancy progresses, the heels on your shoes need to become shorter and broader. Soft, flexible, low-heeled wedges are often the most supportive and comfortable. Choose shoes that are easy to slip on using your feet only, as you will find it increasingly difficult to bend over to tie laces or buckle straps. Also, avoid wearing knee socks with tight elastic bands, which can contribute to ankle swelling.

What helped me rise above that "beached whale" feeling was to glamorize the parts of my body that weren't growing instead of focusing on those that were. I'm a savvy shopper, so I bought two dazzling outfits, got more creative with my accessories, sported a new hairdo, and splurged on my makeup. Whenever my spirits needed a boost, I got all dolled up. I figured I'd have this look for only a few months, so I did my best to enjoy it.

THE THIRD MONTH

❖ ❖ ❖

Emotionally I feel: _____
_____
_____
_____

Physically I feel: _____
_____
_____
_____

My thoughts about you: _____
_____
_____

My dreams about you: _____
_____
_____
_____

What I imagine you look like: _____
_____
_____
_____

Sharing our news. With whom? Reactions: _____
_____
_____
_____

My top concerns: _____
_____
_____

My best joys: _____
_____

My worst problems: _____
_____

VISIT TO MY HEALTH-CARE PROVIDER

Questions I had; answers I got: _____
_____
_____
_____
_____
_____
_____

Tests and results; my reaction: _____
_____
_____
_____
_____
_____
_____

Updated due date: _____
My weight: _____
My blood pressure: _____
When I first heard your heartbeat: _____
My reaction: _____
_____
_____
_____
_____
_____

Feeling my uterus; my reaction: _____
_____
_____
_____

photo at three months

Comments: _____
_____
_____
_____
_____
_____
_____
_____
_____
_____
_____
_____
_____
_____

baby at _____ weeks (ultrasound photo)

Fourth-Month Visit to Your Health-Care Provider (13–16 weeks)

During this month's visit, you may have:

- examination of the size and height of the uterus
- examination for swelling, varicose veins, and rashes
- an opportunity to hear baby's heartbeat
- an opportunity through ultrasound to possibly see baby move and all the organs that are now developed
- a triple-screen test for possible prenatal genetic defects
- weight and blood-pressure check (expect a more rapid weight gain over the next 3 months)
- urinalysis to test for infection, sugar, and protein
- ultrasound screening for possible birth defects, number of babies, and placental location, and to determine baby's age (a standard routine in many practices today)
- an opportunity to discuss your feelings and concerns

The Fourth Month —
Feeling Better

WELCOME TO THE SECOND TRIMESTER! While you probably think about your pregnancy in terms of months, your doctor measures your growth in weeks, and at week thirteen you cross that magic divide into what many women see as the "golden period" of pregnancy. Though some women still have occasional "green" days, especially in the fourth month, most report that in their middle trimester, day-long nausea subsides and their appetite for food — and sex — returns. Most women also get much of their energy back this trimester.

I'm in my thirteenth week and feel I've just returned to life. I now want to eat, make love, go shopping, and even my job is no longer the all-day nightmare of falling asleep at my desk between trips to the bathroom!

The fourth month marks the beginning of rapid growth for you and for baby, as your more rapid weight gain will begin to reflect. This month you will probably begin to look pregnant, and your expanding bust and waistline will mean you are most comfortable in the maternity wear that just a month ago

seemed impossibly big. And, even though the intense emotional and physical challenges of the first trimester have begun to dissipate, the next few months will call for adjustments of their own.

HOW YOU MAY FEEL EMOTIONALLY

Most women find the second trimester to be a more emotionally stable time than the first. The surge in pregnancy hormones that took you by surprise in the early months now levels off, as do your emotions. You'll probably find your reactions to events a bit less dramatic now. Even better, most moms we talked with told us their fourth-month feelings were usually happier.

Relieved. After the twelfth week of pregnancy the chance of miscarriage nearly vanishes, so although the possibility of later miscarriage still exists, fear that you could lose this baby can be put aside. You are also likely to feel relieved to be past the constant nausea and tiredness of early pregnancy. Of course, some women continue to feel these

151

pregnancy symptoms during the next few months, but usually to a much lesser degree.

Ready to tell. Now that you are showing that you have a biological reason for feeling and acting the way you have been, you may be more eager to share the news with friends and relatives. If you previously kept your pregnancy private, the secret is now out — literally. Depending on your body build and the way you carry your baby, you may be showing only slightly at this stage, leading observers to wonder, "Is she or isn't she?" When you begin to show is a good time to tell.

Beginning to bond. Starting to show, hearing baby's heartbeat, seeing him or her on ultrasound, and even suspecting you feel the first kicks make your pregnancy seem more real. These signs will intensify your feelings of closeness with your baby and your realization that this tiny little person inside is really part of you.

When my husband and I saw our baby on the ultrasound screen this month, we were completely blown away. It was somewhat of a visceral shock. I mean I knew I was pregnant, but this was so real and exciting. I've been on a cloud for days.

Ambivalent. Even with all the positive feelings you're likely to experience this month, one day you may be glad you're pregnant, the next day you're not sure. Yes, you're over the hump of first-trimester miseries, but you still have six more months to go. Some women dread the continued uncertainty over how they will feel. Fresh from the throes of nausea, they may nervously anticipate the later stages of pregnancy, when getting around will be more difficult. Other women report

that they are already tired of waiting, that they have the feeling that their lives are on hold while they gestate. One woman we know told us she yearned simply to feel like her "old self" again. Fortunately, this ambivalence generally decreases as the pregnancy advances.

Doubtful. Now that you actually look like a pregnant person, it's normal for those doubts you had on positive-pregnancy-test day to resurface. Are you ready to have a baby? Are you ready to change your lifestyle, career, and marriage? Are you ready to be someone's mother? It's normal to have these feelings at this stage, now that the pregnancy seems more real. Major life changes always bring about what-ifs. Certainly, pregnancy and parenthood bring major life changes, and it would be unusual if you weren't at least a bit concerned about how you're going to cope with them. Thinking about these issues now will make it easier to weather the adjustments after birth. This is time to get worry in perspective. What possible good has worry ever done anyone? If your worrying fits a pattern you are only too familiar with, consider finding someone (a wise friend, a pastor, or a professional counselor) with whom you can talk.

Proud. While some women become anxious, even resentful, about their changing bodies, a great many enjoy their fuller figures and even flaunt them. Growing a baby is a big achievement, and now that you have visible proof of your success, you, too, may feel quite proud. You should! Pregnancy is an important rite of passage for a woman, and it deserves to be celebrated. You are joining your mother, her mother, her mother, and so on, in creating life — it's heady to feel such power. Let your pregnant self-image be a positive one.

Sexy. As your turbulent insides begin to settle and your energy returns, you will probably feel like living again, and for many women that includes sex. Depending on how well you feel physically and emotionally, you may begin to want and enjoy sex even more than you did before you were pregnant. If you experienced the usual sexual low of the first trimester, your heightened interest in lovemaking may be a pleasant surprise for your mate, especially if you are the one doing the initiating. (See "Enjoying Sex While Pregnant," page 120.)

The best part of being pregnant is being able to enjoy sex all the time without worrying about getting pregnant.

Nervous about your appeal. Even if you feel sexy and proud of your changing body, you may be concerned about whether your husband will share your enthusiasm. In fact, many men take a while to get used to the pregnant form. Others find it incredibly sexy. (See "Enjoying Sex While Pregnant," page 120.)

Irritated. Now that you're showing, friends who kept bugging you to play tennis in your first trimester finally believe you when you say you're too tired. Your spouse may be more attentive to you now that he can finally see with his own eyes why you've been dragging or acting so weird. Of course, you would have liked all this consideration last month even more, when you felt so bad.

Now that you are getting more attention from friends, family, and co-workers who cannot help but notice your blooming figure, you

may also find you are not as ready or willing as you thought you would be to receive it. You may even find all the attention irritating. Keep in mind, though, that once people get used to your being (and looking) pregnant, they'll be a lot less likely to comment on your pregnancy unless you encourage it; they'll take their lead from you. The more comfortable you are in your new role, the better able you will be to encourage or discourage the attention paid to your pregnant form.

Now that my pregnancy is becoming public, well-meaning bystanders are becoming inappropriately intrusive. They either accuse me of being overcautious when I refuse to eat my sushi or negligent when I take an occasional sip of wine. It's uncomfortable feeling that no matter what I do, I'm constantly being judged.

People at work are treating me so differently. I feel like politely telling them that I'm the same old me, and I'd rather talk about stock prices than the sex of my baby. Even my mother is lavishing advice about how I should take care of myself and even how I should begin thinking about raising my child. I'm not yet ready for all this advice and attention.

HOW YOU MAY FEEL PHYSICALLY

Just as the side effects of a medication lessen once you become accustomed to the dose, the side effects of pregnancy hormones begin to lessen as your body adjusts to their presence. During these middle months, most pregnant women finally feel better physically, and many feel better than they ever have in their lives.

Back to normal, almost. You're finally feeling like yourself again, at least to some extent. If you're like most women, you're enjoying not having to think about food — if, when, what, and where to eat — all day long. You may even be able to go a few hours between snacks without experiencing empty-stomach nausea.

Beginning to show. If this is your second or third pregnancy, most likely you are obviously showing by the fourth month. If this is your pregnancy, you may still be in that "is she or isn't she?" stage. Whether or not others notice your pregnancy, you will. You may still be in that in-between stage of your regular clothes feeling too tight and maternity clothes looking too large. (For wardrobe advice, see page 142.)

Energized. With the "bed and bathroom" stage of pregnancy behind you (though these will remain important places of refuge throughout your pregnancy), you may find you are now able to resume many of your usual activities. How quickly and to what degree energy returns varies from woman to woman. Most mothers-to-be are not (and should not expect to be) able to function at the same energy level as they did before becoming pregnant. A small percentage of women, however, claim they feel more energetic during this trimester than at any other time in their lives.

Women who suffered through an awful first trimester sometimes want to make up for missed time and plunge back into high gear, trying to do too much. Fortunately, most women find their bodies simply won't let them overdo it. Whatever your activity comfort level, be sure to listen to your body. Don't assume these bursts of energy will last indefinitely, and don't push yourself so hard when you're feeling good that you "crash" later. Pregnant women who try to do too much one day find their bodies make them pay for it by demanding several days of rest in return.

Your mate or your employer may expect you to act like your old self and do all the things your old self used to do once you start feeling better. Remind yourself that you and your baby are growing more during these three months than at any period during your pregnancy; there is only so much energy to go around. Biology will see to it that your baby has first call on your energy, and you will be second. Everyone else must settle for what little is left over.

Needing to urinate less often. The frequent need to urinate that sent you running to the bathroom day and night last trimester will lessen a bit over the next month or two as your uterus rises out of your pelvis and away from your bladder. In the last two months, when your uterus enlarges and baby drops, it's back to the bathroom again.

Warm. You may feel overheated during the remainder of your pregnancy. You are walking around with a body temperature one degree warmer than usual, courtesy of your pregnancy hormones. This phenomenon is similar to the slight increase in temperature that accompanies ovulation during your menstrual cycle. You are like a biological machine in high gear. Your body is working overtime, and it gets hot. Expect to perspire more. It's your body's way of self-cooling.

To help ease the discomforts of overheating, drink extra fluids to replace those lost through perspiration, and wear loose-fitting cotton clothing that breathes. Layer your tops so you can quickly peel off any excess when you find yourself getting too warm. To lessen the discomfort or odor of increased perspiration, treat yourself to more frequent showers and changes of underwear.

I feel pretty warm all the time. I notice I sweat more at even the slightest exertion. I go around in short sleeves even though it's the middle of winter, and sometimes I even want to put on shorts. I also feel warmer at night, so I don't use a blanket. Sometimes I get so hot I even have to put my feet out from underneath the sheet. It's as though I carry around my own personal furnace inside.

Increased vaginal discharge. A milky, slightly odorous vaginal discharge the consistency of egg white is normal during pregnancy and often occurs in increasing amounts as your pregnancy progresses. This mucoid discharge resembles premenstrual vaginal discharge, except that it's heavier and constant. The same mechanisms (pregnancy hormones and increased blood flow to the tissues) that prepare the vagina for the passage of the baby are also responsible for this increase in secretions. Many women change their underwear several times a day or wear panty liners to stay comfortably dry.

While most vaginal discharge is nothing more than a minor nuisance, some types of discharge may signal a vaginal infection. Suspect an infection and notify your practitioner if the discharge becomes pus-like, yellow, green, cheesy, or foul-smelling; if you experience burning or itching; if your labia become more swollen, red, or tender; or if you experience burning pain while urinating.

Here are common types of vaginal infections:

Yeast infections. The most common and most irritating of vaginal infections are caused by a fungus we call "yeast" (e.g., candida, monilia). Yeast is a normal resident of mucous membranes throughout the body, especially in the lining of the intestines and vagina. Under certain circumstances (which can include dietary factors, stress, hormonal changes, or the presence of an antibiotic in the body), this otherwise harmless organism grows into an irritating infection. Because of the high levels of estrogen and the high sugar content of the cells lining the vagina during pregnancy, a pregnant woman is much more likely than a nonpregnant one to get a vaginal yeast infection. Signs of a yeast infection are a relatively odorless but thick and curdy discharge resembling bits of dry cottage cheese; itching; irritation, redness, and burning around the vagina; painful urination; and painful intercourse.

Your health-care provider can usually diagnose a vaginal yeast infection just by noting the characteristics of the discharge, but sometimes she or he may need to take a culture of the discharge to confirm the suspicion and rule out other infections. Candida is easily treated by prescription or over-the-counter vaginal creams, tablets, or suppositories, but not all are safe in pregnancy. Consult your practitioner for the treatment that is right for you.

Vaginal yeast infections can recur throughout your pregnancy. While irritating to you, they are harmless to your baby, although a baby can pick up a yeast infection while traveling through the vagina during birth. Yeast can cause a mild infection of the mucous membranes of baby's mouth called "thrush," which generally appears around a week after delivery and can spread to the mother's nipples and cause pain and tenderness during feedings. Occasionally, a harmless yeast dermatitis may also develop in the newborn; it can be treated easily with over-the-counter antifungal creams.

Fortunately, there are some self-help methods you can use to reduce the frequency and intensity of vaginal yeast infections. Cut down on refined sugar in your diet. Eat yogurt that contains live lactobacillus acidophilus cultures or take oral acidophilus tablets or powder, or drink acidophilus milk. Shower off the discharge — a handheld shower head is useful. (Because of the danger of introducing air into your circulatory system or of damage from high water pressure, douching is not advised during pregnancy.) Avoid using tampons; use a sanitary pad or a panty liner instead. Avoid feminine hygiene sprays, which can irritate vaginal tissues. Wear loose cotton panties until your symptoms are gone. Avoid tight jeans, exercise pants, leotards, and swimsuits. Wear a nightgown and no underwear to bed instead of pajamas. Wear skirts rather than slacks, and skip the panty hose whenever possible. The most irritating symptom of a vaginal yeast infection is the intense itching, which can be relieved by applying cold water compresses and sitting in a warm bath to which a cup of cornstarch and a half cup of baking soda are added. (The over-the-counter soothing bath Aveeno works, too, but avoid soaking in substances like bubble bath and perfumed soaps that may irritate the vagina.)

Trichomoniasis. Trichomoniasis, a sexually transmitted bacterial infection, is less common than candida during pregnancy. Like candida, it is irritating to the mother but harmless to her developing baby. Trichomoniasis is characterized by a yellowish-green discharge with a fishy odor. Your practitioner can diagnose it by observation of the vaginal discharge and confirm his or her diagnosis by culture. Trichomoniasis is treated with an oral prescription or a vaginal gel or suppository. Your mate will be treated at the same time with an oral medication.

Other bacterial infections. Less common bacterial infections that cause a vaginal discharge are gonorrhea and chlamydia, which are usually transmitted sexually. Both are characterized by a yellowish-green discharge accompanied by burning during urination and tenderness throughout the vaginal canal. Your health-care provider will insist on a culture if either of these infections is suspected, because these organisms can infect the baby during passage through the birth canal or can cause inflammation and damage to the mother's reproductive organs.

Congested. Keep your tissues handy. The same pregnancy hormones and increased blood volume that cause increased vaginal discharge also cause the mucous membranes in your nose to swell, secrete fluid, and produce an annoying postnasal drip. Allergic mothers who suffer from asthma and hay fever may find they wheeze, sniffle, and tear more while pregnant, but even women with no history of allergy or sinus trouble often report constant sniffles while pregnant.

Do not take prescription or over-the-counter decongestants, antihistamines, or cortisone nasal sprays without your doctor's advice, since some of them are not safe to take while pregnant. To relieve your nasal stuffiness naturally, humidify your bedroom air any time your central heating is on. (A warm-mist humidifier works well.) Keeping your nasal membranes from drying out can lessen your chance of nosebleeds, another nuisance of pregnancy. Most nosebleeds are mild and temporary enough to be controlled by a few minutes of pressure on the nostrils. Facial steamers (available in cosmetic departments and beauty supply stores) are an easy way to breathe steam in order to loosen secretions and relieve sinus congestion. Over-the-counter saline nasal spray is a safe and effective way to flush out a stuffy nose. Soon after delivery your nasal passages should be less congested.

Bleeding gums (pregnancy gingivitis). Guess what? Those pregnancy hormones that affect the mucous membranes throughout the rest of your body also cause changes inside your mouth. In addition to increased salivation (see page 69), you can expect your gums to be sensitive, swollen, softer, and more apt to bleed easily during brushing and flossing. Have a dental checkup sometime around the fourth month. The dentist, hygienist, or periodontist may be able to help you prevent these gum changes from leading to inflammation of the gums (gingivitis) or gum infections. Because tooth decay and gingivitis are more likely to occur during pregnancy, dental checkups and more vigilant dental hygiene should be part of your overall health-care package. If you need dental cleaning, dental X rays, or a local anesthetic, don't worry. These will not harm your baby. (When you are pregnant, or even if you think you could be pregnant, be sure to inform your dentist, who will drape a protective lead apron over your abdomen as a precautionary measure during X rays.) Should you, because of certain heart valve problems, need to take a couple of doses of antibiotic right before and after having dental work done, make certain your dentist knows that you are pregnant, even though the antibiotic commonly used in this situation is safe to take while pregnant.

Here are some home care tips to help prevent the normal gum changes of pregnancy from becoming more unpleasant and severe:

- Eat more fruits and vegetables that are rich in vitamin C (for more information about vitamin C, see page 95). A calcium-rich diet is good for your teeth, too.

- Rinse with an antiseptic mouthwash several times a day. Spit it out; don't swallow it.
- Use a soft-bristle toothbrush that does not cause your gums to bleed. Brush gently.
- Brush more frequently, and certainly after each meal. Carry an extra toothbrush and tube of toothpaste in your purse or briefcase
- Floss regularly, at least once a day.
- Consider using an ultrasonic toothbrush, which is more effective than a regular toothbrush in removing plaque. It may also be more friendly to your sensitive gums.
- Avoid sticky candy and other sweets. Toffee, figs, and other sticky stuff is likely to collect in the swollen crevices of pregnant gums, so satisfy your sweet tooth with less sticky stuff.

Note: Your gums may also grow tiny nodules that are tender to touch and that bleed easily when brushed. Known as "pyogenic granulomas" (also dubbed "pregnancy tumors"), they are nothing to worry about and disappear shortly after delivery. If you find them annoying or worrisome, they can be drained or removed by your dentist.

Headachy. Headaches, like nausea, are a common complaint of pregnancy. You may experience headaches frequently or only occasionally while pregnant, but chances are you will experience them. Pregnancy headaches often start and stop suddenly and come on without warning. They can throb, pound, feel like a band squeezing around your head, or be like a migraine. Some chronic migraine sufferers find that their headaches get more frequent and severe during pregnancy; others find that their migraines become less intense or less frequent while they are pregnant. Some headaches last a few minutes, some occur off and on all day. Researchers believe hormonal changes are the cause of these headaches, but it is likely that the tremendous emotional and physical changes that accompany pregnancy also contribute to headaches. After all, tension headaches often strike during times of stress and change.

Most headaches that come on in the first two trimesters of pregnancy are simply one more unpleasant side effect of being pregnant, and they usually subside or disappear by the end of the second trimester. *Severe, persistent headaches (especially those accompanied by blurred vision) during the third trimester may be a sign of high blood pressure and should be reported to your doctor.*

The dangers associated with taking headache-relieving medications while pregnant are just another headache to live with. Sometimes, though, not being able to take drugs to alleviate pain can work to your advantage, as it forces you to explore other ways of relieving pain. There are many non-drug therapies you can try to prevent and alleviate pregnancy headaches (see below).

Identify your headache trigger. If you find yourself with a headache, reflect on its most likely cause. What were you doing, eating, or thinking prior to the headache? How often have you said, "This job is a major headache" or "That person is a real headache to be around"? You owe it to yourself and to your growing baby to avoid situations that upset or annoy you.

It's possible to think yourself into a headache. Do not allow your mind to race through a myriad of worries and anxieties; relax, meditate, or sleep.

Change positions slowly. Any movement that changes blood flow to your brain can cause a headache. Normally when you go from lying to sitting or from sitting to standing, your pulse and blood pressure quickly adjust to compensate for the change in gravity in order to pump enough blood to your brain. While you are pregnant, your uterus has "first dibs" on the blood supply, so that the blood flow to your brain is momentarily

ASSOCIATION — TRIGGER	REMEDY	RESULT
Jump out of bed in the morning, feel faint, get headache.	Arise slowly and gradually.	Headache and dizziness don't occur.
Get hungry, get headache.	Snack frequently, don't allow yourself to get hungry.	No more hunger headaches.
Get nervous before dinner party, feel tense, get headache.	Plan several days ahead, invite only good friends.	No tension headache.

reduced. As a result, you may feel dizzy, faint, or have a headache after jumping out of bed in the morning or rising from your easy chair at night. To help your baby-preoccupied cardiovascular system supply adequate blood to your brain, ease into position changes gradually.

Keep your blood sugar steady. Drops in blood sugar trigger hunger headaches that can be prevented by frequent snacking on steady-energy foods, such as complex carbohydrates. Keep a purseful of steady-energy snacks.

Search for fresh air. Stuffy, poorly ventilated, overheated, or pollutant-filled rooms can cause sinus congestion and headaches. Avoid smoke-filled rooms. If you're attending a gathering in a crowded room, station yourself near a door so you can duck out frequently for some fresh air. In the winter months, when the heat is on, sit near a slightly opened window to counteract the drying effects of central heating. If you work in a hermetically sealed office building, take your bathroom breaks near the lobby, and step outside briefly for some outside air. If you can't take frequent breaks to go outside, consider buying an air ionizer. Many women find negatively charged ions vastly improve the air quality in their offices.

Try home remedies. The best way to treat pregnancy headaches is to prevent them in the first place, yet even pregnant women who are calm, eat well, and breathe clean air still get headaches. Many women find that if their headaches are mild enough to be relieved by nonprescription medication, they can also find relief with nonmedical, no-drug approaches. Try these easy-on-the-baby, easy-on-the-body self-helps for headaches:

• A head massage. Lie on a comfortable surface and have your mate massage the site of the pain in a circular motion, firmly enough that the skin moves over the skull. Try various positions, such as lying down with your mate kneeling behind your head or sitting up in a chair with the person massaging you standing above you. If frequent headaches are more than just a nuisance during your pregnancy, consult a massage therapist who is familiar with pressure points for temple and neck massage. Make a consultation appointment at which you and your mate can learn how to use these massage techniques yourselves. (You can try to do a head massage on yourself, but it may not work; you can't fully relax if you're doing the work.)

• A sinus flush. The hormones of pregnancy can increase sinus congestion, which in turn may be aggravated by poorly ventilated, overheated, or stuffy rooms, especially during the winter months. Try a facial steamer, available at beauty supply and department stores. To enjoy your facial steam-bath, place the steamer on a table and lean forward, resting on your elbows while you place your face into or near the steam funnel for twenty minutes. Listening to music or a favorite TV show while flushing your sinuses helps the time pass so you won't be tempted to cut it short.

• A clear mind and closed eyes. As migraine sufferers will tell you, the first line of treatment for headaches is lying down in a dark, quiet room. Try the relaxation and visual imagery techniques listed on page 307, or any you may learn in an early childbirth class.

If you have exhausted all of the above preventive measures and home remedies and still find headaches are a problem, consult your doctor about headache medications that are safe to take while pregnant. At this writing, occasional use of acetaminophen (Tylenol) does appear to be safe during pregnancy, but continuous use of high doses does not. Popular migraine medications, especially those containing ergot, are not safe to take during pregnancy, nor are many common over-the-counter pain relievers, such as ibuprofen (Advil, Motrin). Consult your doctor before taking any medications while pregnant. He or she can advise you on which you can take safely and which you can't.

Dizzy, light-headed, and faint. During the middle trimester, or sometimes earlier, you may occasionally feel woozy and light-headed, as if your head is spinning. These symptoms are one of the normal nuisances of pregnancy and cause no harm to mother or baby, unless they begin to occur more often and more severely.

The dizziness that occurs when shifting too quickly into the upright position is due to a normal physiological quirk that, like many other functions, becomes more quirky during pregnancy. Anytime you get up from a sitting or lying position, gravity immediately pulls the blood from the top of your body to the bottom, but ordinarily your cardiovascular system quickly compensates, preventing your blood pressure from falling and pumping blood back up to the brain. During pregnancy, however, the cardiovascular system does not react as fast; the blood flow to the brain momentarily slows, and you feel dizzy for a moment — a condition called "postural hypotension" (low blood pressure due to change in position). This probably occurs because the uterus is competing with the brain for the maternal blood supply, and sometimes it momentarily wins the match.

Sometimes just standing or sitting for a long period of time allows blood to pool in the lower half of the body, stealing blood flow from the brain and making you prone to dizziness (this condition is called "orthostatic hypotension"). Naturally, this tendency is accentuated during pregnancy as the lower half of the body grows larger. In the third trimester, another cause of dizziness is pressure from the growing uterus on the major blood vessels in the abdomen. This means that blood is slow to return to the upper half of the body, especially when you are lying on your back or right side.

Causes of dizziness or fainting during pregnancy that are not considered normal and should be promptly treated are low blood sugar (which can be corrected by eating healthy foods and snacking frequently) and anemia, or low red-blood-cell count (which can be corrected by eating an iron-rich diet and taking iron supplements). Unlike occasional dizziness, repeated fainting is not normal and should be reported to your doctor, who will search for the cause and prescribe treatment.

To prevent and lessen dizziness during pregnancy, try the following:

- Follow the treatment advice listed above.
- Nibble regularly on nutritious snacks.
- Have regular prenatal checkups; your practitioner will monitor your overall health, check your blood pressure at each visit, and periodically check your blood iron level.
- Avoid sitting or standing in one place for a long time. If you must sit, elevate your legs and don't sit still. Exercise your legs frequently while sitting. (See suggestions, page 181.)
- In the second half of pregnancy, lie or sleep on your left side.

- Move slowly and gradually from lying to sitting, or from sitting to standing, especially when getting out of bed in the morning.
- If you feel lightheaded and need to sit or lie down, do so.
- If dizziness doesn't immediately disappear after sitting down, kneel on one knee and rest your head on the other knee, or on the chair. If possible, lie on a comfortable surface with your head flat and your feet elevated a few inches.

HOW YOUR BABY IS GROWING (13–16 WEEKS)

By the end of the sixteenth week, you can easily feel your grapefruit-size uterus midway between your pubic bone and your navel. During this month, baby doubles her length and nearly quadruples her weight. So, by the end of the sixteenth week she may be around 5 inches long and weigh around 4 ounces.* Her arms lengthen this month, so much so that she can now flex her arms, clasp her hands, and suck her thumb. Her legs lengthen, too, and kicking intensifies, although you will probably not yet feel it. The bones of baby's arms, hands, and legs form and are visible on X ray or ultrasound. Baby has begun to "breathe" amniotic fluid in and out through the developing air passages and tiny sacs in her lungs. She begins to swallow and excrete amniotic fluid; by the end of this month her intestinal tract may begin to collect the beginning of feces, called "meconium." Her external ear folds are becoming

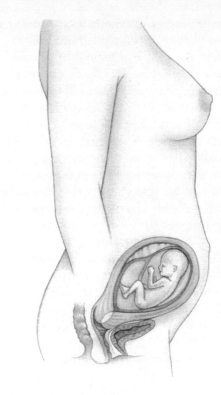

Baby at 13–16 weeks.

more developed, as is her hearing, enabling her to react to sounds. Unique fingerprints develop. Blood vessels proliferate at a rapid rate and show through baby's thin, still-transparent skin. The scant body fat gives baby a lean and lanky appearance. Fine silken hair, called "lanugo," now begins to cover baby's body, and eyelashes start to grow. By sixteen weeks, your little "peach" is about the size of one.

By this month the placenta is a well-developed go-between, linking your circulation to baby's. It transfers oxygen from the air you breathe, nutrition from the food you eat, and infection-fighting substances from the immune cells you make. During each

---

* Fetal length is measured from the top of baby's head to the end of baby's bottom, not including the legs (this is called "crown-rump length").

round-trip passage of your blood and baby's, this magnificent organ, resembling a richly vascularized pancake, selectively picks out the nutrients baby needs from your blood and transfers the waste products baby doesn't need from his blood to yours. Also, during this month the placenta becomes the prime producer of pregnancy hormones you will continually need to nourish your baby and yourself. Baby's umbilical cord, now about the length of his body, looks like a tiny hose, allowing nutrients and oxygen to travel into baby and wastes back out.

Baby now floats freely in her own bubble of amniotic fluid, contained in an amniotic sac. Also, during this month, baby's swimming pool is filled with much more amniotic fluid, allowing baby to float freely in a quart of fluid. By the sixteenth week, there is enough amniotic fluid for doctors to safely enter the fluid-filled sac by a procedure called "amniocentesis."

CONCERNS YOU MAY HAVE

Skin Changes

Some pregnant women are told they "glow" even before they show; their skin gives them away. Most mothers-to-be notice skin changes sometime in the second trimester. These changes may or may not precede the time a woman shows, since that varies so much from woman to woman.

As you might have guessed, the skin changes are due to those hormones, plus the normal stretching your skin must do to cover a larger body. The skin of a pregnant woman looks and feels different because of what's happening beneath it. The increase in blood volume, which peaks during the second trimester, brings more blood to the skin, giv-

ing the areas that are already highly vascular — mainly the face — a rosier appearance. The many glands that lie beneath the skin work overtime in a pregnant body: oil-producing glands produce more oil, pigment-producing glands produce more pigment, and sweat glands cause you to perspire more. The skin changes you see during your pregnancy depend a lot upon the kind of skin you had before you were pregnant. The darker your skin, the more changes you can expect; the lighter the skin, the more visible these changes are. Increased hormones, especially estrogen and progesterone, stimulate pigment-producing cells so that dark areas become even darker.

These changes are not permanent. Shortly after delivery you will get your old skin back, for the most part; some veins and stretch marks linger, but even those fade eventually. Consider these skin changes the mark of motherhood, temporary troubles that the skin goes through in response to all that is going on inside. They are as much a part of pregnancy as nausea or fatigue and are generally temporary. When you stop to think about how much your skin must do to accommodate your changing body chemistry and girth, you'll probably decide that you can put up with these blemishes or marks. Nevertheless, be sure to treat your pregnant skin right by following the pregnancy skin-care basics on page 166.

The pregnancy "glow." The glow that others notice (though you may not) isn't just a sentimental old wives' tale. This facial shine actually has a biological basis. The increased volume of blood causes the cheeks to take on an attractive blush, because of the many blood vessels just below the skin's surface. On top of this redness, the increased secretions of the oil glands give the skin a waxy sheen. The flushed face on many pregnant women is similar to the one nonpregnant people experience when they are excited, cry, or do anything that increases their heart rate (which pregnancy does constantly).

The pregnancy mask. Sometime during the second trimester, you may find yourself gazing at a different face in the mirror. Brownish or yellowish patches, called "chloasma" (also dubbed the "mask of pregnancy"), can appear anywhere on the face but are seen most commonly on the forehead, upper cheeks, nose, and chin. The pregnancy hormones estrogen and progesterone stimulate the melanin cells in the skin to produce more pigment, but because these cells do not produce extra pigment uniformly, your facial skin may acquire a blotchy tan. (If you have ever taken oral contraceptives, you may already have experienced this particular hormonal side effect.) Brunettes and darker-skinned women may notice darkened circles, resembling eye shadow, around their eyes. Chloasma cannot be prevented, but you can minimize the intensity of these blotchy, darkened areas by limiting your exposure to ultraviolet light (i.e., sunshine), which further stimulates melanin production.

Acne. You probably thought your pimple days were over. While the acne of pregnancy is rarely as severe as that of adolescence, you may need to return to some of your teenage cleansing rituals. Fortunately, pregnancy is much shorter than adolescence; the bumps and pimples will subside shortly after delivery. Avoid abrasive scrubs or exfoliants; pregnant skin is too sensitive for these. Milder, oatmeal-based facial scrubs (available at nutrition stores) can help unplug the oily pores and are much kinder to sensitive skin. *Because of the risk of birth defects, the anti-*

acne prescription drugs Accutane and Retin-A cannot be used during pregnancy.

Linea nigra. Many women normally have a faint white line ("linea alba") running from their navel to the center of their pubic bone. It is barely visible before pregnancy; you may not have even known it was there. Sometime in the second trimester a linea alba becomes a "linea nigra," a dark line that is much more noticeable. In some women the line extends upward from the navel as well. The linea nigra is darker in darker-skinned women and disappears several months after delivery.

Dark areas become darker. Little moles and freckles that existed prior to pregnancy may now become bigger, and brown spots or birthmarks become browner. New moles may also appear. (Consult your doctor or dermatologist if these moles seem particularly raised, dark, or have irregular borders.) The areolae and nipples of your breasts will become quite a lot darker; unlike the other darker areas of your skin, which return to their original color after delivery, your areolae will probably always be somewhat darker than they were before you were pregnant.

Red palms and soles. Even as early as the second month of pregnancy, the insides of your hands and the bottoms of your feet may itch and take on a reddish hue, called "palmar erythema." The increased color is nothing more than a curiosity of pregnancy and will disappear a few months after delivery. (To relieve itching, see "Pregnancy Skin-Care Basics," page 166.)

Spider veins. Those much discussed pregnancy hormones, along with increased blood volume, cause those tiny, squiggly red or purple capillaries just below the surface of the skin to branch out and become more visible during pregnancy. It's also common for spider veins (they resemble a small spider web) to pop out on the face or on the sclera (white part) of the eyeballs during delivery; intense, red-in-the-face pushing can break tiny blood vessels. Known as "nevi," these burst vessels can be camouflaged by the appropriate use of makeup (see tips for using makeup, page 167). Nevi take longer to disappear than many of the other skin problems of pregnancy; some spider veins on the legs or torso may not ever go away on their own. A dermatologist can remove them using injections if you feel that's necessary.

Skin tags. Some pregnant women develop tiny polyps, called "skin tags," in areas where skin rubs on clothing or against itself. Commonly found under the arms, between neck folds, or under bra lines on the chest, skin tags are caused by hyperactive growth of a superficial layer of skin. They disappear a few months following delivery, but can be easily excised if they bother you.

Heat rash. You may think that only babies get prickly-heat rash, but pregnant women do, too. Caused by the combination of an already overheated pregnant body, dampness from excessive perspiration, and the friction of skin rubbing against itself or against clothing, prickly-heat rash is pimply and slightly irritating. It is most common in the creases between and beneath the breasts, in the crease where the bulge of the lower abdomen rubs against the top of the pubic area, and on the inner thighs. (To relieve prickly-heat rash, see the advice on page 167.)

Itching. Many pregnant women enjoy a good "scratch down" at the end of the day. Some areas of your skin may itch because they are dry and flaky, other areas may itch because of a prickly-heat rash. Many women find the itching most bothersome in the skin that stretches, mainly over the abdomen, but also on hips and thighs. (To ease the discomforts of itching, see "Pregnancy Skin-Care Basics," page 167, and especially the section on relieving itching.)

Pimply eruptions. Around 1 percent of pregnant women experience itchy, red, raised patches on their abdomen, thighs, buttocks, and extremities. This condition is called "pruritic urticarial papules and plaques of pregnancy" (PUPP). It tends to come and go during the second half of pregnancy and nearly always disappears shortly after delivery. Treat this the same as any other itchy skin eruption.

Hair Changes

Hair is part of the skin system, and, like the skin, its structure is affected by your changing hormones. How hair is affected in pregnancy varies from woman to woman, but by sometime in the second trimester, your hair will probably change.

More hair. Pregnancy hormones lessen the rate at which hair falls out. So during pregnancy you may notice fewer hairs on your brush and more hair on your head. Most pregnant women love this change.

The extra hair that pregnancy gives, the postpartum period takes away. Hair loss will be noticeable from about two to four months after birth, longer if you are breastfeeding. Noticing all that extra hair on your brush or

Stretch Marks

A month or two after they begin to show, nearly all women develop stretch marks, pinkish lines on the skin in the areas that stretch the most during pregnancy: abdomen, breasts, thighs, hips, and upper buttocks. These stretch marks, whose medical name is "striae gravidarum" (stripes of pregnancy), are caused by the tearing of the elastic bands (collagen fibers) in the skin. Some elastic fibers stretch without tearing, some tear yet heal, and others never completely heal. Three factors contribute to tearing and determine how severe your stretch marks will be: hormones, weight gain, and heredity. The pregnancy hormones that relax ligaments decrease the collagen content of the skin fibers, making them more brittle and prone to rupture. The normal growth of breasts and abdomen forces the skin to stretch too far too fast, and excessive weight gain can make this worse. Finally, the skin and body type you inherited will influence the development of stretch marks and how completely they disappear. Some skin types stretch more easily, with little or no breaking of elastic tissue; others do not. Likewise, some skin types heal faster after a fiber tear, and some show tears more than others. No matter what type of skin you have inherited, here are a few ways to minimize how much you stretch and how many marks remain after pregnancy:

- Exercise regularly to keep unnecessary bulges in check.

- Avoid putting on excess weight. Gradually gaining the weight you need helps prevent unnecessary stretching.
- Eat well, taking in sufficient nutrients, especially vitamin C and protein, which aid in building stronger collagen. The skin, including the tissue underneath it, is one of the body's storehouses for nutrients such as protein. If your diet is deficient in protein, your skin is shortchanged, leaving the protein-starved collagen fibers more prone to breakage.
- Oils, lotions, and potions do nothing to keep stretch marks from forming or to accelerate their departure. They may, however, relieve two common annoyances: dryness and itching. There is also some evidence that the daily use of emollients that hydrate the skin and help it retain its suppleness may lessen the severity of stretch marks, and that continuing this massage ritual for three months after birth may lessen the extent to which these marks remain.

Most stretch marks diminish gradually over time. A few months after birth, they fade to stringlike lines of thinner skin, usually slightly indented compared to the surrounding tissue, with a silvery or pearly sheen. They may not even be noticeable in some light. Some never completely fade. Consider these "motherhood lines" a small price to pay for your achievement, and realize that they are not nearly so obvious to others as they are to you.

Pregnancy Skin-Care Basics

The skin of a pregnant woman needs extra care, not only cosmetically, but for comfort. Try these tips for taking good care of the skin that holds you together.

Avoid sun damage. Because of overactive pigment-producing cells, the skin of a pregnant woman is ultrasensitive to the ultraviolet rays of the sun. Don't let your already sensitive skin get sunburned. Avoid unnecessary exposure to the sun in these ways:

- Sit in the shade whenever possible.
- Wear a wide-brimmed hat that shades your entire face.
- Avoid exposure between 11:00 A.M. and 3:00 P.M., when the sun's rays are the strongest.
- Use a sunblock of at least SPF 15. Follow the directions on the bottle. If you are supposed to give the sunscreen time to activate or dry before going outside, ignoring the manufacturer's advice may mean you get less protection. Better to apply it around thirty minutes prior to exposure. A facial sunscreen that we have used and recommend for pregnant women is Aloe-Kote. If you use makeup foundation or a moisturizer every morning, buy one that has a sunscreen built in. Because of concerns over safety, avoid using sunscreens containing PABA.
- Avoid skin-care products that are heavily perfumed or that contain alcohol; these may not only irritate sensitive skin but also increase its sensitivity to sun.
- Avoid tanning salons or artificial tanning lights.

Continue to protect your face from ultraviolet light for a few months after delivery, as your skin may remain ultrasensitive to the sun for around three months postpartum. (Of course, it's a good idea to protect your skin from the sun whether you are pregnant or not.)

Feed your skin. Poor nutrition and a poor complexion go hand in hand. Eat a balanced diet, as recommended in chapter 2. Foods containing vitamin C and vitamin B_6 are particularly friendly to the skin. Taking 25 to 50 milligrams of a vitamin B_6 supplement daily (check with your health-care provider) and using hydrating lotions may help your skin maintain the luster you like. If your skin is very dry you may need to consume more of the liquid unsaturated essential fatty acid linoleic acid (found in vegetable oils and fish).

Hydrate your skin. To counteract the skin-drying effects of pregnancy, drink lots of water and humidify the air in your bedroom during the winter months. If you work in a sealed-window office building, install a humidifier in your office and treat your skin to fresh-air breaks regularly.

Cover your skin comfortably. Wear loose cotton clothing that allows your skin to breathe. Stay away from synthetic fabrics, such as polyester, which tend to trap moisture. Avoiding panty hose may diminish the incidence of prickly-heat–type rash on your thighs, buttocks, and pubic area. Applying some unscented powder or an emollient under your bra straps or on the bottom band of your bra can help minimize irritation.

Be kind to your sensitive skin. When applying emollients, massage in small, circular motions. Stay away from oily, pore-plugging facial creams, harsh abrasives, and skin peelers. Also avoid cleansers that dry the skin, such as those containing alcohol, and highly perfumed or fragranced products, which can increase the skin's sensitivity to sunlight. Before using a new skin product, do a patch test: apply a dab of the product to the inside of your forearm and wait at least twenty minutes to see if you react to it.

If your skin dries out and starts flaking, apply moisturizers and emollients liberally and frequently, especially in areas where your new, larger body rubs against itself or your clothes. If a particular outfit causes discomfort, don't wear it for a week or two until your skin has a chance to heal.

Use skin-care products wisely. Mustela has a line of skin-care products and advice specially tailored for the pregnant woman (800-927-7882). Ask for their booklet "The Wellness Guide to Maternity."

Massage your skin. Treat your body and your mind to frequent massages, either by a trained massage therapist or a dedicated mate. Dubbed "vitamin T," the touch of a caringly performed massage is soothing not only to pregnant skin but also to the pregnant psyche.

Bathe wisely. Water is generally kind to skin, yet too much soaking can irritate it — just think of dishwater hands. Stay in the tub long enough to get clean and relieve the itch, but get out before you "pucker." If your skin was prone to eczema before you were pregnant, too much time in the tub can aggravate this skin problem. Also, since soaps generally dry the skin by removing its natural oils, reduce your use of soap and try using one with a built-in moisturizer. Some of the new cleansing lotions are milder to the skin and do not remove its useful, natural oils. Avoid entirely using soap on your areolae and nipples.

After a bath or shower, seal in moisture by applying moisturizer while your skin is still slightly damp. If you find leg shaving especially irritating to your dry skin, shave with a moisturizing lotion or gel instead of a soap-based product.

Relieve itching. To soothe itchy skin, add a cup of cornstarch and a half cup of baking soda to a half-filled tub of water, or use the soothing commercial compound Aveeno. Soak and soothe your skin. Alternatively, add a tablespoon of cornstarch and a tablespoon of baking soda to a quart of warm water, and use a towel to make a compress to drape over especially itchy areas.

Make up right. Even women who do not usually wear makeup might want to use foundation while pregnant to even out their "glow" a bit. Use mild makeups, preferably water-based ones and those containing emollients. As with skin creams, avoid makeups that clog your pores or dehydrate your skin. And don't forget to do a "make down" at night: carefully remove your makeup every evening to allow your skin to breathe.

pillow may be scary. By a year after delivery, you will have your prepregnancy hair back.

Different hair. Though you are likely to have more hair, it may be different. In pregnancy, dry hair can become drier, oily hair more oily, curly hair may become straight, or straight hair may curl. Individual hairs may become finer or thicker. Hair will take a perm and color differently, too. (See page 55 for safety concerns about hair salons.)

Pregnancy Hair-Care Basics

Here's how you can work your new hair to your advantage while you're pregnant:

- Choose a style to complement your hair and face. For example, if your hair is thicker and your face has become fuller, a longer hairstyle that embraces your face may be becoming. On the other hand, if your already long hair has become drier or more brittle, a shorter hairstyle may be more flattering and easier to take care of. A straight style can show off the luster of oilier hair; a layered look can hide fly-away dryness.
- Experiment with different shampoos. If your hair is dry, shampoo less frequently, and use a mild, low-detergent shampoo that does not wash away the natural oils from the scalp. Also, use a moisturizing conditioner. If your hair is too oily, shampoo your hair more frequently.
- Towel-dry instead of using a blow-dryer.
- While standing in the shower, treat yourself to a gentle scalp massage, using your fingertips to stimulate the circulation in your scalp.
- Electric depilators are safe, but avoid bleaching and chemical hair removal, both of which can irritate your skin.

- When your body image needs a lift, a change of hairstyle can help. But be cautious about color changes. While current research has generally concluded that hair dyes are probably safe to use during pregnancy, they are not advised; some laboratory studies show that coal-tar derivatives in dyes may cause cancer and chromosomal damage in animals. Also, the unique characteristics of "pregnant" hair can make the hair-coloring process unpredictable, and the harsh chemicals used in permanents can damage a pregnant woman's hair much more easily. It seems prudent to avoid exposure to hair dyes during the first trimester, and thereafter to stick to rinses, frostings, or foils that involve minimal scalp exposure and absorption.

  If you can't live nine months with your present hair color, at least use a temporary color rather than a permanent one, and have your hair colored with applications of bleach or dye along the shaft of the hair so it's painted on rather than washed in. (The possibly dangerous dye gets into the bloodstream through the scalp, not through the hair.) Safest while you are pregnant is to enjoy the hair color nature gave you and to promise yourself a new look after you have given birth.

Unwanted hair. Hair may begin to grow in areas women wish it didn't, namely the face, abdomen, back, and legs. Some women notice that their leg hair growth slows down during pregnancy.

Nail Changes and Nail Care

Fingernails and toenails are also considered skin, and, like your skin and hair, they are likely to change during pregnancy. Some changes you may like, some you won't. Pregnancy hormones will help your nails grow faster. On the downside, your nails are likely to break, peel, become softer and more brittle, and form tiny grooves along the base of the nail. Some pregnant women feel their nails get stronger. Here's how to give your nails the special care they need during pregnancy:

• Take gelatin capsules — they're safe during pregnancy.
• Cut your nails frequently and keep them short so they don't get a chance to break unevenly on their own. If you've always loved your long nails, it may help to remind yourself that shorter nails will make it easier for you to care for and caress the sensitive skin of your baby.
• Apply moisturizing and protective creams to your hands and nails at bedtime.
• Avoid nail polishes, which can damage your nails, and acetone-containing polish-removal products, which may not only harm your sensitive nails but give off potentially harmful fumes. If you must chemically treat and color your nails, do so outdoors, or at least in a well-ventilated room.
• Wear protective gloves when washing dishes, using household cleaners, and gardening.

Your nails, like your hair, will be the way they are only for nine months, plus a few more postpartum.

EXERCISING RIGHT FOR TWO

Exercising Safely While Pregnant

There was a time when pregnancy was a time for lying low. It was called "confinement." Today's pregnant women are anything but confined. Because the heart rate increases by 20 percent even in the first trimester, just being pregnant causes a woman's body to perform a low-level of aerobic exercise. Assuming you have a healthy pregnancy, you can generally plan on maintaining an active lifestyle (with time off for frequent naps). Even in your last trimester, when your form may seem to suggest complete immobility, there are satisfying ways to exercise to enhance your feeling of well-being while at the same time being careful of your body and the little being inside.

Consider these tips for ensuring your well-being — and your baby's — during exercise:

1. Consult your doctor. Before you sign up for an exercise program, interview yourself and, in partnership with your health-care provider, determine the exercise program that is right for you and safe for your baby. The following conditions or problems will affect choices you make about an exercise routine:

☐ anemia
☐ heart problems
☐ asthma or chronic lung problems

☐ high blood pressure

☐ diabetes

☐ thyroid problems

☐ seizures

☐ extreme over- or underweight

☐ muscle or joint problems

☐ history of several spontaneous abortions (i.e., miscarriages)

☐ history of previous premature labors

☐ carrying multiples

☐ incompetent cervix

☐ persistent bleeding

☐ placental abnormalities (e.g., placenta previa)

☐ a previously sedentary lifestyle (a serious couch potato)

2. Determine your present fitness level. Prior to becoming pregnant, did you exercise regularly? Did you have an exercise routine? If you were or still are enrolled in a fitness program, did your instructor rate your level of fitness? If you enter pregnancy already fit, you can safely continue your prepregnant level of exercise, although the type of exercise may need to change (e.g., to less jarring movements). But don't expect to continue your prepregnancy level of vigor for long. The little person inside is sharing your energy. If, for example, you are a long-distance jogger, plan to reduce your mileage. Instead of a two-mile jog, a more fitting exercise for you while pregnant would be a four-mile brisk walk. And don't expect that you will walk with the same speed and duration as before when you are carrying an extra 10 to 20 pounds. If you are like many women who never before felt compelled to enter the sweat set, you may find that pregnancy encourages you to join a different crowd (as it

does in so many areas). Notwithstanding your newfound enthusiasm, you will need to begin with light-muscle and joint-friendly exercises and *gradually* build up the time and intensity of the exercises. Finally, exercise to feel good and not to lose weight. Fitness researchers discourage pregnant women from burning off excess weight through exercise because of possible harmful effects on the fetus from the release into the bloodstream of the breakdown products of fat and stored toxins.

3. Dress for the occasion. Wear loose-fitting pants with a loose elastic waistband. To avoid overheating, try the layered look, removing layers as your body warms up. Your clothes should be loose enough to allow sweat to evaporate, thus cooling the skin. Wear supportive shoes that are large enough to allow for swelling feet. To avoid injury to your heel bones, be sure your shoes are well cushioned under the heels. If they're not, insert a ¼-inch shock-absorbing pad. It is best to avoid jogging on hard surfaces. Wear a support bra, or even two if your breasts are very large and heavy. Sport bras that limit bouncing are available in department stores or sporting goods stores. If your clothing rubs and irritates your nipples while exercising, wear a looser top, a special runner's bra, or coat your nipples with a protective emollient such as Lansinoh.

4. Exercise regularly. Short, frequent, consistent exercise routines are healthier than sporadic bursts. Unless you were exercising consistently before becoming pregnant, begin with ten- to fifteen-minute sessions twice daily three times a week and then gradually build up to thirty to forty-five minutes of medium-intensity exercise (cycling, walking, swimming) at least three times a week. Make your exercise routine a priority. "Makeup days" aren't allowed: if you miss a day, you just miss it; don't do double the exercise the next day.

5. Know your limits. The key to exercising safely while pregnant is to work your body without stressing baby's. As a general guide, if the exercise is too strenuous for you, it's too strenuous for baby. Your rising heart rate is an indication of how hard your body is working and of how fit you are. The more fit you are, the more you are able to do while maintaining the same heart rate. Research has shown that baby's heart rate doesn't go up significantly until the exercising mother's heart rate reaches 150 beats per minute. To know when to slow down, observe these monitors:

- *The pulse test.* Take your pulse on your wrist or your neck just beneath the jaw (count the beats for ten seconds and multiply by six to get heartbeats per minute). To avoid accelerating your baby's heart rate, *keep your heart rate below 140 beats per minute.* For adults performing aerobic exercise such as jogging or swimming, exercise physiologists suggest a target heart rate of between 120 and 140 beats per minute depending on age. Not only may 140 beats per minute be too high for your baby, it may be too high for you.

- *The talk test.* If you are too winded to carry on a conversation, ease your exercising to a level at which you can comfortably converse.

- *Listen to your body's stop signs.* If you experience dizziness, faintness, headaches, shortness of breath, hard heart-pounding or palpitations, uterine contractions, vaginal bleeding or fluid leaking, or pain any-

where, stop immediately. The key to exercising wisely is the same as the one you will later use during labor: *listen to your body.*

6. Easy on the joints. Due to the influence of relaxin and other pregnancy hormones, your ligaments loosen, making your joints less stable and more prone to injury if overstretched, especially the joints in your pelvis, lower back, and knees. Avoid sudden hyperextension or hyperflexing exercises, such as back arching and deep knee bends (see "Stretching Exercises," page 178). Gymnastics is out. Five-pound dumbells are safe for toning arm and shoulder muscles. Avoid joint-jarring moves in sports such as tennis and racquetball.

7. Don't shake the baby. Because baby is safely cushioned in his or her own pool, exercise is unlikely to bother baby. Nevertheless, avoid jarring exercises and sudden stops, such as jumping or sudden changes in direction. Go softly on your feet. Avoid running on hard surfaces like cement or asphalt. Upright weight-bearing exercises, such as running, are more likely to bother baby's heart rate than horizontal non-weight-bearing exercises, such as swimming. Avoid hopping and jerking exercises. Swimming and cycling are easier on your body, and baby's, than jogging or basketball.

8. Realize you're off-center. Your enlarging breasts and uterus change your body's center of gravity, increasing your chances of falling during workouts. Avoid risky ventures that require precise balance (e.g., gymnastics and downhill skiing). Dance classes are fun as long as you are willing to grin and bear the fact that your movements may have lost some of their grace.

9. Rehydrate and refuel. To avoid dehydration, drink two 8-ounce glasses of juice or water before and after exercising. Dehydration makes muscles tire more easily. Don't exercise on an empty stomach or when you feel hungry because exercise uses up blood sugar, and pregnancy already makes you prone to blood-sugar swings. A before-and-after exercise snack protects your body and your baby against hypoglycemia (low blood sugar). Try quick-energy snacks, such as fruit, juice, or honey-sweetened whole-grain breads or muffins.

10. Keep cool. In the first trimester, a prolonged body temperature above 102° F can harm your baby's development (see page 56). To keep yourself and your baby from becoming overheated, don't exercise strenuously in hot and humid weather. If you are exercising in one place (e.g., stationary cycling), be sure to ventilate the room. Wear loose clothing to allow body heat to be easily released.

As long as you take these precautions while exercising, you need not worry about overheating baby. Studies show that pregnant women exercising at half of their prepregnancy levels for twenty minutes didn't raise their internal body temperature at all, and raised it only a degree after sixty minutes of exercising.

11. Warm up and cool down. During pregnancy your body's extra blood supply knows its priorities: your uterus and its resident. It takes time for your cardiovascular system to ease into the extra demands of exercising muscles. Don't worry, there is plenty of blood to go around, as long as you are heeding the previous suggestions, but ease into the exercise before going full steam ahead. Take five minutes to *gradually* build up to your peak, then, when you are finished, *gradually* wind down the exercise over five minutes, allowing your cardiovascular system to adjust. Abruptly stopping strenuous exercise may cause blood to pool in the exercised muscles. (Of course, it's all right to stop abruptly if you notice any of the danger signs listed in item 5, above.)

12. Choose the right sport. Swimming is the most body- and baby-friendly exercise for pregnant women (see page 175). Brisk walking is much less jarring to joints and uterus than bouncy jogging. A brisk half-hour walk is an ideal daily exercise for women who are not used to a regular exercise routine prior to pregnancy. Street cycling is excellent exercise in the first trimester but becomes increasingly risky as your center of gravity shifts. When biking, avoid back strain by sitting upright using upright handlebars. Don't bend over to reach dropped handlebars. Stationary cycling is safer in the second and third trimesters. To avoid overheating, use the cycle in a well-ventilated room.

Choose your recreational sport wisely. Because you are carrying an additional 10- to 30-pound load, you just can't do the same sports at the level you are used to. Tennis should be played with caution, since the sudden stops and pivots may stress your pregnancy-changed ligaments. Ditto for racquetball, which has the added problem of overheating associated with any indoor sport. Because of the risk of falling at high speeds, avoid water-skiing. Downhill skiing should be avoided during the second and third trimesters because your changing center of gravity affects your balance. Switch to cross-country skiing on level terrains. Because of the risk of falling, put away your ice skates in the second half of your pregnancy. Competitive basketball and volleyball are too bouncy and stretchy to be played safely while pregnant. Avoid horseback riding as well: besides the risk of falling off the horse, straddling and bouncing in the saddle may overstretch the already sensitive pelvic ligaments, leading to pelvic pain. Heavy weight-lifting is also out, due to the strain on your muscles and ligaments and because of the potentially dangerous breath-holding that accompanies this sport. And because of the possibility of compromising oxygen supply to your baby, scuba diving is an absolute no-no. Try snorkeling instead.

13. Mommy slows as baby grows. In the final months, your baby and your uterus need more of your blood in order to grow, and your heart will have to work harder even when you are resting. There is less reserve blood supply for exercising muscles, so slow the intensity of your exercise routine. Runners, start walking or swimming. Walkers and swimmers, slow your pace. During the last few months of your pregnancy, the combination of increasing weight, general awkwardness, swelling of legs and ankles, and softer joint ligaments calls for a change from weight-bearing exercises (jogging and dancing) to less-weight-bearing ones, such as cycling and swimming.

14. Keep off your back. After the fourth month, avoid exercising while lying on your back. By this stage of pregnancy, your uterus is large enough to compress the major blood vessels (vena cava and aorta) that run along the right side of your spine. Allow your body and your baby to rest after exercise. Lie on your *left* side, a position that prevents your uterus from pressing on the major blood

vessels and promotes circulation to your uterus.

15. Other nuisances that may occur while you are exercising. If you experience leaking of urine during exercise, wear a pad. Since you are likely to get short of breath more easily (see page 256), when you sense that you aren't getting enough air, gradually slow your exercise until you are breathing comfortably again. If your ankles tend to swell later in the day, you may want to get your exercising done earlier in the day so you can have your feet up later on.

I had a pregnancy exercise tape that I used during my second pregnancy. If I did the exercises at least twice a week, I felt great. If I didn't do them, my back would start to bother me. This was all the motivation I needed to get out the tape again. It really made a difference.

Questions You May Have About Exercising While Pregnant

Why should I exercise while pregnant? Will I have an easier birth or a healthier baby?

Studies attempting to relate maternal exercise with pregnancy outcomes yield conflicting results. Some studies show no difference. Others show that physically fit mothers have shorter labors and lower cesarean rates, presumably due to improved muscle efficiency and less fatigue during labor. One interesting study shows that pregnant women who exercise regularly develop a greater cardiac reserve — meaning that the heart operates more efficiently and shunts less blood from the internal organs (including the uterus) when called upon to do so. This could be helpful during the strenuous uterine exertion of active labor and the pushing stage. The general consensus among pregnancy-exercise researchers is that there is no correlation between how much a mother exercises during her pregnancy and the ease of delivery or the health of her baby. Realize, however, that so many variables come into play that there is no completely satisfactory way to study this question. If you are by nature a sedentary person and you are able to maintain a feeling of well-being without adding a three-mile walk to your daily routine, you probably don't need to feel pressure to join the fitness-for-two routine. But it does stand to reason that if you bring a well-toned body into the birthing room, that body is going to labor better for you than if it is not fit.

Regardless of what research shows, common sense tells us that most pregnant women could enjoy their pregnancy more by getting some exercise. Pregnant women we have interviewed feel that a regular exercise routine enhances their feeling of well-being — that immeasurable sense of happy calm in both body and mind that every individual wants. Exercise raises the body's level of endorphins, those hormones that reduce feelings of stress, enhance a person's overall sense of well-being, and lessen the perception of pain and discomfort.

What's different about exercising while pregnant, besides just not feeling like doing it?

Before becoming pregnant, you could roll out of bed, slip comfortably into your exercise clothes, jog to your heart's content and body's limit, and afterward soak leisurely in a hot bath while applauding yourself for having run off the excess calories from last night's eating-out indulgence. Some sweat, no

Safe Swimming While Pregnant

Swimming is a perfect pregnancy exercise if you keep these precautions in mind:

- A water temperature of 85° F is a comfortable temperature for prolonged exercising, yet is cool enough to prevent overheating.
- Be careful getting into and out of the pool and when walking on slippery surfaces. Wearing rubber slip-on shoes into and out of the pool area decreases your chance of slipping.
- Don't hyperextend your joints. In the comfort of water you may not realize you are overstretching.
- Of course, no diving, please.
- Weather permitting, swim in outdoor pools. You are less likely to be irritated by the odor of chlorine. The air around indoor pools can get stuffy and humid, and the chlorine odor can cause nausea. With new pool-filtration technology, namely an ozone system, you can enjoy chlorine-free and cleaner swimming.
- Drink water or fruit juice before and after swimming, just as you would for other types of exercise. Even with all that water around you, you can still get dehydrated while exercising in a pool.
- If you are swimming laps, know when to say when. While water may free the mind of worry, don't forget the precautions listed on page 171. Take the pulse test and the talk test. In water it's easier to be oblivious to exhaustion. If your usual twenty laps becomes too exhausting in the final months, slow your pace and do fewer laps.

Swimming — the Ideal Pregnancy Exercise

Take the plunge. Many women find swimming more relaxing and easier on their pregnant body than any other exercise. Swimming is especially helpful in the third trimester, when exercising becomes increasingly uncomfortable. Swimming actually is easier while pregnant because you are more buoyant. Exercise in water is easier on the joints. When you stand chest-deep in water, the weight on your overburdened knees, hips, and lower back is lessened. Also, the resistance of water encourages smoother movements that are easier on the joints than the jerky movements of land-bound exercises. Swimming is especially friendly to aching back muscles. Lap swimming, water aerobics, or just plain dancing around in the water is great exercise for relaxing both mind and body. Unless given the red light by your doctor, you can swim right up until your membranes rupture.

Being in water helped me appreciate my pregnant body. I felt so free and floaty when I didn't have to worry about my posture or about falling when exercising. It's the only exercise I could do in which I felt being pregnant gave me an advantage.

Besides being more comfortable for mother, swimming is safe for baby, since it's nearly impossible to get overheated while swimming. Besides, as you swim in a pool you can imagine what your baby feels like swimming in hers.

If you don't have a pool but have the means and the space for one, indulge. If backyard space is limited, a "swim spa" (an oblong mini-pool with jets at one end producing a current to swim against, sort of like swimming on a treadmill) is a valuable addition for family fitness. Or try a friend's pool, a public pool, or a local college, or take a swim class tailored for pregnant women, often available privately or at your local YMCA or community center. Be sure the instructor is knowledgeable about the special exercising needs of pregnant women. (See "Safe Swimming While Pregnant," page 174.)

And now a word about swimsuits. Feeling good about your body in a swimsuit is hard for many women, even when they're not pregnant. Putting on a swimsuit while pregnant may require a strong mental commitment to maintaining a positive body image. You'll feel great once you get into the water, so don't let the swimsuit issue become an insurmountable hurdle.

A maternity swimsuit is one garment you may not be able to borrow. Time and pool chemicals tend to destroy elastic, and an old suit may not keep you covered. If you plan to swim during your pregnancy, invest in a new suit, one that makes you feel good and comfortable.

worry. Now, however, you have a different body to carry around the jogging course, one that is challenged by pregnancy. As you and your baby grow, your blood volume increases at least 40 percent and your cardiac output (the amount of blood pumped by your heart) increases by 30 to 40 percent. Your heart rate is automatically increased whether you are exercising or not. In effect, your cardio-vascular system is "exercising" just by being pregnant.

During exercise, the nonpregnant body automatically shifts blood from internal organs that are resting to the muscles that are exercising. One concern about exercise is that some of the blood needed by your uterus and baby might be diverted to fuel your exercising muscles. Another worry is that the same physiological mechanism that causes your heart rate to increase during exercise might cause baby's heart rate to increase, too. The good news is, as long as you exercise sensibly (see above), your muscles don't steal blood from your baby, and your baby's heart rate doesn't go up significantly. A fit mother can exercise sensibly without compromising her baby.

Exercising for an Easier Delivery

Besides conditioning your whole body for pregnancy and birth, it's important to prepare those muscles and joints that are directly involved in pushing out a baby. In our experience, pregnant women like to focus more on the previously mentioned aerobic exercises during pregnancy than on exercises that will benefit them in labor and delivery. Aerobic exercise in pregnancy is important; without it, women tend to gain extra weight, have more discomfort in the last trimester, and have a hard time getting back into shape after pregnancy. But we hope that once you understand the value of these key muscle-conditioning exercises, you will take them seriously too. Even just a few minutes several times a day working your "birth muscles" can make for an easier labor and delivery.

Kegel Exercises

If you do no other conditioning exercises during your pregnancy, do Kegel exercises. Named after the doctor who invented them, Kegel exercises strengthen all the muscles supporting your urogenital tract.

Nature intends the pelvic-floor muscles to relax somewhat during pregnancy to prepare for delivery of the baby. But if your pelvic floor is already weak, you may find you have the problem of leaking urine as your uterus grows and strains the muscles that support it and your bladder. Incontinence can continue after pregnancy, since these muscles are stretched to their utmost when you push out the baby.

Kegel exercises can not only prevent or treat pregnancy incontinence but can also make birth itself easier, because once you have practiced exercising your pelvic-floor muscles, you'll know how to release them. Releasing not only makes labor more comfortable but also helps you avoid tearing these tissues during the birth when baby's head moves through the vagina. As a side benefit, many women who do Kegel exercises report enhanced sensitivity during intercourse, and many of their partners claim greater pleasure as well.

To locate your pelvic-floor muscles, try to stop your urine flow midstream. If you can do it easily and quickly, your pelvic floor is in pretty good shape. If you can't, you'll find a few weeks of Kegels will work wonders. Another way to locate these muscles is to try to clench them around two fingers inserted into the vagina, or around your partner's penis during intercourse.

After childbirth, long-term Kegels will be your ticket to regaining and maintaining a well-toned pelvic floor, thereby avoiding the trouble many women have with drooping pelvic structures. Your main goal during pregnancy is to train these muscles to go into release mode during birth, when your impulse may be to tense up and resist the passage of the baby's head.

There are many different variations on the Kegel, and each one has both a *contract* and a *release* phase. Be sure to practice both. Overemphasizing the contraction part of Kegel muscle exercises conditions women to tighten these muscles, when in fact giving birth requires the releasing of tight and tense perineal muscles. Here are some of the best ones in ascending order of difficulty:

Stop and start. Attempt to stop and start your urine flow four or five times as you urinate. This method of "Kegeling" is sometimes the only one that will work for beginners, since many women don't know how to flex their pelvic-floor muscles. It is a bit tricky because you need to use *only* the pelvic-floor muscles, without assistance from your thigh and lower abdominal muscles. Think of it as "winking" your vagina.

Reps. Contract and release your pelvic-floor muscles. Start with ten repetitions four times a day and work up to fifty reps four times a day. This exercise is great to squeeze in (no pun intended) during TV commercials or when someone on the phone puts you on hold.

Holding. Contract your pelvic-floor muscles for a count of five, then release. Repeat ten times. Gradually increase the length of time you keep the muscles tensed.

Super-Kegels. The longer you can hold your perineal muscles contracted, the stronger

they will be. As you begin your Kegel exercises, you will be in the 5- to 10-second range of holding time. Once you get up to 15 to 20 seconds, you are in the super-Kegel range and are getting the maximum muscle-building power.

The elevator. This exercise takes some concentration, but the results are fantastic. Your vagina is a muscular tube, with the sections arranged like rings one on top of another. Imagine each section as a different "floor" of a building, and that you are moving an elevator up and down by tensing each section, getting progressively higher. Start by slowly bringing the elevator up to the second floor and holding it for a second, then move up to the third, and so on, until you get to the fifth floor. Hold. Now bring the elevator down, floor by floor, "resting" at each floor, to the first floor (the starting point). Then make a trip to the basement, where your pelvic floor is completely relaxed. As you reach the basement, release and push your pelvic muscles down (childbirth educators call this "bulging to the basement") and hold this bearing-down position for a few seconds. This exercise will prepare you to bear down during the pushing stage of labor. (Hold on to how this feels so you'll remember it in labor.) Last, bring the elevator back up to the first floor, your normal state of vaginal tension (the muscles are naturally somewhat contracted without your realizing it). Try to work up to ten elevator rides per session and four sessions a day.

The wave. Some of the pelvic-floor muscles are arranged in a sort of extended figure-eight pattern (like an eight with three loops instead of two). One loop is around your urethra, one around your vagina, and one around your anus. Contract these mus-

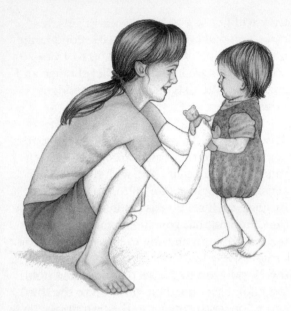

Squatting.

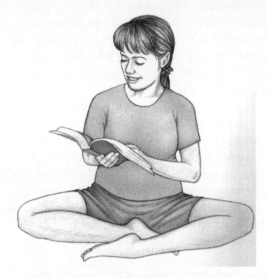

Tailor sitting.

cles from front to back, and release them from back to front.

Positioning. Once you become proficient at Kegel exercises, try them in a variety of positions — lying down, sitting up, squatting, tailor sitting, and on all fours.

Stretching Exercises

You'll have no idea what position will be the most comfortable to deliver in until the time comes, so you'd be wise to make sure that all your birthing muscles are primed and ready to go. Historically, women left to their own devices have used positions that allow gravity to help — squatting or sitting semi-upright with legs apart. Stretching exercises prepare your thigh and pelvic muscles and ligaments for the best birthing positions. But no matter what position you end up giving birth in, spending time in these poses before the big day will help prepare your body by toning the perineal area, stretching ligaments,

strengthening inner thigh and abdominal muscles, and promoting proper body alignment.

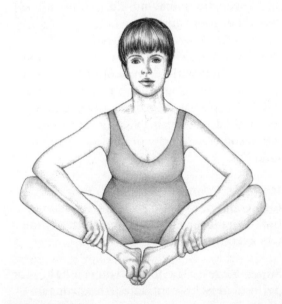

Tailor stretching.

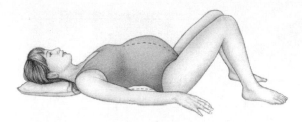

Pelvic tilt position — lying down.

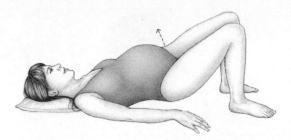

Pelvic rock.

Squatting. Squatting is hard work for most of us, unaccustomed as we are to doing it. Squat for one minute, ten times a day, with the idea of being able to squat for longer and longer periods. Squat to clean out the refrigerator. Squat to change the TV channel (and stay there for a while). Squat to fold laundry. Don't think about how silly it looks. Think about how you are strengthening your legs and conditioning your muscles for birth.

Tailor sitting. Chances are you did a lot of sitting cross-legged on the floor when you were a child. Now you may find it's not as easy as you remember, since it calls for under-used abdominal muscles to keep your back straight to maintain good posture. Nevertheless, spend ten minutes two or three times a day in this position, reading, knitting, having dinner, or doing something else that allows you to remember your posture. Gradually increase the length of time you sit.

Tailor stretching. In this variation of tailor sitting, with your back against a wall (or against the front of a sofa) uncross your legs and put your feet together sole to sole. Then see how far apart you can get your knees. Don't worry — only the most limber women can get their knees all the way to the floor. But you should be able over a few weeks to improve your flexibility by using your hands

and arms to lightly move your knees, one at a time, downward. Don't force them, especially if you have a history of knee problems.

Shoulder rotation. Take the time at the end of a tailor stretch to do a few shoulder circles, bringing your shoulders forward and up, as if to touch your ears, and back around and down. Keep your arms relaxed. The shoulder and neck muscles you stretch with this exercise are ones that easily get overtensed in labor (and when nursing a newborn).

The pelvic tilt. In addition to helping prepare your body for birth, the pelvic tilt is great for alleviating pressure on your lower back during pregnancy. It can be done sitting, standing, on all fours, or in the leapfrog position. In each case, keep your lower back completely flat while you "scrunch in" your abdominal muscles and pull your rear end under you (as discussed in "Pregnancy and Posture," page 181).

When doing the tilt on all fours, take special care not to sway your back. As you inhale, tuck your buttocks under you and hold for three seconds. As you exhale, return to the relaxed, flat-back position. Repeat fifty times, four times a day — more if you have a backache. Some women do their pelvic-floor exercises simultaneously. You might also want to use this position to do a type of

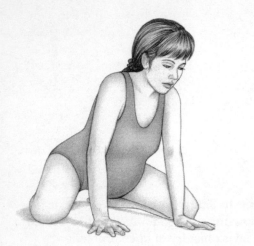

Leapfrog.

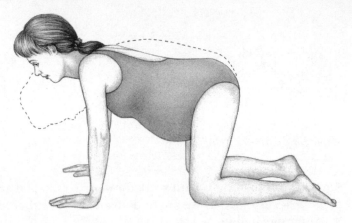

Knees to chest.

pelvic rock in which you rotate your hips around like a belly dancer (some women say this movement reminds them of using a hula hoop) to relieve back pain and develop greater flexibility.

When using the leapfrog position, more of your weight will be back on your legs than forward on your arms. Your knees should be far apart (but not so far as to make you uncomfortable). Do the tilt ten times in this position.

To do the exercise standing, refer to "Pregnancy and Posture," below. Standing correctly, lean your back as flat against a wall as possible (your feet will have to be about 4 inches away from the wall). As you do the tilt, push your lower back "into" the wall (you may have to raise your chest a little to do this). Hold for five seconds; repeat three times or more.

The pelvic tilt can also be done lying on your back, but only if you're in your first trimester. After the fourth month of pregnancy, exercising on your back can be unhealthy for your baby, as the weight of your

uterus in this position could press on the major blood vessels that lie alongside your spine. Lying on your back, bend your knees, keeping your feet flat on the ground. Prop

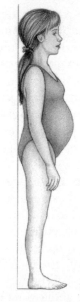

Stand straight.

Don't Sit Still!

It is neither safe nor comfortable for the pregnant body to be stationary too long. Especially in the last three months, when your lower-body circulation is sluggish anyway, sitting still for even a relatively short period can cause your ankles to swell and the veins in your lower legs to expand. Sluggish circulation combined with dangling legs increases the risk of thrombophlebitis (inflammation of the veins), a condition to which pregnant women are predisposed.

To decrease swelling and increase your comfort, try these simple suggestions. While sitting, change position frequently, shifting most of your weight back and forth or from side to side, like a squirmy toddler. Try these exercises, too: flex your feet up and down, point and wiggle your toes, make circles with your legs and feet, lift and kick each leg individually. (Similar exercises with your arms and hands can improve circulation in your upper extremities: stretch your fingers, make fists, raise your arms and hands, and shrug your shoulders.) Stand up at least every two hours and take a nice long walk to the bathroom, around the block, or even just up and down a set of stairs. If you are traveling by plane or train, take a stroll down the aisle at least every hour. If you are traveling by car, stop frequently to stretch and walk around.

your head up a bit (a throw pillow works well). Take a deep breath; then, as you exhale, push your lower back against the floor. After a few repetitions, try the tilt with the pelvic rock (described above) by elevating your hips slightly and rotating them in a circle. You might also want to do the "buttocks curl," in which you first do the pelvic tilt, then gradually bring your knees up toward your chest and hold for three seconds before putting your feet back on the floor.

The knee-chest stretch. This position is terrific for relieving lower back pain and is one of the positions favored by laboring mothers. Assume an all-fours position on hands and knees, then gently lower your weight onto your elbows and forearms, supported by a pillow or two. Now lower your head, cradling it within your forearms. Keep your hips up, directly over your knees and supported by your stomach muscles. Practice staying in this position for five minutes at a stretch.

Pregnancy and Posture

If, despite your mother's admonitions, you've never quite learned to stand up straight or sit without hunching over, now might be a good time to heed her advice. Before you dismiss posture as one of those pregnancy niceties you don't have the time or energy for, remember that the loosened ligaments, added weight, and new proportions of the pregnant body can lead to back discomfort, hard-to-break habits like a swayback posture, and even injury if you do not learn correct muscular support. For best results, start early in pregnancy to give your muscles time to catch up to your growing body. Note that good pregnancy posture is the same as good basic posture for the nonpregnant person.

Stand straight. Keep your chin level with the ground. (Imagine a string attached to the middle of the top of your head is being pulled upward toward the ceiling.) Some women, out of habit or to minimize a double chin, jut their chins upward; others tend to turn their gaze downward. Either extreme throws off your balance. Next, check your shoulders to be sure they are dropped naturally. Throwing your shoulder blades too far back strains your lower back. (You will notice that if your head is positioned properly, your shoulders will automatically drop into the correct, relaxed position.) Continue down your body to your abdomen, which should be gently pulled in, not pooched out with your back swayed. Your buttocks should also be pulled in, as if you were tucking a tail between your legs. This posture gives your pelvis the correct tilt and shifts your weight so that your center of gravity is directly over your hips. Practice this posture against a wall, feet 6 inches out, pulling and tucking so that the small of your back is flat against the wall. Now for the legs: don't lock your knees, which can put yet another strain on your lower back. Instead, stand with your feet about shoulder-width apart and flex your knees just a bit to let your thighs support more of your body weight. Also, make sure your weight is spread out over your entire foot, not just your heels. Though this posture may feel awkward at first, remind yourself to use it as much as possible. After a while it will become second nature. (By the way, most women find it difficult to achieve correct posture in high heels; in later pregnancy it's practically impossible; see page 195 for footwear guidelines.)

Standing for too long when pregnant can impede proper circulation and cause uncomfortable swelling of the ankles and feet. If you must be upright and stationary, rest one foot on a low stool for a time, then switch. And keep your blood flowing by moving your calf muscles; stand on your toes every now and then, or lift one foot off the ground in order to do foot exercises: rotate your foot around in full circles clockwise and counterclockwise, using your ankle as the pivot point. If you have a job that requires you to stand throughout most of your workday, ask for a transfer to a position that requires less time on your feet. Studies show that women with stand-up jobs throughout their pregnancy are more likely to deliver smaller babies. (See also how to care for your feet, page 195, and prevent backache, page 260.)

Sit smart. Choose a hard, straight-backed chair. Position a throw pillow behind your lower back if you need additional support. Many women find using a footstool takes further pressure off the lower back. If you do not have a footstool, at least make sure your chair is low enough for you to place both your feet squarely on the floor. Under no circumstances do you want to cross your legs; this common habit contributes to poor circulation and promotes varicose veins. To increase circulation when sitting, do the foot exercises mentioned above. If you work in an office where you must sit most of the day, make sure you get up and walk around for a few minutes at least once every half hour. Keep a low stool, or even a stack of books, under your desk to elevate your feet.

If you must sit in a car for any length of time, get as much leg room as you can so you can have your legs less bent and your feet supported. Use a small pillow to maximize support of your lower back, and be sure to flex your calf muscles regularly. Get out and stretch as often as you feel the need.

Sleep right. Your body will normally let you know what is the most comfortable sleeping position. Standard pregnancy advice is that after the fourth month, sleeping on your back should be avoided, since lying on your back puts the whole weight of your uterus on the major blood vessels that lie to the right of your spine. Since some women find themselves unable to sleep on their left side, the advice to avoid both back- and right-side lying is distressing for them. There is a theoretical advantage to sleeping on your left side, as it enhances circulation to the placenta. For women with placental problems, the advice to sleep on their left side only is of utmost importance. But for some women, sleeping on the left side aggravates regurgitation and resulting heartburn. Most women move around during the course of the night and probably whatever position is comfortable for you is all right. Realistically, by the time you should not be sleeping on your stomach, you will find it is very uncomfortable to sleep on your stomach; and by the time you should not be sleeping on your back, you will find it is very uncomfortable to sleep on your back.

Don't forget to use care when getting out of bed. Roll onto your side and use your arms to slowly push yourself up to a sitting position, and then put your legs over the side of the bed. Plant your feet firmly on the ground, then use your arms to push yourself into a standing position. These precautions may sound silly, but your back and abdominal muscles are resting as you sleep and may need "warming up" before you can depend on them as you would during the day.

Shift slowly. When shifting from standing to sitting, lower yourself gently. Extend your arms behind you, bend your knees, and let your thighs do most of the work. Resist the temptation to simply fall into a chair. While it certainly won't hurt the baby, it could, in later months, cause you to strain some already

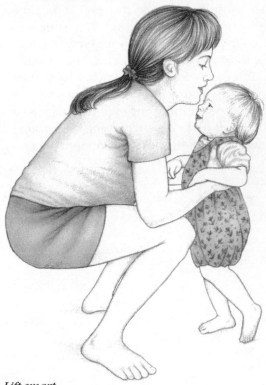

Lift smart.

loose ligaments. To stand from sitting, once again make the most of your leg muscles. With your feet well under you, push up from your calves. Take care not to jerk yourself forward; it may be faster, but it can wreak havoc on your lower back. In fact, any kind of movement while pregnant is best done a bit more deliberately than you're used to.

When walking, wear sensible shoes that evenly distribute your weight. Remember the elements of good standing posture, and watch where you are going. Your ankles, knees, and hips are looser than they were before you got pregnant and may not be as able to compensate if you lose your balance. They may also not be as resilient if you fall.

The principles are the same for lifting. Bring yourself down to the level of the object being lifted; don't bend over from your waist. Hold the object close to your body, making the most of your arm muscles. Then, using your leg muscles more than your back, stand up. One way to tell if you're lifting properly is to note whether your back is straight as you lift. If it's bent, you're using the wrong muscles. Do not, under any circumstances, strain to lift something heavy (women have different fitness levels, but probably anything over 35 pounds is too heavy); you could do serious damage to your back and abdominal muscles.

If you experience any discomfort as a result of or when engaging in any physical activity, tell your doctor or midwife. He or she may recommend rest, physical therapy, or chiropractic care.

THE FOURTH MONTH

❖ ❖ ❖

Emotionally I feel: _____

_____

_____

_____

Physically I feel: _____

_____

_____

_____

My thoughts about you: _____

_____

_____

My dreams about you: _____

_____

_____

What I imagine you look like: _____

_____

_____

_____

My favorite exercises: _____

_____

_____

My top concerns: _____

_____

_____

_____

My best joys: _____

_____

_____

My worst problems: _____

_____

_____

VISIT TO MY HEALTH-CARE PROVIDER

Questions I had; answers I got: _____
_____
_____
_____
_____

Tests and results; my reaction: _____
_____
_____
_____
_____
_____

Updated due date: _____
My weight: _____
My blood pressure: _____
Feeling my uterus; my reaction: _____
_____
_____
_____
_____
_____
_____

How I feel now that I am starting to show: _____
_____
_____
_____
_____
_____
_____
_____

photo at four months

Comments: _____

_____

_____

_____

_____

_____

_____

_____

_____

_____

_____

_____

_____

_____

_____

Fifth-Month Visit to Your Health-Care Provider (17–20 weeks)

During this month's visit you may have:

- examination of the size and height of the uterus
- examination of your abdomen to feel the top of the uterus
- examination of your breasts and skin
- examination for swelling of hands, legs, and enlargement of veins
- weight and blood-pressure check
- urinalysis to test for infection, sugar, and protein
- an opportunity to hear baby's heartbeat
- an opportunity to see baby on ultrasound, if indicated
- an assessment of fetal activity — how often your baby moves and what it feels like
- an opportunity to discuss your feelings and concerns

The Fifth Month —
Obviously Pregnant

MANY WOMEN FEEL THIS MONTH OF PREGNANCY — from the seventeenth week through the twentieth — is one of the most rewarding. You're probably feeling pretty good, and it's now obvious to the whole world that you're growing a baby. Anyone who was still wondering "Is she or isn't she?" now knows for sure. Expect to be on the receiving end of the perks of being pregnant as well as the unwanted advice. You go public in your lead role in the most awesome drama of life. Better yet, you can now probably feel your little co-star moving. And this month you reach a milestone in your pregnancy — believe it or not, you are halfway there!

HOW YOU MAY FEEL EMOTIONALLY

At the beginning of your pregnancy, your endocrine system worked feverishly to make the hormones your uterus and baby needed to grow. Around halfway through your pregnancy, your placenta takes over the production of most of these hormones. This explains why you feel better physically: placental hor-

mone-production does not have as many side effects for mother as maternal hormone-production does. Nevertheless, you are still likely to find that your emotions are more intense than before you were pregnant. Many moms-to-be are surprised at how easily they weep — even a McDonald's commercial can make them cry. Luckily, month five typically is filled with many good feelings, or at least less ambivalence.

Special. Now that it's obvious to the world that you are growing a baby, you can enjoy the perks that may come with your status. The clerk at the supermarket may offer to help you load your groceries into the car. Passersby may glance your way with admiration. It's pretty heady stuff to be letting the whole world in on your own personal miracle. And, it may seem to you that you've gone up a few notches in the eyes of many people whose respect, admiration, awe, and tenderness suggest they know you are doing the most important job in the world — growing a baby.

I'm enjoying this stage so much, feeling so queenly and elegant with my new maternal profile. The biggest boost comes from my husband, who doesn't miss a day of coming

189

up and putting his hands on my belly and telling me how beautiful I am to him.

Awestruck. Last month, hearing the swoosh of baby's heartbeat and perhaps also seeing the tiny body on the ultrasound screen were reassuring signs that there really is a baby inside you. Now finally you feel baby move — unquestionable proof that you really are going to be a mother.

I remember the first time I felt my baby really move — I had a visceral reaction: there's someone in there! Even though I'd known intellectually that I was pregnant, feeling such clear evidence of another person's presence was a thrilling shock.

Wanting to stay in your nest. The nesting instinct, so much a part of the folklore of later pregnancy (see page 254), often shows itself for the first time around the fifth month. Along with a spurt of energy, you may have a sudden urge to clean house, even going to extremes you've never tackled before (wall washing, anyone?). The desire to prepare your nest will grow stronger over the next few months.

You may also find your social life beginning to change. Once you see, hear, and feel the life inside you, your nesting instinct might just urge you to retreat into the comfort of your home and the company of a few favorite people. While many women find that keeping busy helps them get through their pregnancy, even the busiest pregnant woman will have times when she yearns to be among familiar things and people. Even if you are usually outgoing, you may now prefer to keep to your nest, like a brooding hen.

People keep telling me, "Go out now while you can to a movie or dinner. Once the baby's born, you'll be stuck at home." But I just feel like staying at home these days.

Introspective. Just as your body is focused on nourishing a new life, your mind may become preoccupied with the little person you share space with. You may want to be alone to meditate or just think about your baby. You will probably enjoy long periods of doing nothing more than feeling baby's kicks. You might zone out into motherly thoughts and baby imaginings at inappropriate times, such as in the middle of a conversation or during a meeting. These mental digressions are normal and necessary, as they help you prepare for the reality of being somebody's mother.

Mentally fuzzy. Martha has laughed with many women over "mommy brain" — you can't quite get a fix on what you want to say; you fight harder for simple vocabulary sometimes; you can be forgetful or "spacey." If you don't know about this phenomenon beforehand, it can be quite alarming, especially if you aren't sure you will get your old brain back later (you will, although mental fuzziness extends well into the postpartum period). If you do know about it, you can make allowances for it, even laugh at it. These momentary memory lapses rarely interfere with a pregnant woman's ability to carry on her job. Mothers-to-be in positions of responsibility manage to compensate for this problem quite well.

Overwhelmed with advice. The whole world wants to help you grow your baby. Seeing a pregnant woman seems to bring out the busybody in everyone. (Wait till you have a new baby — it gets even worse!) At times you may enjoy the extra attention; at other times you may find it disturbing, especially when the conversations dwell on the what-if and the "what-went-wrong-with-my-cousin-Faye." Be ready with a few quick retorts that silence your advisers, such as, "Thanks, I'll think about it." Or use your doctor as a scapegoat: "My doctor says . . ." Your already touchy emotions will probably make you hypersensitive to even well-meaning suggestions that somehow there's more you should be doing for your health or the health of your baby. As irritating as these unwanted commentaries are, they are but a pale prelude to all the critical mothering advice that you can count on later. This is a good time to learn to ignore unhelpful advice and become more discerning about whose opinion you value.

Panicky. For unknown reasons anytime during pregnancy, and especially during the middle trimester, some women have panic attacks: they gasp for air, have difficulty breathing, experience a fast heartbeat (palpitations), and feel like their chest is closing up. An attack may awaken you in the middle of the night. If one of these comes on, check into relaxation mode, and convince yourself, "I'm OK." These episodes pass quickly, reassuring you there's really nothing to panic about.

HOW YOU MAY FEEL PHYSICALLY

As in the fourth month, both you and your baby grow rapidly during month five. You will probably gain around 5 pounds, and your baby's weight will nearly double. Naturally, you will feel these physical changes. Referring to their abdomen and breasts, women during this month often exclaim: "All of a sudden I've popped out."

Showing more. Many factors go into how early and how much you show: your body type, your weight gain, the size of your baby, how many babies you are carrying, the position of your uterus (see figure, page 117), and whether this is your first or a subsequent pregnancy. Much of your look while carrying a baby reflects the body type you inherited from your mother and father. Tall, slim women tend to show later and higher; short and wide women tend to show earlier and lower. Long-waisted women have more room for the uterus to grow up before it has to grow out, so they tend to show later. By the end of this month, however, no matter what your body type, you will no longer be the recipient of those doubting "is she pregnant or is she getting fat?" looks. Even in the fifth month a few mothers will still try in vain to squeeze into their previous size 8 dress. Most will begin to flaunt their showing body and take on a proud and pregnant pose.

Itchy and sensitive belly. Stretching skin itches. That is a dermatological fact. Massage a soothing emollient into the itchy areas. Beginning in the second half of your pregnancy, you may not want to wear anything that binds your belly, and you may not wish to lie on your stomach, as you begin to embrace your bulge lovingly and cherish the person inside.

Navel discomforts. Around twenty weeks your expanding uterus presses outward beneath your belly button. It may hurt slightly when you walk. You may now experience occasional minor discomforts in the area beneath your navel, and the navel itself may suddenly pop and become an "outie." (It will return to normal after delivery.)

Breast changes. Your nipples may be more sensitive than ever, especially when you are

Feeling First Kicks

Those first kicks you've been longing for are coming! When you feel them and what they feel like varies from mother to mother and from day to day.

When. Your baby has been stirring since the end of the second month, but the fetal movements have been too faint and the baby too small for you to feel them. But by eighteen weeks, baby's arms and legs can reach out and touch the wall of the uterus. Most mothers will first feel these movements — called "quickening" — sometime during the fifth month of their pregnancy (between the eighteenth and twenty-second week). A few moms may feel their babies move earlier than the eighteenth week, some not until the twenty-fourth. A veteran mother is likely to feel first kicks earlier, since her uterine muscles and her memory are primed. Thin women may experience fetal movements earlier and more distinctly than well-padded mothers. If your baby's movements come earlier or later than expected, your practitioner may wish to reevaluate your due date.

When the kicks begin, only you can feel them. They are too gentle to be shared, a delicious secret for you alone. Usually by twenty-four weeks, anyone else can share the excitement with you. (Some dads refer to their first feels as the "kickoff.") From here on in, each little kick will add a little more cement to the mother-baby bond.

What you may feel. Don't expect to feel the hard thumps right away. First kicks are not nearly so distinct and obvious. After all, a ½-pound baby with 2-inch limbs doesn't pack much of a punch. Your first suspicions may be wishful imaginings, easily confused with gut rumblings. Then the flutters come more frequently and feel like nothing you've ever felt before. These first movements are so miniature and so precious. The sensation will be unique to you and often indescribable to anyone else. Mothers use words like "flutters," "bumps," "flicks," "twitches," "bubbles," and "little nudges."

When I lay on the beach with "the bulge" pressed into a hollow in the sand, I first became aware of the little movements inside.

Baby's kicks gradually strengthen from flicks to pokes to punches over the next two months. As those little limbs grow and become more muscular and the womb becomes more crowded, the frequency and intensity of these jabs increase. Late in pregnancy, the kicks will be strong enough to wake you up.

How often. The frequency of kicking increases steadily each month, reaching its peak during the seventh month; the frequency diminishes then, but the intensity increases during the last two months. In the twentieth week, the amount of kicking a baby does is extremely

lying on them during sleep or when they rub against your clothing. You may also notice leaking colostrum, a golden yellow substance that is the first milk for your newborn.

variable, ranging anywhere from fifty to a thousand kicks in twenty-four hours, with the average being two hundred in twenty-four hours. You are most likely to feel your baby move when you are resting. (In the next month you'll even be able to see the movements.) Studies show that babies in the womb move the most between the hours of 8:00 P.M. and 8:00 A.M.; during the day they are lulled to sleep by mother's movements. Also, in the beginning when you are busy or preoccupied, you may not notice many kicks. But next month little thumper will catch you by surprise even during busy times, as if to say, "Stop what you're doing and pay attention to me."

I started to feel him moving. It felt like butterflies flitting in my abdomen. I was so excited. My husband felt him soon after that. Since then I have felt him every day. I love to put my hands on my belly and feel him kicking. I can't wait to get bigger and bigger because I know the more I grow, the more strongly I will feel the baby kicking. It's one of my favorite parts of being pregnant.

While the movements of most babies are unaffected by what their mothers eat, some mothers report baby moves more within a half hour of a high-glucose (sugar) meal or snack or after a glass of orange juice. Some mothers notice their babies kick more within an hour of drinking a caffeine-containing beverage. Perhaps they woke their baby up.

My friend said, "Cola will get 'em moving every time."

Where. In months five and six, kicks occur randomly, anywhere in your abdomen. There's still plenty of room for baby to turn around in the womb. In late pregnancy, if your baby is head down (as most are), you will probably feel jabs most often toward the center or in your ribs to the right; most babies settle in with their backs to your left. Some mothers can best feel their baby's feet under their right rib cage while lying on their left side. Some rarely feel rib-cage kicks, but instead feel kicks a lot lower, side and front. As an added show, you may begin to feel baby's hiccups, which sometimes feel stronger than baby's kicks.

Record in your journal those situations that bring out your baby's kicks and explain what makes them easier to feel each month. These kick stories will prove to be some of your favorite pregnancy memories (like when the bowl of ice cream you're resting on your abdomen jumps around all by itself). Later, it's fun to compare these prenatal behaviors with what you see baby doing outside the womb.

In the previous months there were plenty of signs to tell you that you were pregnant — a positive pregnancy test, hormonal havoc, hearing baby's heartbeat, and seeing baby on ultrasound — but none so strongly convinces you of the reality of motherhood as feeling your baby move.

Cramping. As early as the fifth month, some women, especially those in their second or a subsequent pregnancy, experience abdominal discomfort similar to, but less intense than, menstrual cramps. These itty-bitty contractions are a prelude to warm-up contractions

Bringing Out Flat Nipples

Flat or inverted nipples can make the early days of breastfeeding more challenging. If you're worried about nipples that seem flat, or even inverted, consult a lactation specialist or call a La Leche League leader. She can help you determine what to do. Most women do not have to worry about nipples that seem flat before birth. After birth, a breast pump, in addition to baby's sucking, can help bring them out. If necessary, wearing breast shells (plastic cups that fit inside your bra) for several hours a day during the last three months of pregnancy can help draw out nipples that are truly inverted, making the early days of breastfeeding easier.

that are more frequent and more noticeable during the third trimester (see "Braxton Hicks Contractions," page 223).

Round-ligament pain. The tissue surrounding and supporting your uterus has more work to do now that your uterus is bigger and heavier. This brings new physical sensations. Large ligaments, called "round ligaments," on each side of your uterus attach your uterus to your pelvis. Round ligaments must stretch as your uterus grows. This slow and steady stretching does not itself cause discomfort, but stretching with normal activity can send shooting pains that catch you by surprise and stop you in your tracks. The most common offender is a sudden change of position. When you twist or get out of bed in the morning, for example, round-ligament strain can cause a gripping pain along one or

both sides of your lower abdomen or even toward your back. While not harmful to baby, this pain can sometimes be excruciating for you. Some women report this ligament pain from exercise, even from walking. Round-ligament pain is usually sharpest and most uncomfortable between fourteen and twenty weeks, when the uterus is big enough to exert pressure on the ligaments and not yet big enough to rest some of its weight on the pelvic bones. Women can experience round-ligament pain anytime during pregnancy, depending on how they are carrying baby, especially in the final month, when baby's head is pressing downward.

To prevent or lessen round-ligament pain, try leg-lift exercises, as described on page 116. Avoid sudden changes of position, especially from sitting to standing and when getting out of bed. Try lying down on your side, either on the side with the pain or on the opposite one — whichever brings you more relief. If you need more relief, try a hot water bottle. Round-ligament pain tends to subside quickly with rest and usually lessens as your pregnancy progresses and the ligaments adapt to uterine growth.

Changes in your vision and eye moisture. Pregnancy and the hormones that run it affect every organ in your body, and the eyes are no exception. Sometime during the second trimester, many women find their vision changes, usually for the worse. The increased fluid retention throughout your body actually changes the shape of your eyeballs, and with it your vision. Some women become more farsighted, some more nearsighted, during pregnancy. You may feel you need a change in the prescription of your glasses, or your contact lenses may become uncomfortable, as if they no longer fit. After delivery, as your whole body regains its shape, so will your eyeballs, and your previous vision should return. If you find three or four months of hazier vision intolerable, see an eye doctor about changing your glasses or your contacts, or consider wearing glasses if you haven't before.

Another cause of vision changes in pregnancy is the drop in estrogen, which decreases the moisture available to your eyes (dry eye syndrome) and can lead to blurred vision, sensitivity to light, and red, burning eyes. A severe form of dry eye can cause damage to the cornea. The only treatment for dry eye is to use one of the over-the-counter "artificial tears" products to restore moisture to the eyes. Don't confuse these with eyedrops for bloodshot eyes. You may not be able to wear your contact lenses at all, and you should use sunglasses to protect your vulnerable eyes in the sunlight.

While slight and gradual visual changes are normal and only a temporary nuisance of pregnancy, sudden, drastic changes may signal a serious problem, such as high blood pressure. Notify your practitioner immediately if you experience severely blurred vision, blind spots, increasing dimness in your vision, or double vision.

Foot changes. If you feel your feet are getting larger and heavier as your abdomen does, you are right. That's because fluid collects in your ankles and feet, especially after a day of standing. Feet also feel the effects of the normal ligament loosening that develops throughout your body, causing weight-bearing joints to stretch and widen and arches to fall. The extra body fat you are accumulating doesn't help any either. Put all these changes into a shoe, and it's no wonder that it no longer fits. Most women require at least a half-size-larger shoe in the second half of

their pregnancy, and around 15 percent of moms permanently require footwear at least a half-size larger. Try these ways to be kind to your feet:

- Elevate them as much as possible.
- Avoid standing for long periods without a break.
- Do foot exercises: flex your toes and then pull them toward you as you point the heel away from you. Extend your leg, point your toes up, and make a circle with your toes, rotating your whole foot and ankle. This is also good for exercising the calf muscles (see page 181) after you've been standing or sitting for a long time.
- Get a foot massage: the masseur holds the aching foot in both hands, places his or her thumb just under the ball of the foot, and moves along the arch, massaging in slow circular strokes.
- Nurse swollen, painful, day's-end feet in cool water.
- Wear cotton socks to allow your feet to breathe.
- Wear proper footwear. Choose shoes with wide, low heels (no higher than 2 inches) or wedges. Nonskid soles make you more surefooted. Try soft leather or canvas shoes, preferably without laces, since sooner or later you won't be able to bend over to tie them. Shop for new shoes at the end of the day, when your feet are most swollen. Unless you are very knowledgeable about shoes, ask a salesperson's advice on proper fit: too tight, and your feet will hurt; too loose, and you won't be able to walk safely in them. Be sure the front of your shoes is wide enough to allow your toes to fan out comfortably. Remember, pregnancy relaxes all of your ligaments; your feet and ankle ligaments are no excep-

tion. Be sure your shoes support your feet, even if you have to sacrifice looks for support. If loose ligaments are causing your ankles to roll, you may have to stick to shoes that lace up (versus slip-ons), since the open areas on the top decrease overall support. Pregnancy is not a good time to sprain an ankle.

If your arches are painful at the end of the day, take it as a signal to stay off your feet more or try orthotic inserts — plastic arch supports that fit into your shoes. These are available at most shoe stores and pharmacies or can be custom-molded by a podiatrist. If you had flat feet prior to pregnancy, they are likely to feel even flatter in the coming months; this might be a good time to treat your feet to proper-fitting orthotic inserts.

My feet took a real beating during pregnancy. My increasing weight and the stresses of chasing and often carrying a toddler produced heel pain and other foot discomfort. As long as I wore my sturdy running shoes with the well-padded heel, it was bearable, but a Sunday morning in pumps guaranteed the afternoon and evening would have to be spent in very sensible shoes. And there was no going barefoot that summer. My feet needed constant protection.

HOW YOUR BABY IS GROWING (17–20 WEEKS)

By the end of this month you can feel your cantaloupe-size uterus at the level of your navel; baby weighs around ¾ pound and measures between 8 and 10 inches long — about half the length baby will be at birth. Baby's legs, now around the size of your little finger, continue growing, become more muscular, and make their presence felt as tiny flutter kicks. He waves his growing but still tiny arms and may be seen on ultrasound sucking his thumb or making a fist. First baby hair is beginning to appear on his upper lip, eyebrows, and head. His skin, previously thin and transparent, now begins to accumulate fat deposits. Baby's oil glands start to secrete a waxy substance that mixes with his dead skin cells to form a cheesy coating, called the "vernix caseosa," which acts like a sort of wet suit protecting the little swimmer's skin from chapping. Fine, temporary hair — called "lanugo" (meaning "wool") — covers most of his body and helps to hold the vernix on the skin. Baby's digestive system functions better

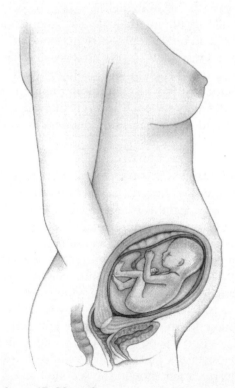

Baby at 17–20 weeks.

now, and he regularly swallows amniotic fluid and urinates into it. By this month, baby's middle ear structures have formed, enabling baby to hear sound. The main reason your baby cannot yet survive outside the womb at this stage is that his lungs are still undeveloped.

CONCERNS YOU MAY HAVE

Now that you are bigger, you may have a whole host of new fears. Feeling the baby move and perhaps seeing the clear evidence of baby's presence tend to make mothers acutely aware of the little life they're protecting. With this awareness comes new, and very real, concerns. How will you be physically able to handle everything — job, home, older children? How will you be able to stretch yourself emotionally? How will your relationship with your mate change now that you are so preoccupied with your pregnancy? What about the baby? The fear of bearing a deformed baby crops up now and then. Here is a look at the most common concerns women have during the middle trimester.

Falling

In the first trimester, your baby is shielded by a thick, muscular uterus and an even more protective pelvic bone, so it is nearly impossible to injure her if you trip and fall. By the fifth month, however, your uterus grows beyond the protective shell of your pelvic bone. While the chances of injury from a simple fall are still very unlikely, you will naturally worry more. And there *are* reasons that you are now more prone to falling. If your expanding breasts don't yet obstruct your view of your feet, your abdomen soon will, and so you can't always look down to see where you are stepping. Since your body is changing rapidly, your balance will not be as secure or as graceful as it used to be. In the months to come, you will become not only less graceful but also less agile.

There is no need to worry unduly about minor falls. Your baby is well protected by the natural shock absorbers of your abdominal muscles, uterine muscles, fetal membranes, and the amniotic fluid, all of which cushion any outside blows. It would take an accident that seriously injures mommy to have even a remote chance of injuring baby. To see how well your baby is protected by the amniotic fluid in the amniotic sac, fill a mayonnaise jar with water, place an egg in it, shake it up, and see how well protected the egg is. And amniotic fluid is actually even thicker and more protective than water.

While baby is unlikely to be hurt by a fall, you may be. A sprained ankle or twisted knee is no cake walk without painkillers and might necessitate X rays or other medical interventions you would rather avoid. And walking on crutches while you are pregnant is a real bummer. So, for your own safety, be extra-cautious when navigating unfamiliar or hazardous terrain. Take special care when walking on ice or along unfamiliar paths or sidewalks and sidestep toys on the playroom floor. Hold on to railings when going up and down stairs and plant your whole foot firmly on each step. Realize the natural limitations that your new body imposes.

Deformities

It is inevitable that you will be afraid that your baby will be imperfect; that's why moms and dads count fingers and toes with such delight right after birth. Minor imperfections like birthmarks, skin tags, or an oddly shaped head (it will look nice and round in a day or two) often alarm new parents the day of birth. Major deformities, such as clubfeet, cleft palate, heart defects, and digestive abnormalities, are possible, but they are extremely rare. Firmly tell yourself to stop worrying. Nothing is gained by borrowing trouble, as our grandmothers used to say. Medical science is so advanced that it can correct or alleviate most infant problems. If you can't stop obsessing to the extent that it disturbs your ability to be a wife and enjoy your pregnancy, seek professional help.

Driving and Auto Accidents

Now that there are two people in the driver's seat, you may worry about driving. You may even worry more about car travel in general. As mentioned above, your baby is well protected by your body; just be sure your body is well protected in your car. Remember, you are driving under the influence of pregnancy hormones, which may make you prone to fatigue, diminished concentration, or falling asleep at the wheel. If you are prone to dizzy spells (see page 160), you may want to leave the driving to someone else. If possible, drive at off-peak traffic hours and at times of the day when your mind is most alert. Keep trips short. *Above all, wear your seat belt.* You don't want to go flying forward in an accident. (See "Safe and Comfortable Car Travel," page 232.) Not only would your baby come between you and the wheel, the extra weight of your baby would greatly increase the force with which you would be propelled forward. You have a much greater chance of getting hurt if you are not properly buckled up.

Infants in the womb are rarely injured during car accidents. They are well protected by the muscle of the uterus and the amniotic fluid. The main risk to baby during a high-impact accident is separation of the placenta from the uterine wall. Following such an accident, signs of possible danger to your baby, which warrant immediate medical attention, are vaginal bleeding; leaking of amniotic fluid; severe pain or tenderness in your abdomen, uterus, or pelvis; onset of contractions; or a change in the amount and characteristics of fetal movements. In the event of an automobile accident, contact your doctor. Your health-care provider will often do an exam, mainly for reassurance, which may include a monitored tracing of baby's heartbeat, palpation of your abdomen, and possibly even an ultrasound.

Most women, by taking extra precautions for the extra "passenger," can drive quite safely throughout their pregnancy.

Coping With and Involving Your Children

Being pregnant while you have a toddler in tow can be both challenging and exhausting. Involving preschoolers and older children in your pregnancy is easy and often fun. There are ways to involve both age groups in the "family pregnancy" and prepare them for the facts of life with a newborn.

Show and Tell

Younger toddlers won't have a clue about a baby "growing in your tummy." Because they can't see it, they won't be able to understand much of the explanation. Even when you are in your ninth month, big as a house, your older baby won't take much notice of the bulge, except to realize that it is harder for her to sit on your lap. Arrange to be around very young babies a lot so that your older baby will hear how they sound, see what they look like, observe you holding one now and then, notice that they need comforting, and learn about nursing. Once your belly is really big (around 8 months), talk about the new baby, letting your child know the new baby will belong to her, too: "Susie's new baby." Let her feel the baby's kicks, and help her talk and sing to baby and encourage her to stroke your belly. Show her simple children's books about new babies. Show her pictures of when she was a tiny baby and tell her about all the things you did for her. Say things like, "Mommies hold tiny babies a *lot* because they need that."

Once a toddler is older, closer to two years, most families elect to let him in on the big news much sooner. As a general guideline, the older the child, the sooner you can tell him; very young children may be confused or disappointed when the baby fails to arrive the next day. With an older toddler or preschooler, try all of the suggestions above, and, in addition, use the diagrams in this book to talk about how the baby is growing, month by month. You'll be surprised by questions like, "What part did baby grow today, Mom?" Depending on the age and level of understanding, tell your child why you are feeling so tired, grouchy, short-fused, impatient, or whatever else you are feeling: "Baby needs a lot of energy to grow, and that's why Mom is tired and sleeps a lot" or "The hormones baby needs to grow make Mommy feel funny." Show your child pictures of what the baby looks like inside, especially once you're big enough to make the baby seem real. Expand on what newborns are like: "They cry (some cry *a lot*) and like it when you talk to them and make funny faces. They can't do anything for themselves for a long time, and they can't play games until they grow bigger. They need to be held a whole lot, just like I held you when you were little." Include them

in baby-related activities: "You can help me change the diaper, bathe baby, and dress baby."

One day four-year-old Matthew saw me lying down and asked me if I was giving the baby a rest. How neat that when he looks at me he sees baby, too.

When you are feeling grouchy, short-fused, impatient, and irritated, be sure you take care of those feelings yourself and don't let them spin out onto your family. Exercise, take a hot bath or a nap, read a book, eat a delicious, nutritious snack, go for a walk, or chat with a helping friend. Do whatever you have found helpful in the past to vent your emotions. Your toddler didn't ask for this baby; your preschooler is not supposed to take care of you. Many a crisis (money, a new job, a move, the death of a grandparent, or a problem pregnancy) has to be kept from young ones. True, it's a good lesson in life for the older children to help mommy and be sympathetic to her, but you have to strike a balance. Don't let them feel that they are bad children because they can't keep you happy.

A time to let go. Growing a baby while raising a toddler can be doubly exhausting. It's good for your toddler or preschooler to learn to be less dependent on you. Though he may be frustrated, not being the center of attention all the time helps him mature. This is called "individuating," a necessary childhood developmental stage in the normal process of going from oneness to separateness. Your child learns he can wait his turn, soothe himself when you are busy, help you with the new little person, and help you with your needs. As he moves into this next stage of development, you'll experience an important aspect of parenting — the gradual releasing of the child to whom you have been so attached. These transitions can be scary for you, so it helps to know you've given this older one what he needed when he was little. Remember, if you are anxious about letting go, your child will also be anxious.

Enough love to go around? Every mother expecting her second baby wonders how she'll ever be able to love another child the way she loves her first. She fears there could never be enough to give that much to someone new. Or, she fears that the new baby will somehow come between her and that very special toddler or preschooler. Set your mind and heart at ease about these fears. Yes, of course, you'll have enough love for your second baby (and third . . . and . . .), and you won't understand how it happens until it does. Love just seems to multiply — the more you give, the more you have.

Kids visit the doctor, too. Children close to age three should not only be able to behave well at visits to your health-care provider, they may even get a lot out of it. Take them along as often as possible. For older children already in school, include them on special visits, such as the three-month visit, when you are likely to hear baby's heartbeat, for the first time, as well as any visits that your practitioner has told you will include an ultrasound and several visits toward the end, so they'll catch the excitement and be more tuned-in. Prenatal bonding cannot be overdone for siblings old enough to understand.

Offer kids a hands-on demo. Usually by the fifth or sixth month, older children can feel their baby brother or sister move. During the times of the day or evening when your baby typically moves the most, lie down and invite your children to feel the show. Let them guess which body part they are feeling.

Encourage baby bonding. Invite your children to talk to and about the baby. If you already know the gender and have chosen a name, encourage them to use it when referring to the baby. Or, you can welcome the baby nicknames your child invents. Babies can hear at around twenty-three weeks, so this is a good time for the kids to start talking to the baby so he or she will get to know them. After about three months of this, their voices will be very familiar to the baby still in utero, and bonding will already be under way. Studies show that babies tend to turn toward voices they recognize right after birth.

Tyler sang three songs to the baby every night. After birth she recognized the songs. We enlisted his help with choosing names — suggestions only, leaving the final say to mom and dad. Tyler wanted to call his sister Hunca Munca.

Know your limits. Realize that while you're pregnant it's impossible to give other family members the same degree of attention they are used to. Sooner or later the children will realize that they must share mom with another tiny taker in the family. Fortunately, pregnancy provides you with plenty of time to prepare your older children for what life will be like after the baby arrives. Getting them used to helping you while baby brother or sister is still inside is actually another good tool for bonding. The children will have invested their time and energy even before baby comes, and the baby will have more personal value to them.

As your pregnancy progresses, and especially in the third trimester, you will naturally become more preoccupied with your pregnancy and less willing to put up with the antics of your children. This is a good time for your spouse to take over much of the child-care. Alternatively, employ a teen helper. Most teens are great with kids. They like to play and act goofy, and they work for minimum wage.

The farther I got along in my pregnancy, the less tolerant I was of what I would otherwise have regarded as normal childhood behavior. I learned to address this problem on two levels: first, I made more time for myself to rest and relax, limiting my work to what had to be done; and second, I placed limits on the behavior I no longer wanted to tolerate. When my limits were defined clearly (for myself and for my children), we were all happier.

We're in this together. If your child is included in many of the practical preparations for baby, this time of waiting can be a way of deepening your bond with him even as you help him get connected prenatally with the new baby. Picking out new toys together and buying clothes for baby ("these are just the ones baby will like") will get your child thinking of baby as a person who will have preferences. Getting out his old stuff can be nostalgic for you and reassuring for your child: "Oh, I remember you used to love this toy." Extra cuddle time is a great way to ease any guilt you may be feeling and any worry your child may be having. Try to nap together, since you both need the rest anyway. A retreat into your arms can go a long way toward settling insecurity.

Getting a Distant Dad Involved

When, if, and how much mates get involved in the pregnancy varies greatly from man to

---

Be a Positive Model for Your Children

Be positive. While you have every reason to make excuses for how you act and feel, try not to overdo it. You want your children to look upon your pregnancy as a joyful family enterprise, not as a scary time when mom is secluded in the bedroom and bathroom. Even older children can be frightened by mom's unavailability, and seeing her sick can exacerbate their natural worries about a new baby. You want your daughters especially to understand that pregnancy and childbirth are normal and not medical conditions to be treated.

I would catch myself complaining and sometimes put on a happy face even though I felt miserable. I didn't want my daughters to grow up in fear of growing a baby.

I hope to be able to convey the same attitude toward birth to my daughter that my mother conveyed to me. Since I was an older sibling, I got to watch what a joy being pregnant and giving birth were to her. So, when my daughter comes to me and asks, "What's it like?" or "Is it scary?" I will tell her that pregnancy is the most special thing her body is designed to do and to trust that design.

---

man. Some fathers-to-be focus on what they gain during the pregnancy. They become supersympathetic and superattentive from the minute their wife breaks the news, want to be deeply involved in the pregnancy, and espouse the joys of expectant fatherhood. Other dads dwell on what they've lost. In the first half of the pregnancy, they've lost their wife to day-long nausea; in the second half, they fall to number three on the priority list as their wife becomes preoccupied with the little life inside and how she herself will be as a mother. Add to these ambivalent and overwhelming feelings worries about living on a lower income (or about ever being a couple again), and you have the makings of a mixed-up mate.

Many men get excited by the changing pregnant body and marvel at the growing life inside. Others regard pregnancy as mysterious, complicated goings-on to which only women should be privy. These men seem put off by pregnancy and shy away from what they don't understand. They become even more frustrated when a pain or a problem occurs that they can't fix. Many mothers report that their husbands were very involved in the first pregnancy but less involved in subsequent pregnancies.

I kept thinking that once my abdomen started to grow, my husband would show more interest in the baby, but he still acts as if everything is the same as it was before. It's really putting a strain on our marriage, as I feel we're going in different directions. How can I get him more involved in the pregnancy?

The fact is, this pregnancy is something that is happening to *both* of you. Here are ways to help him share the joy:

Share the pregnancy. Include your significant other when talking to family and friends about the pregnancy. "We're having a baby" is a better boast than "I'm pregnant" if you want to win over a mate who is feeling left out.

Go gradually. Don't overwhelm a less-than-bubbly mate with all the decisions you have to make and the stuff you need to buy. Take baby steps instead. Talk about major decisions and lifestyle changes one issue at a time, and don't do it all within the same conversation. Examine your husband's past history of handling change. If he's the cautious type, respect this trait and give him time to warm up to these big changes.

Be positive. Try to find something to be cheerful about even when nausea and fatigue get your body down. Look at yourself. What do you reflect? What kind of pregnant person does your husband see? While some "green" days are a fact of pregnant life, weeks of complaining are bound to put off even the most sympathetic partner. Are you happy to be pregnant? If so, let your mate catch the spirit. Unfair as it seems, it might be better to unload your misery on more sympathetic female friends than to overload your husband with more problems than he can handle. It is well known that most men are slower to mature in the area of interpersonal relationships, and his behavior may at times feel incredibly unfair to you: you worry about him even when you're feeling sick, but he doesn't seem to care about what you're going through. Take heart! There's nothing that matures a man faster than becoming a father.

Make decisions together. Involve your mate in all of the important obstetrical decisions: choosing a health-care provider, childbirth class, and birth place, and all the decisions about routine (and not so routine) procedures. He loves you and your baby and wants the best for you and will probably relish the chance to do something concrete to ensure you both get proper care. Note, however, that involving him in decisions about tests and technology can be a mixed blessing. On the one hand, you may find your mate contributes valuable insight into the safety and necessity of a procedure. On the other hand, some males are enamored of the medical technology used in pregnancy and childbirth because it takes much of the mystery out of baby-growing and fits in nicely with their take-no-chances mind-set. Thus, you may find your husband nudging you into accepting more testing (and other interventions) than you want or feel you need. Be that as it may, the more involved your mate is in these decisions, the more likely he is to be involved in the rest of what's going on in your pregnancy.

Go to school together. Attend childbirth classes together. Your mate will be amazed how much there is to learn about the miracle that is taking place under the bulge. Seeing pictures and videos and getting feedback from veteran dads will open the eyes of even the most reluctant husband. With appreciation of pregnancy and birth usually comes a respect for the mother-to-be and involvement in her care.

An additional benefit to attending childbirth classes is that your husband will have the chance to share the pregnancy experience with other men. Getting together with other couples going through pregnancy can be very helpful. However, pick these couples carefully. You want men who are good role models for your mate. Avoid couples who insist on overdosing you and your spouse with their scary birth stories.

Do your homework together. Help your husband understand why you feel and act the way you do. Study together. Read this book together. He needs to know that those same hormones that make you moody support the growth and development of his future Little Leaguer.

Enjoy a photo shoot. You can really get creative and have fun with this. A series of as-you-grow portraits, artfully highlighting your blossoming belly, is a treasure well worth capturing on film. Don't let your pregnancy progress too much farther before finding the perfect piece of maternity lingerie that will both adorn and reveal. Such a picturesque opportunity is too special to pass up — and if the photographer wishes to put these pinups on a wall to admire daily, don't be surprised.

Invite hands-on care. Ask for a daily rubdown from your mate-turned-masseur. Show how much you like and need his touch. Make these sessions special with soothing music, soft lighting, and an attractive setting, such as in a room warmed by natural sunlight. Your mate may be ecstatic over what all this extra touch could lead to. But also make sure you get some thoroughly relaxing rubdowns that don't lead to excitement.

What's in it for him? As you round the halfway mark, there are bound to be days when you feel totally alive and sexier than ever. You may even feel like surprising your lover by flaunting your more generous endowments. These days are usually the exception rather than the rule, so don't waste them in front of a mirror or at a shopping mall if there's romance to catch up on.

Make him feel needed. Many men feel left out of the inner world of the expectant mother, since they believe there's really not much a man can do except drive the woman to the hospital on time. A fact he should know: women who have less stressful pregnancies are more likely to deliver healthier babies. He also needs to know that, while you can nourish a baby without him, his baby is likely to grow better if he nourishes you.

Try a bedtime ritual. At around twenty weeks, most dads can feel the baby move. Hearing the heartbeat and seeing baby on ultrasound don't win over all dads, but feeling baby move is enough of a thrill to hook even the most distant father-to-be.

Martha notes: A nightly custom we enjoyed with our pregnancies is one we called the "laying on of hands." Beginning around the sixth month, before going to sleep, Bill would lay his hands on my abdomen each night to feel baby move. He would also talk to our baby. This made a double impression on me: I felt his commitment both as a mate and as a father.

Dr. Bill notes: These were precious moments for me — to feel our baby kicking inside Martha. Initially, I felt kind of foolish talking to a tiny baby whom I couldn't see and could barely feel. Then after a while I got to enjoy this nightly ritual, and somehow I feel baby did, too. I shall never forget those sensual bonding sessions.

Ask and you shall receive. While a few husbands instinctively know their wives' desires before they have to ask, most need to be told. Besides sending him on odd-hour treks to the supermarket to satisfy your food cravings, let your mate know specifically what you need from him: help with housework, shopping, or the other kids on days when you have barely enough energy for yourself and baby. He needs to know you need him. You're not a superwoman, and pregnancy is not just another "extra job" added to your routine chores. While you do baby work, he can do housework. Many men, like kids, are more willing to help if you give them specific requests. Instead of a general "I need your help," try "I need you to do the grocery shopping today."

Work out for three. Try exercising together. A brisk, half-hour morning or evening walk is not only a time to tone your body, it's also an opportunity to tune your communication.

Break habits together. If you are both involved in any of the big three (smoking, excessive alcohol drinking, or drug abuse), it's unfair for your mate to continue his habit while you quit. Not only do you need his support to replace unhealthy habits with healthy ones, he owes it to his baby to be a healthy father. The same goes for healthy eating. Be aware that one or both of you may need professional help for breaking addictions. (See "Kicking the Smoking Habit," page 46.)

Make a date for your next prenatal visit. When you visit your practitioner, especially on visits that include exciting procedures like hearing baby's heartbeat (usually the third- or fourth-month visit) or seeing baby on ultrasound (usually the fifth- or sixth-month visit), invite your mate along to share the experience. Ask for a souvenir ultrasound photo for him to put up at his workplace.

Share feelings. While you don't want to play amateur psychologist, it's important to share your feelings about the pregnancy. Listening in a nonjudgmental, accepting, and caring way helps your husband explore some of the feelings that may be putting a distance between him and the baby or between the two of you. Also, be careful not to let a controlling mate keep you from expressing your feelings. Developing a solid, trusting, comfortable pregnancy dialogue is a good warm-up for the couple talks you will later need when you become a threesome. If you find it difficult to share feelings, it may be an indication that a professional counselor should help you learn to do so. Time and energy spent in counseling now (even just a few sessions) can make a difference in how the two of you move into parenthood together.

When all is said and done, what baby needs most is two happily coupled parents who are committed to each other and to her. It is well worth the effort it may take to draw your husband out and lead him into an involvement he would otherwise not manage on his own. Then prepare to watch your husband's face light up when his newly born baby recognizes his voice and turns toward it — he'll be a *daddy*.

TESTS AND TECHNOLOGY

Ultrasound

Ultrasound technology has revolutionized the practice of obstetrics. By providing a window into the womb, ultrasound allows the doctor to detect actual and potential problems, and to rule out others, and it gives parents an early glimpse of their baby. Diagnostic ultrasound enables mother and doctor to arrive at labor and delivery with fewer unknowns. It is often reassuring, and sometimes even lifesaving, but, like any technology, it must be used wisely.

Why is it done? Ultrasound yields information that could influence how your pregnancy is managed and also improve its outcome. Besides yielding medical information that can be valuable for your health-care provider, ultrasound allows parents to see their baby on a monitor and have photos (often hazy and confusing as to which parts are what) to post on their refrigerator. The first views of baby may leave you in awe, but it may require a leap of faith to believe the tiny white blur your doctor points out is really

baby's head. By eight weeks the image resembles a lima bean with a pulse. Seeing this blip of a pulse will reassure you that you really do have a live baby in there. By fifteen weeks the ultrasound image can show baby's major organs. For many parents, an ultrasound sparks the sudden realization that they truly are pregnant and triggers a sort of space-age prenatal bonding. Another perk is that you can share the photo with grandparents who may be having to bond long-distance. The further along in your pregnancy, the more detailed the viewing. Usually by the twentieth week, ultrasound pictures confirm the presence or absence of a penis, so the sex of your baby may be apparent (though sometimes this is subject to misinterpretation, and your doctor may not yet want to put it in writing). If you don't want to know your baby's sex, be sure to tell your doctor or ultrasound technician beforehand, in case the image reveals all. You may even see your preborn baby sucking his or her thumb. And, as you and your doctor are counting heads, you may even count more than one.

Ultrasound is useful to:

- verify whether or not a woman is pregnant when pregnancy tests and the usual signs of pregnancy are unclear.
- detect a possible ectopic pregnancy.
- obtain a more precise determination of baby's gestational age when there is a discrepancy between uterine size and estimated due date. Precise dating will be needed in case a preterm delivery or a post-term induction becomes necessary for the well-being of mother or baby. Ultrasound is also useful, but not necessary, to determine gestational age when mother is unsure of the date of her last menstrual period. In the first half of pregnancy, ultrasound can accurately date baby's gestation

within seven to ten days. In later months it is not as accurate, and it is useless for dating the pregnancy; this fact argues in favor of doing an ultrasound early in pregnancy.

- evaluate baby's growth if other signs, such as uterine size, suggest a problem. It is more accurate if later ultrasounds can be compared to earlier ones.
- determine the cause of unexplained bleeding.
- confirm how baby lies in the uterus (breech, transverse, vertex) if the clinical signs are unclear late in pregnancy.
- detect suspected multiple pregnancies if mother's uterus is growing faster than expected.
- detect problems with the placenta, such as placenta previa (the placenta being positioned too low or over the cervix) and abruptio placentae (the placenta is separating prematurely, causing bleeding).
- measure the amount of amniotic fluid if mother is losing amniotic fluid or not replenishing it at a normal rate.
- detect abnormalities of the uterus, especially in women with a history of previous miscarriages or problem pregnancies.
- detect abnormalities in the baby, such as spina bifida.
- detect developmental abnormalities in the growing baby that would influence where baby should be delivered and what preparations need to be made beforehand. Abnormalities of heart, lung, and intestinal development can, if detected early, alert parents and health-care providers to deliver the baby in facilities equipped to begin management immediately after birth. Oftentimes, early recognition and early treatment can be lifesaving.
- assist in medical or surgical procedures, such as amniocentesis (see page 131), chorionic villus sampling (see page 133),

turning a breech baby (see page 294), fetoscopy (visualizing baby in the womb), and intrauterine transfusion (injecting needed blood into baby).

Ultrasound enables parents and doctor to enter the labor room with fewer "surprises," a fact that increases your chances for having a safe and satisfying birth.

When is it done? Ultrasound can be done at any time throughout the pregnancy, right up through delivery. It is used at different times for different reasons. (See "Why is it done?" page 205.)

How is it done? As the name implies, this technology employs sound waves at frequencies higher than the human ear can hear. Ultrasound may be performed transabdominally or transvaginally. In a *transabdominal ultrasound,* the doctor or technician runs an ultrasound transmitter across your abdomen. Aided by a gel substance that improves sound conduction, the sound waves bounce back off your baby, much like sonar waves locating a submarine. The echoes are detected by a receiver, and a computer translates the sounds into a picture of your baby on a screen. The Doptone device used for detecting your baby's heartbeat also uses ultrasound; in that case, the echoes are translated into the "swish-thump" you hear every month at your checkup. Other terms that refer to ultrasound include "scan," "sonogram," "Doppler" (after the physics term "Doppler effect," for the relationship between waves and the distance they travel), "echo," and "electronic fetal monitoring."

In the case of a *transvaginal ultrasound,* a tubelike transmitter is inserted painlessly into your vagina just beneath your cervix. Because the transmitter can be placed closer to the uterus, it can visualize intrauterine structures more clearly than a transabdominal transmitter. It can also visualize these structures a week to a week and a half earlier than by the transabdominal method. A vaginal ultrasound can visualize the sac of a growing embryo in the uterus as early as two and a half weeks following conception and can detect a fetal heartbeat as early as four weeks after conception, approximately a week and a half earlier than abdominal ultrasound.

Is it safe? Every test, like every pill, has benefits and risks. Tests should be performed when the benefits outweigh the risks, and in the case of ultrasound, the benefits clearly seem to outweigh the risks. Twenty-year follow-up studies of thousands of mothers and babies who received diagnostic ultrasound have shown no apparent harmful effects. Depending on the information desired, ultrasound can be performed at any time during your pregnancy, and repeated ultrasound exams appear to have no harmful effects. Ultrasound is certainly safer than X rays.

The other side of the safety question is a theoretical concern about what happens when these sound waves strike growing fetal

Knowing Your Baby's Gender Before Birth

The modern technology of ultrasound and amniocentesis makes it possible for you to know your baby's gender before birth. But do you want to know? It's up to you to decide if you can't wait and must know, or if you want to be surprised at the moment of birth.

Knowing beforehand. Knowing your baby's gender ahead of time cuts the name-choosing task down by 50 percent. Some couples feel that knowing baby's gender promotes prenatal bonding. By giving baby a specific name (rather than "the baby" or "the bulge"), they find it's easier to relate to the baby and imagine what he or she will be like. Knowing baby's gender makes your daydreams more meaningful. This knowledge also makes decorating the nursery and outfitting baby's layette easier.

My husband had his heart set on having a boy. I wanted to know our baby's gender beforehand because if our baby turned out to be a girl, I couldn't bear to see his look of disappointment at the *moment of birth. Ultrasound showed we were having a girl, and this gave Daddy a few extra months to look forward to holding a daughter.*

Waiting to be surprised. Other couples prefer to wait until delivery to know their baby's gender. They enjoy the mystery and the surprise and feel it gives them something to look forward to, an added bonus at the moment of birth. If you're having an ultrasound or amniocentesis, be sure to tell your doctor or the technician ahead of time that you don't want to know whether you're having a son or a daughter. Sometimes a health professional may give the secret away by referring to your baby as a "he" or "she." But even that slip of the tongue can be covered up.

I know I'm going to deliver a baby, but I don't know whether it's going to be a boy or girl. I like the joyful anticipation of being surprised.

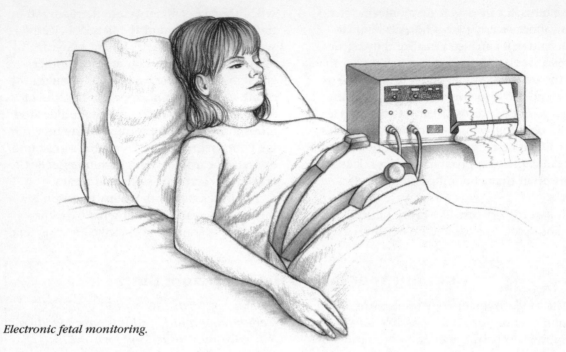

Electronic fetal monitoring.

tissues. When sound waves bombard laboratory tissues at high frequencies, they shake
up the molecules, heat them, and produce microscopic gas bubbles in the cell called "cavi-
tation." Whether this heat or these bubbles
damage the cell is unknown, but studies suggest that the changes demonstrated in research test tubes are insignificant in babies.
However, this uncertainty was enough to
prompt the National Institutes of Health Task
Force on Diagnostic Ultrasound to conclude,
"We could find no evidence to justify the recommendation that every pregnancy be
screened by ultrasound. In the face of even
theoretical risks, where there is no benefit,
then the theoretical risks cannot be justified."

Health-care providers use the term "diagnostic ultrasound," implying there should be a
reason for doing the test. It's important that
every parent approach every test wearing

two hats: the scientist hat, in which you read
or ask about all the benefits and risks of a
particular test and try to weigh them against
each other; and the parent hat, in which you
consider your feelings about the test, the information that is sought, and how the test
will affect the course of your pregnancy. Parent and health-care provider both participate
in the final decision. Curiosity about the sex
of your baby, the desire to have a prenatal
photo to pass around to family members, or
the wish for prenatal bonding are not good
enough reasons for having an ultrasound.
Also, avoid commercial ultrasound "photographers" who offer color pictures of the baby
in the womb. Color exposes the baby to
much more ultrasound wave energy and is
definitely a case where you owe it to your
baby not to satisfy your curiosity.

If you want a replay for home-movie night,

bring along a blank videotape and ask for a copy. When you first see the ultrasound pictures you will have difficulty identifying all the black-and-white blurs as baby parts. During the ultrasound, ask the technician to point out the features of your baby: the arms and legs, chambers of the heart, the head and spinal cord; and watch baby's heart beating. Play the tape or show the ultrasound pictures to your spouse so he can see his baby grow. Ultrasound has been a boon for encouraging fathers-to-be to bond with their children.

I was absolutely relieved and elated. You looked so adorable. You were moving all over the place, kicking your legs, waving your arms all around, moving your fingers, doing somersaults. You looked happy and active. Now I really feel pregnant.

Seeing our baby grow on ultrasound was just the pep talk I needed to get me through this high-risk pregnancy and continued bed rest. It was reassuring to see that everything was so perfectly formed. It made me feel less high-risk.

I had no idea ultrasound could show us so much. We saw your spine, your vertebrae; we looked at your little heart with all its chambers perfectly formed, and we saw the blood flowing through them and circulating back. We saw all of your organs. I put your ultrasound pictures in my journal.

Glucose Tolerance Test (GTT)

Many women normally spill some sugar in their urine from time to time during pregnancy. This biochemical overflow happens because the hormones of pregnancy normally suppress insulin release, allowing a mother's blood sugar to be higher during pregnancy in order to provide more glucose to nourish her baby. Your growing baby depends on a steady supply of glucose, which is why it's important to eat frequent, small meals and not skip meals. In a small percentage of pregnant women (2 to 10 percent) the blood sugar is higher than average for pregnant women — a temporary condition called "gestational glucose intolerance" (a less alarming and more accurate term than the older tag "gestational diabetes"). Gestational glucose intolerance is detected during pregnancy with the glucose tolerance test.

Why is it done? The theoretical fear that has prompted doctors' concern over high blood sugar during pregnancy is based on the belief that long exposure to high blood sugar causes the fetus to grow excessively large, resulting in more birth complications, such as prematurity, respiratory problems, and difficult deliveries. This worry is based upon the observation that diabetic women, especially those whose blood sugars are poorly controlled during their pregnancy, deliver excessively large babies with these complications. Another concern is that continual exposure to high blood sugar may prompt baby to manufacture too much of his or her own insulin, causing the baby's blood sugar to drop quickly and dangerously immediately after birth. When gestational glucose intolerance is identified during pregnancy, the mother can alter her diet to keep her blood sugar from getting too high. Gestational glucose intolerance is more common in overweight women, older women, those with a family history of diabetes, or women who have previously delivered a baby weighing more than nine pounds.

How is it done? In her doctor's office, the woman drinks a glass of sweet liquid called "glucola" (it tastes like extra-sweet Coke or

Pepsi) on an empty stomach. Her blood-sugar level is checked one hour later with a blood test. (An alternative to drinking the sugar-loaded liquid is to measure the blood-sugar level one to two hours after a big meal.) The result of the GTT should be available within a few hours. After ingesting the test "meal," it's important to stay active (e.g., walking) so your body will have a better chance of metabolizing the sugar load than if you were just sitting there waiting to have your blood drawn. If this one-hour screening test turns out to show high blood sugar, the doctor may recommend a more accurate three-hour test. Only around 15 percent of women with an abnormal one-hour GTT will have an abnormal three-hour GTT test. If the three-hour test is abnormal, the doctor may recommend a diabetic diet throughout the rest of the pregnancy.

When is it done? The GTT is usually recommended between twenty-four and twenty-eight weeks and may be repeated around thirty-two to thirty-four weeks in mothers with high-risk pregnancies.

Is it safe? Not all obstetricians agree on the necessity or safety of the GTT, and new research questions the value of routine screening for gestational glucose intolerance. A 1990 study of 1307 women (533 of whom were not screened and 774 who were screened) showed that screening resulted in more tests and worry during pregnancy, and there was a significantly higher cesarean rate among the screened mothers. It did not decrease the number of large infants, however. These researchers concluded that the routine use of GTT caused more worry than benefits.

Another concern is the physiological wisdom (and possible safety) of the GTT. Pregnant women seldom drink a 50-gram slug of glucose solution on an empty stomach. This is unnatural eating; therefore, the test could show unnatural results. And a 50-gram glucose dose is more of a load for a 100-pound woman than it is for a 250-pound one. Some women who are not in the habit of ingesting sugar to this extent develop side effects from the glucola, such as headaches, nausea, and bloating. Because of these concerns, the routine use of GTT is being reconsidered by many practitioners. Discuss with your practitioner whether or not the GTT is necessary in your particular pregnancy.

Tests that are reserved for rare and risky circumstances during pregnancy are discussed in the glossary. If you need to have one of those tests, your doctor will discuss it with you first. Whatever the test, be sure you understand why the test is necessary, how it is performed, when it is performed, what the risks are, and how the results of the test will affect your care.

THE FIFTH MONTH

❖ ❖ ❖

Emotionally I feel: _____
_____
_____
_____

Physically I feel: _____
_____
_____
_____

My thoughts about you: _____
_____
_____
_____

My dreams about you: _____
_____
_____

What I imagine you look like: _____
_____
_____
_____

My top concerns: _____
_____
_____
_____

My best joys: _____
_____
_____
_____

My worst problems: _____
_____
_____

VISIT TO MY HEALTH-CARE PROVIDER

Questions I had; answers I got: _____
_____
_____
_____
_____
_____

Tests and results; my reaction: _____
_____
_____
_____

Updated due date: _____
My weight: _____
My blood pressure: _____
Feeling my uterus; my reaction: _____
_____
_____

How I feel now that the whole world can see I'm pregnant: _____
_____
_____

How I felt when I first felt you move: _____
_____
_____

How I feel now that I am wearing maternity clothes: _____
_____
_____

What I bought when I went shopping: _____
_____
_____
_____

photo at five months

Comments: _____

_____

_____

_____

_____

_____

_____

_____

_____

_____

_____

_____

_____

_____

_____

_____

Sixth-Month Visit to Your Health-Care Provider (21–25 weeks)

During this month's visit you may have:

- examination of the size and height of the uterus
- weight and blood-pressure check
- urinalysis to test for infection, sugar, and protein
- oral glucose tolerance test, screening for gestational glucose intolerance, if indicated
- vaginal culture, screening test for beta strep infection, if indicated (see "Group B Streptococcus," page 412)
- an opportunity to hear your baby's heartbeat
- an opportunity to see your baby on ultrasound, if indicated
- an opportunity to discuss your feelings and concerns

The Sixth Month — Feeling Baby Move

DURING THE SIXTH MONTH (twenty-one to twenty-five weeks), the fun of pregnancy is in full bloom. You will continue to grow at a rate of about 1 pound a week. That would be a bit alarming if you weren't also growing a baby. Expect to gain 4 to 5 pounds, with one whole pound of that going directly to the baby. Your uterus reaches above the level of your navel this month, and the bulge shows in all its glory. As you gaze at your new profile in a mirror, you'll be amazed at how much you've expanded in a month. You'll feel stronger and more frequent kicks, and your mate and children will be able to feel them now, too.

HOW YOU MAY FEEL EMOTIONALLY

As you see yourself grow larger and feel the baby's kicking, wiggling presence much of the time, the reality that you are responsible for another human being's life sinks in. This realization may awaken deep feelings about yourself and the rest of your life.

Wanting to Heal the Past. The natural turning inward of pregnancy often brings with it a journey to the past. You may rerun scenes from your childhood, pleasant and unpleasant, and wonder how your mother's mothering will influence yours. You may even begin to think about unhappy incidents in your past — unresolved problems or other "baggage" that was never properly unloaded. Pregnancy gives many women deeper insight into themselves, and many women regard pregnancy as a window of opportunity for healing their psychological selves. While pregnancy is a good time to consider the blessings and challenges in your life and how they will affect your parenting, it's not a time to be consumed by a problem past. Try not to dwell on gut-wrenching psychological problems to such an extent that they overshadow the joy of your pregnancy.

For some women, pregnancy is not a good time for plumbing the depths of their psyche. While many can use heightened emotional awareness to their advantage (for career changes, for example, or shifting priorities), some find that pregnancy causes their emotions to play tricks on them, even to the point where they imagine problems where there are none. If you feel yourself getting in too deep, discuss your concerns with your practitioner and seek professional counseling if necessary.

215

One area where a thorough soul-searching can reap some constructive change in your life during pregnancy is family relationships and dynamics. Moving toward assuming the adult role of parent, for example, opens the door for making new connections with your own mom or dad. If you've been estranged from your parents, this may be the time to make up. If you have a good relationship with your parents and in-laws, you may find that it deepens as you share your pregnancy with them. This is also the time to learn to stand fast if you've previously been a pushover with relatives; a controlling mom or a competitive sister will have a lot to say about your mothering choices, but those choices should be made by you, not by your family. This brings up another important area that may need some attention: Just what will your mothering choices be? Giving some thought now to this issue will help you determine ahead of time what kind of parent you want to be and what kind of childhood you want your baby to have. You'll be surprised how much of a difference this can make in the months and years to come.

Impatient. While more than half of your pregnancy is behind you, there are still nearly a hundred l-o-n-g days ahead. There will be many times when you will truly enjoy everything about being pregnant; there will also be days when you just want to get it over with. Along with this impatience may come a bit of boredom. Any slowdown in your usual activities — from job to hobbies to sports — may leave you with time on your hands. Take advantage of this slower time to read, go for walks, or just rest.

Pregnancy brings a season in which busy women can learn to enjoy a more contemplative lifestyle. While you can keep yourself busy catching up on photo albums or studying a foreign language, remember that you are entering a new, rather unintellectual, phase of life. Practice listening — to the wind or to your own heart. Or consider learning to meditate. Sooner than you think, you will have an infant to feed, a crawling baby to watch, a toddler to play with. If you are able to have a peaceful pregnancy, you and baby will be healthier because you will have learned to be content with a slower pace.

Frustrated with having to share your body. During pregnancy you've had to be so vigilant, watching everything you eat, not taking your usual headache medicine or cold remedies. And there's still a long stretch of more of the same. Your body is being taken over by another person. You may delight in the privilege of carrying this person, yet wonder why you have to endure many discomforts. You're tired of conking out at night, leaving you with precious little time for yourself let alone for your mate. You're probably even tired of being noticed and fawned over — it can be irritating to be talked to all the time as if your only function in life were to gestate. And you are overwhelmingly amazed at all the changes you've undergone physically and emotionally — perhaps even a bit scared by the way nature has taken over your body.

Martha notes: I marvel at the incredible changes my body has gone through to accommodate this pregnancy. It's as though my whole abdominal structure is being remodeled, forced by relentless inner changes. My body is not my own anymore — it has been taken over by a process and a presence that draws everything it needs without regard to how that would affect me. I can only stand by and watch it happen and re-

alize the consequence of sharing my body with someone else. The takeover is far from pleasant at times. Yet these discomforts are a small price to pay for the prize to come.

HOW YOU MAY FEEL PHYSICALLY

Toward the end of the middle trimester most women continue to feel delight in being big enough to look pregnant but not yet so large that their bodies become unwieldy. They usually feel relatively well. Nevertheless, as you round the bend into the last trimester, you may begin to get a hint of the discomforts to come.

Needing to slow down. Not only will your mind tell you to slow down by the end of the second trimester, your body will force you to do so. On the days you overdo it, you will know it. After a busy day, you will need some catch-up rest that evening or the next day. Exhaustion is your body's reminder that there is just not enough energy, emotional or physical, to continue a busy lifestyle *and* grow a baby. If you feel you need to keep busy to get through your pregnancy, try to balance physical exertion with rest; mental stimulation with mindless relaxation; work that makes the time fly with leisure that allows your mind and body to catch up.

More kicks. If the origin of those faint little flutters was previously in doubt, now there's no question. You are feeling *life*. The gentle, butterfly-wing kicks of the last month now become definite jabs. If you feel the baby kicking several places at once, just remember little thumper has shoulders, elbows, knees, and hands that may all stretch out at once in a uterus in which there is still room enough to maneuver.

If your children have not yet felt baby move, get ready for those curious little hands on your abdomen. Once your children feel the kicks, they will continue to get a "kick" out of it and may eagerly anticipate baby's active times — usually before you go to bed or upon awakening in the morning. To help your child feel baby move, place his hand where you last felt a lot of movement and hold it there with some pressure for a while. If your child does not show particular interest in the kicking, don't worry. It may be too abstract to her; it doesn't mean she won't adore the baby.

Each night George and I looked forward to lying next to one another and watching and feeling our baby move. Soon after we went to bed, the kick show would begin. Sometimes my belly button would pop out with each kick.

Tom and I enjoyed falling asleep with me curled around him. He'd feel the baby gently thumping him on the back. It was a nice experience for the three of us to be all cuddled up together.

Our baby moved most when I was quiet, so we had a before-bed ritual we called the "night show." We'd lie in bed together and watch and feel our baby make his presence known.

I love waking up to your gentle nudgings. I reach for your daddy's hand and put it on where you are nudging. A smile breaks out across his face as he says, "My baby."

When my husband first felt our baby kick (week twenty-three), he finally made the connection with our baby that I had waited for so longingly. Now our baby makes himself felt in our lives literally, and to be able to feel movements highlights the reality of baby's presence in such a beautiful way. When baby starts to move, I suddenly realize that he is awake and conscious on some level that we are only starting to understand. If he is awake, can he be aware of us, too — our voices, our movements, our hands pressing over the place where he kicks? Will he be getting a message back from us?

Besides feeling more movement, you can now see it. You may be sitting at your desk and look down periodically to see something jump beneath your clothes. If you lie on your back you can watch areas of the bulge "bubble up" from beneath. It's natural to respond to these movements by placing your hand above the punch site, acknowledging what you felt. Next month this magnificent sight will be even more noticeable.

Leg cramps. Toward the end of the middle trimester and throughout the last one, many women are awakened by knotlike cramps in their calf muscles or feet. These cramps are sometimes blamed on an electrolyte imbalance of calcium, phosphorus, magnesium, and potassium. An additional explanation is the decreased circulation to the most active muscles in your legs. Pressure of the uterus on major blood vessels, as well as standing, sitting, or lying for a long time, can slow blood supply to these muscles, causing them to cramp up.

Preventing leg cramps. You can lessen your leg cramps by improving the circulation to your leg muscles in these ways:

• Wear support stockings during the day. Avoid standing or sitting for long periods.
• Exercise your calf muscles before going to bed: try the foot exercises described on page 181. Pulling the toes up toward your leg while pushing your heel away from you stretches the calf muscles that are most likely to cramp up. The cramp relief exercises described below are also good preventive measures. Do them about ten times on each side.
• Have your partner massage your calf muscles before you go to bed.
• Elevate your legs on a pillow at night.
• Lie on your left side in the sleeping position shown on page 225.

Relieving cramps. Leg cramps can be extremely uncomfortable and often awaken you with a painful startle. When the cramp occurs, you can massage the cramped muscle or have your mate rub it to promote circulation, but getting up and moving around works best. Walk if you can, or do the following stretching exercises in the standing or against-the-wall position. If the cramp is severe, lie in bed, grab the toes of your hurting leg, and pull them back toward your head while keeping your knee straight and as close to the mattress as you can. Remember to stretch *gradually,* avoiding lunging or bouncing movements, which only aggravate the cramp and may even injure the muscles. If your tummy bulge prevents you from bending forward enough to grab your toes, simply straighten your leg, pressing the back of your knee into the mattress and flexing your toes toward your head.

The following exercises will help relieve cramps when they happen and, if you do them faithfully, may prevent them.

STANDING CALF STRETCH. Place the leg with the cramped muscles one foot or so behind your other leg. While keeping your back straight, gently bend the knee of the non-cramped leg so that you are leaning forward while keeping the cramped leg straight and its heel to the floor. (The forward leg also keeps its heel to the floor.) Without bouncing, stretch gently. You may find it easier to balance if you press your hands or forearms against the wall while doing this stretching exercise.

WALL PUSH-UPS. Place your hands flat against the wall and step back until your arms are fully extended. Keeping your feet flat on the floor and your back straight, lean in toward the wall while bending your elbows. You should feel your calf muscles stretch comfortably. If it's too much of a stretch, stand closer to the wall.

SITTING LEG STRETCHES. Sitting on the floor, stretch one leg out to the side, foot flexed. Fold your other leg in, foot toward your crotch. While keeping your outstretched leg straight, bend forward and reach toward your toe. Hold this stretched position for a few seconds. Switch sides and repeat. Don't point your toes straight out and pull your heel toward you since that contracts the muscles that are already cramped.

An electrolyte imbalance is unlikely to be the cause of your leg cramps, but if exercises aren't working, you might want to give calcium supplements a try. Consult with your health-care provider about taking extra potassium or calcium tablets (calcium carbonate) that do not contain phosphorus. In a recent study women who took magnesium tablets daily experienced fewer leg cramps. Unless your practitioner advises it, it is not safe to eat a low-phosphorus diet while pregnant.

Numbness and tingling in your hands. Another occupational side effect of pregnancy is numbness or tingling in the hands. This pins-and-needles or burning sensation usually involves the thumb, first two fingers, and half of the ring finger, and may be accompanied by pain in the wrist that can shoot all the way up to the shoulder. Sometimes you may feel soreness when you press the inner

surface of your wrist. This condition is known as "carpal tunnel syndrome." The extra fluid that seems to accumulate everywhere in the pregnant body also settles in the sheath beneath the ligament running across your wrist. This excess causes swelling, which pinches the nerve beneath this ligament that leads to the hand, causing the hands to feel numb or tingly.

Carpal tunnel syndrome is a repetitive-strain illness (RSI) and is common in persons, pregnant or not, who work with their hands. People who use their hands and wrists a lot (e.g., when typing, checking groceries at the supermarket, or playing the piano) are more likely to experience symptoms; women who work on keyboards are particularly prone to RSIs. But you may suffer from the syndrome even if you're not in a high-risk group: a full 25 percent of pregnant women experience tingling in their hands toward the last half of their pregnancy. For pregnant women this condition is particularly annoying and sometimes even disabling. Carpal tunnel syndrome symptoms are most likely to occur during the night, after a day-long accumulation of fluid in the wrists, or when you wake up in the morning, especially if you sleep with your arm under your head.

To ease carpal tunnel syndrome discomfort, try resting your hands more during the day. Avoid activities that aggravate the tingling, such as turning your wrist to pour, or anything that involves repetitive wrist movements. If you work on a computer, type with your wrists in the neutral position, flexed slightly down, rather than with your wrists curved up. Use a wrist rest to help you maintain this position. At night elevate the affected hand or hands on a pillow. Wearing a plastic splint at night to immobilize your wrist in a neutral position should alleviate the pain. (Look for these in drugstores. If needed, your doctor can prescribe a splint that is custom-fitted to your wrist.) If the pain is particularly severe and persistent, a specialist can immediately relieve the discomfort with periodic cortisone injections, which are safe during pregnancy.

As with nearly all the muscle aches and pains during pregnancy, carpal tunnel syndrome goes away after delivery. Some breast-feeding mothers need to continue to use their splints (or wind up getting one) until the body's fluid balance adjusts to lactation, in about four to six weeks. The use of the wrists is important for positioning the baby properly at the breast, and long periods of time spent holding the baby in one position for nursing may aggravate carpal tunnel syndrome. A lactation consultant can help you with special positioning tips, such as the use of pillows to help you hold baby correctly without stressing your wrist.

Abdominal-muscle separation. No, you don't have a hernia. There are two large bands of muscles that run down the middle of your abdomen from your ribs to your pelvic bone. As your uterus grows, it stretches these muscles and pushes them apart, and you may notice that your skin "pooches out" in the area where these muscles have separated. If you run your fingers along the middle of your abdomen between the muscles, you may feel a soft gap where the muscles have separated, and this separation may become more pronounced in the next trimester. Be advised that sit-ups are inadvisable during pregnancy, even early on. Your abdominal muscles simply don't have the strength once this separation starts, even though you may not notice it until your uterus gets large enough to make the separation obvious. Several months after delivery, your rectus muscles come back together and fill in the gap, but most women have less and less abdominal tone with each subsequent pregnancy.

Leaking urine. You may notice that every time you sneeze, you have to cross your legs or else you wet your pants a bit. Don't worry — this problem will go away after the baby is born. When you sneeze, cough, or belly-laugh, your diaphragm contracts and pushes your abdominal contents and uterus down onto your bladder, causing you to dribble urine if your bladder is full or your pelvic-floor muscles are weak. To avoid this nuisance, keep your bladder as empty as possible. Urinate frequently and get into the habit of triple voiding: every time you urinate, bear down three extra times to empty your bladder as completely as you can. Also, to lessen the force on your diaphragm, be sure to open your mouth when you cough or sneeze; keeping your mouth closed causes pressure to build up in your chest and aggravates the problem. As soon as you deliver the little person who takes up space in your abdomen, your bladder will have more room to expand. In the meantime, a napkin or panty liner may be necessary.

To strengthen the muscles that control urination, practice Kegel exercises (see page 176). Contract and release these muscles between urination times as if you were trying to stop urinating. If you use Kegel exercises while urinating, be sure to empty your bladder completely; otherwise you might worsen pregnancy incontinence.

My mother told me to bend my knees and lean forward slightly if I have to sneeze or cough while standing. A big help.

Rectal pain and bleeding. Hemorrhoids, which are varicose veins in the rectum, cause rectal pain and bleeding. The increased blood volume of pregnancy and the pressure of the enlarging uterus on pelvic structures can cause the veins in the rectal wall or around the anal opening to enlarge into pea- or grape-size clusters that bulge out, bleed, itch, and sting, especially during the passage of a hard bowel movement. Swollen blood vessels that occur inside the rectum — internal hemorrhoids — may bleed but are usually not painful. Besides rectal discomfort, one of the first signs of hemorrhoids is fresh red blood on the toilet tissue you wipe with. Although rectal blood is nearly always nothing more than a sign of harmless but irritating hemorrhoids, you should report this symptom to your health-care provider, who can confirm the diagnosis with an exam. Though they can occur at any time, hemorrhoids usually appear toward the end of the second trimester and worsen during the third trimester. They are often at their worst immediately postpartum, after the pushing during delivery, but they shrink after that.

Preventing hemorrhoids. While these "pains in the butt" for many women are just part of being pregnant, there are things you can do to minimize them.

- Avoid sitting for long periods of time, especially on hard surfaces, and sleeping on your back, because the weight of the uterus presses on the major blood vessels behind it, causing the blood return from these rectal veins to be even more sluggish.

- Practice your Kegel exercises (see page 176) at least fifty times a day. Tightening your pelvic-floor muscles, especially those around your rectum, will strengthen the anus and the tissue around it and prevent the stagnation of blood in this area.

- Keep your bowel movements frequent and loose. Eat a fiber-rich diet, drink a lot of fluids, and ask your health-care provider to recommend a stool softener, if necessary. See the tips to avoid constipation on page 70.

- Use soft scent- and dye-free toilet tissue. Use a baby wipe when necessary. (They're cheaper than adult towelettes.)

- Avoid putting undue pressure on your rectal muscles by straining during a bowel movement. Wipe gently, using more of a patting motion than a rubbing one. When bathing, cleanse your rectal area with a handheld shower instead of rubbing vigorously with a washcloth.

Treating hemorrhoids. If these swollen blood vessels appear, here's how to manage them:

- Apply cool or cold compresses: crushed ice in a clean sock will shrink the vessels and alleviate the pain. Lie on a thick towel to keep water from soaking your sheet.

- To relieve itching, take a short soak in a warm bath to which a half cup of baking soda has been added. (While warm water can soothe an itchy bottom, it can also dilate blood vessels and further aggravate bleeding, so don't stay in more than a few minutes.)

- Place a cotton ball or gauze pad soaked in cool witch hazel (or a medicated pad recommended by your health-care provider) against the hemorrhoid to help shrink it and ease the discomfort.

- If you find the hemorrhoids extremely irritating or painful, assume the knee-chest position (see illustration, page 180), which takes pressure off the swollen blood vessels momentarily while you await relief from the witch hazel or other remedy.

- If you must sit on a very sore bottom, buy a rubber doughnut to place on your sitting surface. Some women, though, find the pressure the doughnut puts on the buttocks aggravating. Alternatively, sit on a pillow, or lean to one side while sitting.

- Check with your doctor before using an over-the-counter medication. Though there is little evidence that these ointments are dangerous to baby, some of them can be absorbed through the rectal tissue and into the bloodstream.

Shooting pains in your lower back and legs. You may occasionally feel shooting pains, tingling, or numbness in your lower back, buttocks, outer thighs, or legs. These occur when your relaxing pelvic joints, the baby's head, or your enlarging uterus press on the major nerves that run from the backbone through the pelvis and toward each leg. Sudden, sharp pain that begins deep in the buttock on one side and travels down the back of that leg is due to pressure on the sciatic nerve in your lower back; hence the name "sciatica." Sciatica is aggravated by lifting, bending, or even walking. Tingling numbness and pain along the outer thigh is caused by stretching of the femoral nerve to the leg. Rest and a change of position (try the knee-chest position; see illustration, page 180) that shifts the pelvic pressure away from these nerves should alleviate the pains. Try a warm bath, ice packs to the site of the pain, or lying on the affected side. These pains can be very debilitating for some women. They vary so greatly from woman to woman because of individual differences in pelvic bone structure and shape.

Enlarged veins. Varicose veins are just another of the many side effects of being pregnant. The hormones of pregnancy relax the muscular walls of your veins, causing them to enlarge. These vessels need to expand to accommodate the extra blood volume of pregnancy. The legs are particularly likely to host varicose veins, because the expanding uterus presses on the major blood vessels beneath it, and this puts pressure on the veins of the pelvis, sometimes causing blood to pool in the legs. But veins enlarge all over; you may notice little knots in the bulging veins along the sides of your neck or even along your vulva. These are due to the normal accumulation of extra blood in and near the veins' valves. Hemorrhoids are also a type of enlarged vein (see page 220). Whether or not you develop varicose veins during pregnancy is mostly a matter of heredity.

Do not knead or vigorously massage varicose veins, as this could cause further damage to the veins and might even cause a blood clot. If you notice that an area around the visible veins of your lower leg has become increasingly painful, red, swollen, warm, or tender, a vein may have become infected, a serious condition called "thrombophlebitis," which could lead to a blood clot. Elevate your leg and notify your health-care provider.

Most of the unwanted, but inevitable, venous changes of pregnancy subside within a few months after delivery. To lessen the appearance and the annoyance of varicose veins:

- Avoid standing or sitting for long periods of time. Don't cross your legs while sitting. If you must be stationary, promote circulation by doing the leg and foot exercises described on pages 181 and 182, and walk around periodically to encourage circulation in your legs.

- Elevate your feet as high as possible when you sit. Lie and sleep on your left side, as shown on page 225.

- Wear loose-fitting clothing. Avoid tight pants, tight waistbands, garters and socks, and any other clothing that may restrict your circulation.

- Wear support hose. Put them on even before you get out of bed in the morning, before gravity gives your veins a chance to pop out. Avoid knee-high support stockings, since the band at the top may constrict blood return.

HOW YOUR BABY IS GROWING (21–25 WEEKS)

By the end of this month, baby weighs around 1¼ to 1½ pounds and is around 1 foot long. Increasing fat deposits beneath the skin cause her to take on a more plump, though still wrinkly, appearance. Her fingernails and eyelashes develop, scalp hair increases, and her face is more babylike. The vernix caseosa now covers the skin completely, like a layer of thin, whitish paste. By the twenty-fourth week, baby's nostrils open

Braxton Hicks Contractions

Don't be alarmed when you suddenly feel your uterus tighten. You are not going into labor. Your uterus has been flexing its muscles since the third month, even though you may not have been able to feel the contractions. Even when you think your uterus is resting, it is contracting several times an hour.

The point at which mothers-to-be begin feeling these contractions varies — some claim to feel them as early as the fourth month. Most women begin to feel them in month six or seven. Called "Braxton Hicks contractions" (named after the doctor who described them in 1872), they are typically felt as short periods (usually less than forty-five seconds) of uterine tightening. Braxton Hicks contractions are usually painless, but may feel at first like mild menstrual cramps. They occur at irregular intervals and often happen more frequently when you are tired, such as at the end of the day. Some women report breathlessness with the contractions. Braxton Hicks contractions are reported to be felt more

strongly in subsequent pregnancies than they are the first time around; or perhaps mothers just notice them more in their next pregnancy.

These "practice contractions" are thought to tone up the uterus for the strenuous work it will soon have to do, sort of like prenatal exercise for the uterus. As your uterus grows, the contractions will gradually increase in frequency and intensity until they become strong enough to push baby out. In the eighth or ninth month, they may become frequent and uncomfortable enough to make you wonder if "this is it." (See page 264 for how to tell the difference between labor and prelabor contractions.) Use these strong Braxton Hicks contractions to your advantage by practicing your relaxation skills when they occur. As soon as you feel one coming on, click into the relaxation mode you are learning in childbirth classes. Remember, though, this is only a rehearsal; these contractions bear little resemblance to the ones that do the real work later on.

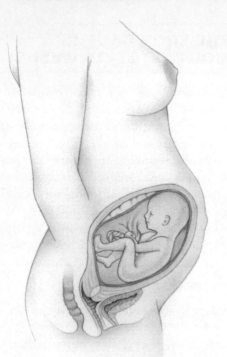

Baby at 21–25 weeks.

and her lungs begin to develop air sacs, called "alveoli," though not enough of them to sustain breathing outside the womb. If she were born now, her breathing would have to be assisted.

CONCERNS YOU MAY HAVE

Bonding with Your Preborn Baby

As you probably suspected, you don't have to wait until you hold your baby in your arms to begin communicating with your son or daughter. New research supports what mothers have long believed, that babies in the womb hear what's going on outside. Even more intriguing, there is evidence that babies may share their mothers' emotions. The influence mothers have on their preborn baby's developing body is obvious; what is less obvious, but perhaps just as important, is the influence mothers have on their baby's developing mind. Mothers often wonder if their thoughts, actions, and words are perceived by their baby. New studies suggest babies may hear and feel more than we think they do.

For centuries in many cultures, people believed that some sort of emotional network operated between mother and baby, and for this reason mothers were admonished to keep their minds and bodies pure during pregnancy. There is much superstition and folklore built around possible connections between what's in mother's mind and what goes on with her baby. Apparently, practitioners of traditional wisdom were on the right track — they just didn't know how this communication happened. In the past twenty-five years, the new field of prenatal psychology has sprung up. Using new technology that provides various windows into the womb, prenatal psychologists have found much that is credible about these superstitions. When mother is happy, baby is happy; when mother is anxious, baby is, too.

Stories mothers share. There are many anecdotal tales in which babies recall in later life sounds they heard while in the womb. Orchestra conductors have claimed they feel an unexplained familiarity with music their mothers played while pregnant. Toddlers have been heard reciting phrases their mothers uttered frequently during their pregnancy: one two-year-old loved to repeat "breathe in, breathe out," which his mom had rehearsed in her Lamaze class. Adults under the influence of medication to draw out

Sleeping Comfortably

If your increased bulk makes getting comfortable difficult, try this nighttime-proven sleeping position that is most restful to mothers and safest for baby: lie on your left side and support yourself with at least five-pillows — two under your head, two supporting your top leg, and one wedged between your back and the mattress. (Sometimes a smaller pillow wedged between your abdomen and the mattress is also comfortable.) If you feel off-balance lying on your side, roll slightly onto your stomach, moving your top leg forward so that it is completely off your lower leg, and let your abdomen snuggle into the mattress.

Dr. Linda notes: I used anatomy texts and heavy research journals to help me sleep. The more I tried to concentrate on some particularly boring and obscure point, the more soundly I would fall asleep.

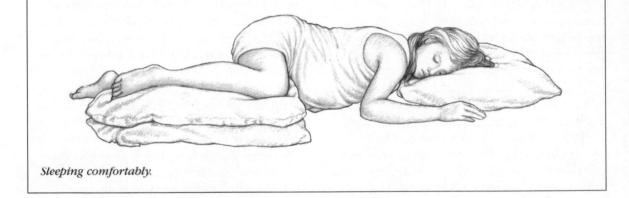

Sleeping comfortably.

buried memories have accurately recalled voices or sounds they heard during the last few months in the womb. One man vividly described the sounds of a carnival his mother attended in her ninth month. Dismiss this anecdotal evidence if you wish, but new studies suggest there may be a physiological basis for these observations.

What babies can hear. Concertgoing mothers report their preborn babies jump at the sudden sound of drums. In fact, from at least the twenty-third week on, a preborn baby's hearing is developed enough to enable him to respond to outside noise. Prenatal re-searchers believe that from at least six months of pregnancy, the preborn baby is aware of and influenced by what's going on in the outside world. (From the twenty-eighth week, the cortex of the brain is developed enough for thinking, which is one of the reasons twenty-eight-week-old premature babies can often survive outside the womb.) Babies seem agitated by rock music, kicking violently when they hear it, and are calmed by some classical music. Even the five-month-old fetus has been found to have discriminating musical ears. In one study, kicking babies calmed to the sounds of Vivaldi but became agitated in response to Beethoven.

Studies also show that a six-month-old fetus can move his body to the rhythm of his mother's speech. Perhaps most astounding, preborn babies can be taught when to kick. Researchers stimulated babies to kick by making a loud noise. After these babies were used to kicking with the noise, the researchers placed a vibrator on mother's abdomen immediately following the noise. Soon these smart little babies learned to kick in response to only the vibration. In other words, they learned to associate the noise with the sensation.

At least one study has shown that babies in the newborn nursery are calmed by tape recordings of heartbeats. And there is endless anecdotal evidence that babies and adults are naturally soothed by rhythms resembling resting heartbeats, meaning sixty to ninety beats per minute. This suggests that womb sounds are imprinted on the mind before birth.

What else baby can sense. Not only can a preborn baby react to sound, he or she can perceive different tastes and sights. Add sweetener to the amniotic fluid, and the fetal gourmet doubles his rate of swallowing; add a sour substance, and baby slows his swallowing. Even as early as the fourth month, baby frowns, squints, and grimaces in response to experimentally produced outside stimuli. At five months the fetus can startle in response to a light blinking at mother's abdomen.

What babies think. Can a fetus form attitudes about life even before birth? Prenatal psychologists claim yes. If so, do a pregnant woman's thoughts influence the emotional life of her preborn baby? Prenatal researchers believe that there is indeed some connection between what a mother thinks and how her baby feels, and that from six months on, a preborn baby can share mother's emotions via the hormones associated with them.

While babies can't understand actual words, perhaps they do react to the tone of mother's voice. Soothing tones calm baby; angry or anxious sounds upset baby. Mothers' positive and negative feelings also appear to affect their babies. One study showed that babies' heartbeats increased each time their mothers even thought of lighting a cigarette, regardless of whether or not they smoked one.

The long-term effects. One of the most controversial areas of prenatal research is the study of correlations between a pregnant woman's emotional life and the personality of her child. Is an anxious mother more likely to produce an anxious baby? Studies relating maternal attitudes to the emotional development of the offspring do indeed reveal a tendency for anxious mothers to produce anxious babies. They also show that mothers who resented being pregnant and felt no attachment to their babies in the womb were more likely to have children with emotional problems. Mothers with less anxious pregnancies, whose babies were wanted and loved, tended to have emotionally healthy children.

Before you worry that every anxious or negative thought that flashes through your mind might leave a permanent emotional scar on your baby, be reassured that neither common sense nor scientific study supports this alarming assumption. In fact, studies suggest that the short-term emotional upsets and quickly resolved anxieties that occur in all pregnancies do not harm the baby emotionally. Major emotional disturbances, however, and unresolved stresses throughout the pregnancy may lead to emotionally troubled children. (Extreme maternal distress even poses a risk of hurting baby physically, as it has been linked with increased risk of prematurity and low birthweight.) Statistical studies show that the babies at greatest risk of developing later emotional disturbances are born to mothers who are the victims of disturbing marital relationships and who throughout their pregnancy regarded their baby as unwanted. The good news is that even mothers who were besieged by months of personal and medical problems, by maintaining a happy attitude about their pregnancy and thinking loving thoughts about their baby, have gone on to have children everyone likes to be around.

Hormones form this emotional link.
What could cause this fascinating correlation between maternal thoughts and fetal personality development? Certainly, mother's emotions don't cross the placenta; her hormones, on the other hand, do. Researchers believe that a stressed mother produces an abundance of stress hormones called "catecholamines," which in turn have been shown to affect the emotions of the fetus. When catecholamines are taken from frightened animals and injected into other animals, the recipients act frightened as well. Scientists theorize that these chemical stressors cross the placenta and "frighten" the developing nervous system. If it happens often enough, the fetus actually gets used to feeling chronically stressed. His system is prepared to overreact to stimuli. Babies who are born with an already overcharged and possibly disturbed nervous system show more emotional disturbances and gastrointestinal upsets, which will earn this baby the label "colicky."

Responsibility for the physical *and* emotional health of a baby is a heavy burden to place on a pregnant mother already worried about keeping her baby safe in a confusing world. Not only must she abstain from polluted foods and try to avoid polluted air, now she must guard against polluted thoughts! Relax. Don't let worry over your emotional state become yet another stressor in a busy life. Take reasonable measures to rid your life of tension, take time to rest and revel in positive emotions, and understand that there is reason to be concerned only about emotional problems that are serious and that last throughout the pregnancy. Nature can certainly compensate for life's normal ups and downs. Besides, the field of prenatal psychology and prenatal bonding is truly in its infancy, and its study methods are imprecise. For example, one of the ways that researchers make judgments about fetal thoughts is to note changes in baby's movement. They assume that a quiet baby who starts to move quickly in response to a stimulus must be disturbed by the stimulus. But who is to say that the baby is not simply being awakened and that fetal movements are not actually a response to emotional disturbance? Also, it's difficult to evaluate all the different factors, such as heredity and parenting style, that influence personality development. Use your common sense in how you regard prenatal psychological research.

Still, you might as well do whatever you can to be sure your baby gets the best emotional start. Remember that emotions, positive and negative, are more intense during pregnancy. Resolve stresses quickly, in a positive fashion; seek professional help if necessary. Talk to, sing to, and share affectionate thoughts with your baby. If nothing else, it will make your pregnancy nicer for you. At best it will have a happy effect on baby.

The new and somewhat speculative area of prenatal psychology does not let fathers off the hook either when it comes to a baby's personality development. While a father's emotional state doesn't directly affect the baby, dad can indirectly influence the emotional health of his baby through his relationship with the mother. In fact, as we have previously mentioned, studies show that unhappy marriages pose a risk to the emotional development of the preborn baby. How a man feels about his wife and preborn baby is one of the greatest influences on how secure and content the woman feels. Even prenatally, he can nurture his child by emotionally nourishing the mother.

Traveling While Pregnant

If your work or your pleasure requires travel, you may have concerns about traveling while pregnant. Most routine travel, even air travel, should pose no problem, but check with your health-care provider just in case.

Questions You May Have About Traveling

Here are some of the most commonly asked questions regarding travel.

Before our baby comes, my husband and I want to take a romantic trip alone. When during pregnancy is the best time for a vacation?

By all means treat yourself to a fling before baby arrives; after baby comes, candlelight dinners intended for two and even your bed may have to accommodate an added guest. Your best odds for a safe and satisfying vacation are during the fourth through the sixth month of your pregnancy. In the first trimester, you are likely to be too tired or too nauseated to enjoy your vacation; in the last trimester, you may be too uncomfortable.

I go cross-country on business once a month, so I have to fly. What can I do to be more comfortable? What precautions should I take for my baby?

Since you are traveling for two, take measures to ensure both your baby's safety and your own comfort:

In the last month of your pregnancy, keep your feet on the ground. Domestic-airline regulations prohibit air travel in the last four weeks of your pregnancy (from thirty-six weeks). Foreign airlines prohibit air travel after thirty-five weeks. Don't count on flight attendants being trained midwives. If you look obviously pregnant, airlines will request a note from your health-care provider stating your estimated date of delivery. If you are at risk of delivering your baby prematurely after you are twenty-five weeks along, it's safest not to travel to any place that is not equipped with newborn intensive-care facilities.

Position yourself for comfort. Request a seat as far forward on the aircraft as possible. Not only is the air circulation better in front, it's easier to get on and off the aircraft. Some women find a window seat helpful for minimizing early pregnancy queasiness; others prefer an aisle seat, which makes it easier to get to the bathroom. Many mothers-to-be ask for the bulkhead seats, which have the most leg room. (However, their armrests are stationary, which can restrict your sideways mobility and prevent you from stretching out should the adjacent seat be vacant.) Pregnant women are not allowed to sit in exit rows, because the occupants of those seats are expected to assist with opening a heavy door in an emergency. If you want to be near an emergency exit, choose a seat in the row behind the exit row; seats in the row in front of the emergency exit don't recline. If you are traveling with a companion, request the aisle and window seat, and ask that the middle seat be left vacant if the flight is not full to give you some extra space for maneuvering. If you can afford to upgrade to first-class, now is the time to pamper yourself. Air circulation is usually better in the first-class cabin, too. Cushion your growing body with extra pillows. Elevate your feet as much as possible and walk frequently during the flight to lessen leg swelling. On long flights, expect your feet to expand a size no matter what you do. Once you remove your shoes, you may not be able to get them back on, so be sure to take along a roomier pair, or even a pair of slippers.

Sit in clean air. Absolutely avoid flights where smoking is allowed. (While smoking is not permitted on domestic flights, some foreign carriers still permit smoking.) Even though aircrafts are divided into smoking and nonsmoking sections, trying to keep the air in one section smoke-free is like trying to chlorinate half a swimming pool. (For a discussion of the harmful effects of cigarette smoke to you and your baby, see pages 44 to 48.)

Drink to your thirst's content — and more. Airline air dries the mucous membranes of the mouth and nose and can contribute to dehydration. Drink plenty of caffeine-free, nonalcoholic fluids before, during, and after the flight.

Humidify the air. The humidity of cabin air is only around 7 percent. Besides being uncomfortable to your nasal passages, dry air can contribute to dehydration. In addition to drinking extra fluids, prevent your nasal passages from drying by breathing the steam from a cup of hot water. You can also take along a bottle of saline nasal spray (available without a prescription at any pharmacy), and spray some of the salt water into your nose every hour or so.

Eat comfortably. If you're planning to travel during your first trimester or are still experiencing morning sickness, calling ahead to request a vegetarian meal can increase your chance of getting the airline food that is most friendly to your queasy stomach. Better yet, pack your own already tested munchies. Take special care to avoid gassy foods; the low cabin pressure can cause intestinal gas to expand and contribute to uncomfortable bloating. In flight, nibble frequently to keep your stomach settled. Alert the flight attendant to any special needs.

Avoid nonpressurized high-altitude flights. As you probably know, most airline cabins are pressurized to compensate for the lower levels of oxygen available at high altitudes. Once you get to 7000 feet above sea level, oxygen levels decrease as altitude increases. Be especially careful with commuter flights. Most commuter crafts are not pressurized, since they usually fly at low altitudes, but pilots may have to change flight plans (and exceed 7000 feet) once in the air. While a short time spent in an unpressurized cabin above 7000 feet is unlikely to harm your baby (baby's oxygen level in the womb is already lower than mother's), it can reduce the oxygen in your blood, causing you to feel light-headed, and impair your thinking and ability to move. Oxygen levels can fluctuate even in a pressurized cabin, so ask for some oxygen if you feel lightheaded or disoriented. (Pregnant women should avoid vacationing at altitudes greater than 7000 feet. Some studies show a statistical correlation between living in high altitudes and having lower-birthweight babies.)

Seek assistance. Pregnant women, like senior citizens, should always be given a seat on public transportation or assisted with their luggage. Many people, however — perhaps wishing not to insult a woman's independence by offering aid — do not voluntarily relinquish their seat. Don't be afraid to ask! Be especially careful to avoid stretching and reaching into overhead compartments for heavy luggage. You don't want to overtax any muscles unnecessarily; pregnancy is not the time to strain a muscle. Take advantage of your pregnancy and avail yourself of what manners are left in our society. You deserve a helping hand.

Consult your health-care provider before you travel. Check with your doctor to be sure you do not have any complications of pregnancy that would put you at risk of a preterm delivery or other dangers: preeclampsia, high blood pressure, diabetes that is poorly controlled, a multiple pregnancy, incompetent cervix, repeated miscarriages, previous multiple premature births, or a baby who is not growing optimally in the womb. Many obstetricians encourage women with these complications to avoid airline travel or any long trips in the last three months of their pregnancy.

I worry that passing through airport X-ray security machines may harm my baby. Are they safe?

The handheld security scanners and walk-through security machines in most airports emit low levels of either ultrasound waves or nonionizing radiation, not the potentially dangerous ionizing radiation that comes from hospital X-ray machines (see page 53). While the type of radiation and ultrasound used in these scanners is probably safe, the correct answer is that no one is absolutely certain. As a precaution, instead of being exposed to these machines, you can

ask for a personal search by a female security guard.

We want to take a cruise before our baby arrives, but I'm afraid I'll get seasick.

Cruising can be one of the most relaxing — and romantic — vacations for a pregnant couple. All your dining and entertainment are just an easy walk away, and you don't have to pack and unpack as you would going from hotel to hotel on some land tours. To make your days and nights at sea more comfortable, try these cruising tips:

• Choose your itinerary wisely. If this is your first pregnancy and your first cruise, a long ocean voyage may be a bit unsettling. Try a shorter voyage in calmer waters.

• Choose a large and new ship. The larger and newer ships have stabilizers, which lessen their side-to-side rolling. In fact, the larger the ship, the less likely you are to sense the craft's up-and-down motion and side-to-side roll. On many new ships you may even forget you are at sea.

• Motion is less mid-ship, so choose a cabin in the middle of the ship.

• Choose a balcony cabin. Most of the newer cruise liners have cabins with sliding glass doors that open to a balcony. Access to space and fresh air helps you avoid feeling cramped or confined.

• Ask to be seated as far as possible from the smoking area in the dining room. As often as possible, dine outdoors.

• Take along a pair of acupressure bands (see page 21) in case you do experience seasickness.

I tend to get diarrhea when I travel, but I'm afraid to take anything while I'm pregnant.

Traveler's diarrhea, besides being unsettling to mother, is potentially harmful to baby. Diarrhea depletes your body of necessary nutrients, salts, and fluids, all of which you need more of during pregnancy. If severe and prolonged, diarrhea can dehydrate mother and lessen blood flow to baby. To avoid the foods and germs that cause diarrhea while traveling, take the following precautions:

• Drink only boiled or bottled water. Bottled water is safest, since high doses of iodine, used in some water-purification processes, can be harmful to baby. Use ice cubes made only from bottled water.

• Consume only pasteurized dairy products.

• In countries with a reputation for traveler's diarrhea, avoid uncooked fruits and vegetables. Eat fresh fruit and vegetables only if you wash them in clean water yourself and then peel them.

• Avoid undercooked meat and fish. Don't eat fish from waters known to be mercury-contaminated.

• Dine only at hotels and restaurants that appear to have high standards of sanitation.

If despite many ounces of prevention you still get traveler's diarrhea, your main goal is to keep yourself from getting dehydrated. Here are ways to treat your diarrhea:

• If the diarrhea is severe (more than six watery stools per day), drink small, frequent sips, adding up to a quart or two a day of an oral electrolyte solution. (This is a sugar solution that replenishes the salts and minerals you are likely to lose during diarrhea. It is available without prescription at a pharmacy.) Call your doctor.

• Some over-the-counter antidiarrheal medicines are safe during pregnancy, some are not. Antidiarrheal agents that contain salicylates and bismuth (e.g., Pepto-Bismol) are not safe to take while pregnant, as some animal studies have shown them to be harmful to fetuses. Prescription antidiarrheal medications containing atropine and narcotics are certainly not safe. Consult your doctor about what antidiarrheal medicines are safe to take while pregnant.

• Be prepared. Consult your physician before your trip about what antidiarrheal medications you can safely take during pregnancy, what medications to take along, and what you should do to prevent dehydration.

I'm four months pregnant and have to travel to a foreign country. I'm worried that the required vaccines may harm my baby.

Fortunately, vaccines are no longer required when traveling to most countries. In fact, vaccines are rarely required by law; they are simply suggested. But because the requirements for vaccines frequently change according to the disease prevalence in the area, contact your local health department for up-to-date information, or call the Centers for Disease Control International Travelers' Hotline at 404-332-4559. State that you are pregnant and ask what vaccines are recommended or absolutely necessary for travel to a particular country at this time.

You may have to weigh the risk of getting a particular disease against the risk of harm from the vaccine during pregnancy. If possible, avoid immunizations during the first

three months of pregnancy; avoid live vaccines, and, if possible, avoid typhoid and
cholera, measles, yellow fever, or rubella vaccines. If absolutely necessary, pregnant
women can be given the following vaccines:
tetanus, diphtheria, rabies, and injectable po-
lio. Gammaglobulin and hepatitis B vaccines
are also safe vaccines during pregnancy if absolutely indicated. Since malaria is particularly harmful to pregnant women and their
babies, it's best not to travel to areas where
malaria is prevalent.

*I'm six months pregnant and want to
take a two-week European vacation. But
I'm afraid that I won't have access to
medical treatment should a problem occur. What precautions should I take?*

First, ask your health-care provider for advice
on any special precautions you should take.
Better to know before you go. Then, research
the medical facilities available at your destina-
tion by contacting the U.S. Embassy in the
countries you plan to visit. Information on
English-speaking doctors and hospital facilities can also be obtained from the International Association for Medical Assistance to
Travelers (IAMAT), 417 Center Street, Lewis-
ton, NY 14092 (716-754-4883). You might
also want to check with your insurance carrier to see if you're covered while traveling.
Many insurance companies require a supplemental fee for coverage during travel to a foreign country. Last, if you have had special
complications during your pregnancy, take
along pertinent medical records.

When traveling during pregnancy, you'll
want to continue as much as possible the
healthy living styles you follow at home. Eat
healthy, appealing, and low-risk foods. (See
food precautions, page 231.) Listen to your
body's signals: urinate when you have the

Safe and Comfortable Car Travel

To travel safely and comfortably by car,
try these tips:

- Wear your seat belt. Don't worry that the
seat belt will squeeze your uterus and
harm your baby in the event of a crash.
The amniotic fluid will help to protect the
baby, and studies have shown both mother
and baby are more likely to survive a crash
when secured in a properly positioned
seat belt. Buckle up properly.
- Raise the headrest on the back of the seat
to reach the level of your head. Not only is
it nice to be able to lean back, but the
headrest also helps prevent whiplash in
the case of an accident.
- Stop, stretch, and stroll at least every two
hours during long trips. Make frequent
bathroom stops.
- Move the seat back and stretch your legs.
- Practice "sitting still exercises" (see page
181).
- Use pillows.
- Take along a snack pack.

Place the lap belt as low as possible
below your uterus, underneath baby
and snug across your upper thighs
and hipbones. If the belt presses
uncomfortably on your protuberant
pelvis, insert a small pillow or pad
between the belt and your lap. Place the
shoulder belt above your uterus and
between your breasts, but not so high as
to chafe your neck.

urge to go (bathroom availability may not be as convenient in other countries) and avoid constipation. Don't give in to the urge to relax your vigilance as you relax your body. Avoid taking unwise risks: accidents can be more common on strange turf. Now you have another life to consider, so travel wisely — you're traveling for two.

MORE CHOICES IN CHILDBIRTH

Choosing a Childbirth Class

You should take a childbirth class for the same reason you are reading this book: the more informed you are, the more satisfying your pregnancy and delivery are likely to be. And a satisfying birth will get your parenting career off to a confident beginning. Besides, the class provides a social group where you will feel comfortable talking about your pregnancy.

When to enroll. Most childbirth educators gear their regular classes toward women nearing the end of their second trimester. These classes generally run from six to twelve weeks and ideally end a week or so before your due date, so the knowledge you gain will be fresh in your mind when you deliver. As we advised on page 74, consider taking an "early bird" class in the first month or two of your pregnancy.

What you will learn. Besides helping you explore the many birth options available to expectant couples and work out your own personal birth philosophy, a complete childbirth class should cover the following:

• *What's going on in your body in each month of pregnancy.* By the use of illustrations and charts, you will learn the anatomy and physiology of the miracle that's going

on inside you, and about the miracles to come. (In Martha's early days of teaching childbirth education classes one night a week, our living room was regularly filled with pictures of the various stages of pregnancy and delivery. You can imagine the questions we got from our curious children!)

• *Good nutrition throughout your pregnancy.* For many couples, this is the first time in their lives that they have had a course on nutrition, and it may also be the first time in their lives that they have been motivated to eat right.

• *The wise use of tests and technology.* A good class should teach the expectant couple to be wise consumers: to know what tests are available, when and why they are used, and how to decide whether to have them. The class should teach you what questions to ask your practitioner and how to be sure your questions are answered to your satisfaction.

• *Exercise during pregnancy.* You'll learn when, what, and how much to exercise.

• *Stages of labor.* You will learn how to recognize your body's signals at each stage of labor.

• *Relaxation and pain-management techniques.* A painless birth is a promise on which no childbirth class can deliver. You will learn that pain has a purpose in birth: it's a signal to do something. Pain means you need to make a change. A good childbirth class will explore not only relaxation skills and self-help methods, but also medical methods of pain relief, so that you go into labor armed with a whole menu of pain-management strategies and the knowledge to enable you to choose and use the ones that are right for you. A wise child-birth educator does not present birth as a contest to see how much pain a woman can withstand. Rather, she advises women on using both natural and medical pain re-lievers wisely. Parents should not be made to feel that opting for medication means they have failed. Some women find child-birth classes too lenient about medication; other women find childbirth classes too dogmatic about the risks of medications. Best is a balanced approach.

• *The role of your labor coach, usually your mate.* Many fathers, when asked at the first class why they are there, honestly say, "To please my wife." Don't worry if your hus-band is initially reluctant to participate. In our experience, once dads appreciate what's going on inside the body of their pregnant wife, they become more sympa-thetic and helpful. They also learn a lot from the give-and-take with other pregnant couples in the class.

• *The how-to's of breastfeeding.* Successful breastfeeding depends on a good start; the more you know before you begin — especially the importance of proper posi-tioning and latch-on techniques — the eas-ier it will be.

• *Postpartum issues.* You'll cover whether to leave your baby intact or have him circum-cised, how and when to introduce the new baby to the whole family, what to expect from your postpartum body, even the basics of newborn care. A good childbirth class not only helps you have a safer and more satisfying birth, it helps prepare you to ad-just to the many changes a baby brings to your family.

Perhaps the most valuable lesson you will learn in childbirth classes is how to break the fear-tension-pain cycle. Dr. Grantly Dick-Read, a pioneer in the field of unmedicated birth, identified this cycle as a key reason many women need drugs during childbirth. By eliminating the fear of childbirth (especially the fear of the unknown), by telling women how their bodies work in labor and why they feel the way they do, by teaching relaxation techniques to reduce the tension in minds and muscles produced by that fear, and by showing women how to work *with* rather than against their bodies in labor, Dr. Dick-Read demonstrated that most women do not have to choose between suffering greatly or being heavily drugged to give birth.

Childbirth classes can also provide a ready-made support group to help you through your individual questions and introduce you to friends you can call on after your birth. You may also learn from experienced moth-ers in the class who share their previous birth experiences and what they want to do differently this time around. A fun part of the childbirth class was what we called the "show-and-tell" night. A month or so after the last couple delivered, everyone gathered for a reunion to show off their babies and swap birth stories.

How to choose a class. Your reasons for choosing a class should be better than which one is closest to your home or offered at the most convenient times. It's worthwhile to change your schedule so that you can take a class that supports your birth philosophy. It's helpful to have at least interviewed yourself about a preliminary birth philosophy (see page 256) before you sign up for a class. At the very least, do some reading and talk to veteran mothers. Attending an early-bird class is another way to work out a birth philoso-phy before choosing a class to take during the last weeks of pregnancy. Doing your homework before you choose a class will enable you to select a class that fits your needs.

Just as one mother chooses an obstetrician for her birth attendant and another chooses a midwife, different women will choose different approaches to childbirth education. There are three prominent schools of thought in childbirth education, and many types of classes are spinoffs or combinations of these three. One type of class is not better than another; each offers a different approach and will meet different needs and support different birth philosophies. Childbirth education philosophies differ on two main points: their approaches to pain management and whether they prepare women to fully accept the currently available medical system — to work with the current system — or to seek alternatives outside the system.

ASPO/Lamaze

Now the most popular method with North American couples, ASPO/Lamaze had its beginnings in Russia as a spinoff of the teachings of Dr. Ivan Petrovich Pavlov, who conditioned dogs to salivate at the sound of a bell. A French obstetrician, Fernand Lamaze, brought these conditioned-response exercises to Europe, added breathing patterns and a *monitrice* (a highly trained labor support person), and created the package that became known as "The Lamaze Method." It was originally called "psychoprophylaxis" because it focused on preparing the mother to use her mind to condition her body's response to pain; its practitioners in the United States founded the American Society of Psychoprophylaxis in Obstetrics (ASPO). The organization is now known as ASPO/Lamaze, and its teachers are known as ASPO-certified childbirth educators, or ACCEs. There are more ASPO/Lamaze classes offered in this country than any other kind of class.

One major difference between Lamaze and other methods of childbirth education is its approach to pain management. Through learned breathing patterns, dubbed "paced breathing," and by focusing on imaginary or real diversions, Lamaze classes teach a woman to divert her attention from her pains in order to convince her mind that her body really doesn't hurt. Originally these breathing patterns were quite contrived and varied, with several types of tempos being used in each of the four distinct phases of labor. Unless a woman practiced religiously and trained herself to focus and breathe like a robot, the breathing patterns often became counterproductive, producing tension rather than relaxation. In the past decade or so, ASPO has been teaching a wider variety of techniques for pain control and emphasizing relaxation skills. Lamaze students are also taught the advantages and disadvantages of all medical options of pain relief. The Lamaze graduate is then equipped to choose either no medication, an injection of pain reliever, or epidural anesthesia without feeling that any judgment is being placed on her choice. Some women choose Lamaze because they do not want the "full experience" of birth; they just want to be informed and reasonably comfortable, and to take home a healthy baby.

The other distinctive trait of Lamaze, and one of the secrets of its success, is that its teachers tend to be less "radical" than teachers of other methods. The medical establishment generally backs Lamaze programs, since most ASPO classes are hospital-based and focus more on preparing their clients to deliver within the medical system that is available in their community than on arming their students to shake up the obstetrical-hospital world. (Not all ASPO instructors are hospital employees, and some do teach independently.) To find out more about ASPO and which classes are available in your community, contact the American Society for Psychoprophylaxis in Obstetrics (ASPO), 1200 19th Street NW, Washington, DC 20036 (800-368-4404).

The Bradley Method®

Also called "Husband-Coached Childbirth," this method was developed in the 1940s by Denver obstetrician Robert Bradley. Central to the Bradley approach is a more physiological rather than a psychological approach to pain. Dr. Bradley believes that it is healthier for a woman to be involved in the sensations of her labor than to try to escape from them; that pain, rather than being a problem to get rid of, is a signal to be listened to. The Bradley philosophy and the people who teach it are passionate about instructing women to trust their bodies. They believe that nearly all women, given proper education and support, can have a safe and satisfying birth without medication — and over 90 percent of Bradley grads do. Rather than using diversions to try to control or cover up their birth sensations, Bradley laborers are encouraged to relax themselves, listen to their basic instincts, and work with their bodies (mostly by position changes during labor and delivery) to find their own way to labor most comfortably and efficiently. Bradley recommends breathing techniques that are more natural and less conditioned than those promoted by Lamaze. Bradley courses tend to be more detailed and longer (usually twelve weeks) than most other methods. The classes not only help women to be informed participants in their birthing decisions, they also equip them to be wise consumers.

Because it teaches women to question childbirth policies, Bradley is often perceived as being at odds with the current maternity health-care delivery system and is therefore not embraced with open arms by many obstetricians and hospitals. Opponents claim that Bradley prepares couples better for "alternative" out-of-hospital births than for traditional births. However, in our experience, if a mother truly wants to have a natural birth in a hospital, Bradley gives her the best chance of doing so. It is true, however, that Bradley pupils are more likely to get an earful from their instructors about their personal obstetrical biases; in some instances this approach serves no useful purpose and only undermines the trust between a mother and her chosen practitioner. For information about Bradley, contact the American Academy of Husband-Coached Childbirth (AAHC) — The Bradley Method®, PO Box 5224, Sherman Oaks, CA 91413-5524 (800-423-2397; in California, 800-42-BIRTH).

The International Childbirth Education Association (ICEA)

This organization trains and certifies teachers who incorporate the best of several methods into their instruction, in keeping with the organization's motto: "Freedom of choice through knowledge of alternatives." The ICEA is a credible source of information for expectant couples and childbirth educators. Members hold national conventions, operate a mail-order bookstore for parenting and pregnancy resources, and put out some of the best and best-researched childcare pamphlets in the business. For more information on resources from the ICEA or on how to find your nearest ICEA instructor, contact the International Childbirth Education Association (ICEA), PO Box 20048, Minneapolis, MN 55420 (612-854-8660).

All of the Above

Many childbirth instructors incorporate the best of Lamaze, ICEA, and Bradley, add what they have learned from their own birthing experiences, and formulate a unique educational package. Because they are not locked into one method, these "independents" enjoy the flexibility of tailoring their classes to the individual needs of their clients. In teaching her childbirth classes, Martha has found the most useful approach is an integrated one: taking the best of each method and offering a more balanced curriculum.

Before you make your final choice, interview or sit in on a class led by various instructors. Ask the following questions:

- Has the instructor experienced birth herself? Have her own personal birth experiences become an asset to her teaching? Does she have some personal biases or chips on her shoulder that could cause you to project an adversarial attitude onto or toward your practitioner?

- Is she familiar with the local hospital routines, especially those of the hospital that you have chosen?

- Does she keep her classes small enough (preferably no more than eight couples) to be able to give you individualized attention? Does she make learning easier through the use of visual aids: dolls, posters and charts, movies and videos, handouts?

- Does she offer her experience, opinions, and guidance yet remain open-minded enough to help you achieve the birth you want?

- Does she emphasize relaxation and self-help techniques? Does she spend a good portion of the class helping participants practice them? While relaxation is the key to a drug-free birth (also dubbed a "pure" birth), it is also essential in a medically assisted birth. One of the most useful parts of any childbirth class is practicing various positions for labor and delivery, especially ones that emphasize a more vertical position and downplay the traditional horizontal ones.

- Does she provide adequate time for group discussion and for answering questions?

To increase your chances of having a satisfying birth experience, do a lot of book work, leg work, and phone work to pick the childbirth class that is best for you. Ask any prospective childbirth educator for names of her previous clients and check her references. Ask yourself if you feel comfortable with both her style and her course content. Talk to friends, not only about their childbirth educators, but about what they wish they had known (or done differently) at the time of their baby's birth. Realize there will be a huge range in the cost of a series of classes. Some hospital classes may be included in the cost of your birth package or be quite inexpensive, because the number of couples will fill up a whole lecture room. In other cases, where class length and content may be double that of others, expect the price to be at least double, especially if the number of students is low. Find out what you will be getting for your money. A good class is worth every penny.

The best thing I learned from childbirth class was how to become a better decision maker.

Choosing a Birth Place

As you assemble the right team to help you birth your baby, you also need to choose the right place for this special event to happen. Oftentimes, the birth attendant and the birth place go together as a package. The doctor

The Coach

Both Lamaze and Bradley have in the past emphasized the role of the father as labor coach. Few men are comfortable with the role, and few women find their mate's play-by-play strategizing helpful. Most childbirth methods, while still emphasizing the important function of the father at birth, have redefined the father's role as one of psychological supporter and reassigned the coaching task to a professional labor assistant (see page 273).

Dr. Bill notes: I am a very good Little League baseball coach, but I don't feel comfortable as a coach for laboring women. My first experience as birth coach was twenty-nine years ago, when, even after rehearsing all those breathing and stopwatch exercises, I panicked at Martha's first contraction. At the height of her labor, I totally forgot what I had learned in the classes and did what I naturally did best — loved my wife. Once I dropped the role of coach and took on the role of lover, the whole process became more natural for me and better for Martha.

you choose may deliver at only one hospital. Many times, however, you have a choice of hospitals, so it's back to doing your homework, or, in this case, leg work.

Liz, a friend of ours, was very happy with her midwife-assisted birth:

My husband was really nervous about a home birth for a first pregnancy, but I really wanted a midwife. Luckily, we live in a big city with several midwife groups affiliated with hospitals. My midwife arrived at the hospital just after I did. My water had broken, and my contractions were coming on too fast. I wasn't dilating at all, and I was vomiting like crazy. When she suggested medication to slow things down, I felt like a failure at first. I wanted no intervention; that's why I had chosen a midwife in the first place! But the fact that a midwife and not a doctor suggested medication made it easier to accept, somehow. She was right. My contractions became productive and soon I was propped up, one foot on the hip of the midwife and one on the hip of a nurse, pushing. Perineal massage really helped, too. Five minutes later my son was born and placed right into my arms. The midwife and the nurses helped me breastfeed him. I held him while I delivered the placenta, and we stayed cuddled for over an hour while I rested.

Choosing a Hospital

Women of the '80s and '90s have influenced how business is done in many fields — and the birth business is no exception. Over the past decade hospitals have become more family-friendly. In fact, the obstetrical ward in most hospitals has undergone a name change: now it's the "family birth center" or "family-centered maternity care" — whatever marketing term will convince today's savvy birth consumer that a particular hospital is a nice place to have a baby. Gone are the days when maternity wards looked like surgical wards, when mother labored in one room, was wheeled into another room to have the baby, and was then shuttled into another room to recover from the procedure while her baby went into still another room, the nursery, and dad was stuck in the waiting room.

Nowadays every hospital that plans to stay in the baby business offers the "LDRP concept": mother *l*abors, *d*elivers, *r*ecovers, and spends her *p*ostpartum stay in one room, and baby and mother are together unless a medical complication requires them to be separated temporarily. (Some places have LDRs; in these hospitals, mother spends her postpartum time in another area.) Interior decorators have outdone themselves, creating a homelike atmosphere in these rooms. In fact, most birthing rooms, as they are sometimes called, look very much like a comfortable hotel room. They are pleasant and inviting, with a rocking chair, curtains, an attractive bedspread, maybe matching wallpaper, and a cradle. There may even be a tub, and a bed for your mate. At first glance, the birthing bed resembles any other bed, but it is adjustable and will accommodate many different labor-friendly positions. All the obstetrical equipment is unobtrusively but efficiently placed around the room. At the push of a button, a huge light can descend from the ceiling, and cupboards can be opened and all the necessary emergency equipment wheeled over. Mother and father, and often siblings, if desired, are present as mother begins labor in this room and delivers the baby in this room, and they all spend their entire postpartum stay in this mother-and-baby-friendly place (or go to a postpartum room if it is an LDR). Of course, baby rooms-in with mother. Father's presence during labor and birth is no longer considered optional; he is expected to be present and to participate.

When you are selecting a hospital, don't be oversold by the appearance of the birthing room. The skills and attitudes of your birth attendants matter much more to the health and well-being of you and your baby than whether or not the bedspread and draperies match. When selecting a hospital, consider this rating system:

5-star hospital. While a 5-star birthing facility may exist only in the realm of fantasy now, history shows that hospitals will eventually supply what mothers demand. Here is an ideal that we hope many hospitals will shoot for:

☐ A family-centered maternity unit with LDR suites. A nice place to labor, deliver, and enjoy the first day of your life with your baby.

☐ Oversized labor tubs. The newest innovation among the many natural methods to ease labor pains (see page 309).

☐ A birthing bed that is comfortable to labor and sleep in, yet adjusts to many positions to accommodate different stages and styles of labor.

☐ The latest noninvasive technology, especially the new electronic fetal monitoring by telemetry, in which baby's heart-rate changes can be monitored without mother having to stay in bed or be tethered by wires to a bedside machine.

☐ Up-to-date intravenous technology and policy: saline or heparin-lock devices, which allow mothers to walk and roam around (instead of the older intravenous equipment that requires mother's IV to be attached to tubing all the time, forcing her to remain in bed) should be used when medically necessary.

☐ A "level-3" special-care or newborn intensive-care unit. A level-3 facility has all the equipment and personnel essential to provide top-quality care to a sick newborn, including assisted ventilation for respiratory problems and twenty-four-hour access to on-premises neonatologists. An on-premises neonatologist is crucial should the baby need specialized care at the moment of delivery; having essential equipment nearby also saves transferring a sick newborn to another facility and separating mother and baby.

☐ Access to anesthesia specialists. The hospital has an anesthesiologist or nurse-anesthetist residing in the hospital twenty-four hours a day in case an emergency cesarean section or other obstetrical emergency occurs.

☐ Nurse-midwives. Midwives are intricately involved in the obstetrical facility, either as head nurses, labor support persons, or as the primary attendants at low-risk, uncomplicated births.

☐ A certified lactation consultant (or obstetrical nurses with such certification) on staff to help breastfeeding mothers get the right start.

☐ A flexible birthing philosophy. Wearing both a "natural" and a "medical" hat is difficult, if not impossible, for most obstetrical units. Nevertheless, a 5-star hospital operates with the knowledge that 90 percent of births are uncomplicated. Attendants assist mothers with walking during labor, encourage delivering in whatever position is most comfortable for mother and most healthy for baby, and are open to following

a mother's birth wishes and birth plan as long as these are in the best medical interest of mother and baby. On the other hand, the staff is able to click into the medical mind-set should an unanticipated complication arise or a high-risk patient be delivering.

A hospital is able to wear both hats well only by employing midwives on the obstetrical unit or by allowing certified midwife deliveries in the hospital. Few, if any, medical doctors think like midwives do, and midwives are not trained as doctors. The two professions reflect their different styles of training. In the right environment they complement each other beautifully.

4-star hospital. A 4-star facility has all of the services of the 5-star ideal except midwife involvement. There are now 4-star hospitals that provide an excellent standard of obstetrical care in nearly every major city.

3-star hospital. The obstetrical units in a 3-star hospital, many of which are found in smaller communities, do not have a level-3 nursery or twenty-four-hour in-hospital anesthesia coverage. Anesthesiologists are on call should an emergency arise, but there is usually at least a twenty-minute delay. For many uncomplicated, low-risk deliveries, a 3-star facility is just fine — and it may be the only level your community can support. Many of these facilities have level-2 nurseries that can care for sick newborns; some have newborn specialists on call.

2-star hospital. A 2-star facility has a nice LDR room but no special-care nurseries for newborns or in-house anesthesia, and it may or may not have new technology such as telemetry that allows mothers the freedom to walk while being monitored.

1-star hospital. It has no LDRP facility, no new technology, no new birthing philosophies, and looks like a surgical unit. Shop around.

Choosing a Birth Center

The main difference between a birth center and a hospital is not so much what the birthing room looks like (birthing rooms are beginning to look a lot alike), but the birthing philosophy. Birth centers are a women-run show, and midwives usually attend all the normal deliveries, with obstetricians available as consultants (and backups in case transfer to a hospital becomes necessary). Birth-center midwives focus on supporting the mother and the birth she wants. Birth centers trust nature, are cautious about technology, and assume that most of the time everything will go right (whereas hospital philosophy assumes that something may go wrong). Opponents of birth centers fear that the pregnant woman places herself and her baby at unnecessary risk, since emergency care that can be given only in a hospital is not immediately available at a birth center. Proponents of birth centers counter that because a mother is allowed to labor and deliver in a more natural way, she is less likely to need emergency care.

A professionally staffed, properly accredited birth center is a safe alternative to a hospital birth. In 1989 one of the most reputable medical journals, the *New England Journal of Medicine,* reported a study of twelve thousand women admitted for labor and delivery to eighty-four birth centers in the United States. The cesarean section rate for women

in this study was 4.4 percent, far below the national average. There were no maternal deaths, and the neonatal death rate was well below average. Twenty-five percent of first-time mothers had to be transferred to a hospital, and only 7 percent of women who had had a previous birth needed to be transferred. The study concluded that a birth center offers a safe and acceptable alternative to hospital birth for low-risk expectant mothers. So if you are low-risk and have a "proven pelvis" (i.e., you have previously delivered a baby vaginally), delivering in a birth center is an alternative to consider. If you are a low-risk, first-time mother, you might consider a birth center, but do your homework about hospitals and get to know your backup obstetrician in case a transfer is necessary. This way, you can combine the environment and birthing philosophy of a birth center with the option of having a satisfying birth in the hospital should it become necessary.

Choosing a Home Birth

In 1900 at least 95 percent of births took place at home; in the 1990s more than 95 percent of women deliver in hospitals. Whether or not this represents progress depends on whether you ask an obstetrician, a midwife, or seek the opinion of various childbirth reform organizations. For most women, especially in today's maternity-care delivery system, a home birth is neither a desirable nor realistic alternative, but some women do want to explore this option. We wish these women to be informed and discerning about home birth, and to make this decision with at least as much, if not more, care than they would about other birth place alternatives.

Checking Out a Hospital

It's the rare hospital that will have everything a mother wants, and, unfortunately, your choice of hospital may be limited by what is available in your area, by your insurance plan, or by your own needs (especially if this is a high-risk pregnancy). If you do have a choice in hospitals, use this checklist to compare them; if not, use it to determine what you can expect from your birth experience, and which important items you may wish to negotiate. The more you know ahead of time, the better you will be able to enjoy your experience.

- Is there a birthing bed or an old-fashioned delivery table?
- Is there an LDR suite that you will be comfortable birthing in and living in for a day or so?
- Who can use the LDR room? Years ago only "low-risk" women could use the LDR room. Studies have shown, however, that many "high-risk" mothers have lower-risk deliveries if they are able to deliver in the homelike and unintimidating environment of the LDR room. (Studies have also shown that a mother who is at higher risk for having a cesarean is more likely to need an operation if she is put in a birthing room that looks like an operating room.)
- Are there enough LDR rooms, or might you get stuck in a regular delivery room if you're the last one in on a busy night?
- Does the birthing philosophy of the staff match the attractiveness of the LDR room? Does the administration support individual birth plans? Are the nurses friendly and unintimidating? Are they eager to know what mothers want and willing to help them get it?
- Is there an anesthesiologist in the hospital twenty-four hours a day or just someone on call outside the hospital?
- What is the level of newborn nursery care? A level-3 facility has a full-service intensive-care unit with full-time, in-hospital neonatologists; seldom is there a reason to transfer a sick newborn to another hospital. Level 2 means the hospital has the staff and facilities for less serious illnesses, but more serious cases must be transferred. The neonatologist may be in the hospital or on call. Level 1 means there is no neonatologist on staff (though one may be available for consultation) and no facilities to

Questions You May Have About Home Births

Here are common questions women have about home birthing.

I'm considering a home birth, but I'm worried about what would happen if something goes wrong. Are home births safe?

A more important issue is whether or not a home birth is right and safe *for you*. Studies from European countries where home births are the rule rather than the exception show that if a mother has been properly selected (i.e., she has been deemed "low-risk" by a qualified obstetrician or midwife) and the home birth has been expertly attended (by a qualified doctor or midwife), home birthing is safe. In North America, the safety of home birth is another issue. It's not that home birth in itself is unsafe; it's that the current maternity-care delivery system in North care for an infant with respiratory distress. Most sick infants are transferred to a level-2 or -3 hospital.

- Are there midwives on staff?
- How much labor support will the obstetrical nurses provide during your labor? What will they do? Are they open to your employing your own professional labor support person? Do they have a list of such persons from which to choose?
- Are you encouraged to move around as you wish during labor and to deliver your baby in whatever position works for you? Does the staff allow vertical birthing?
- What are the policies concerning the use of intravenous? If you need an IV, will they use a heparin lock so that you can move around?
- What are the policies concerning electronic fetal monitoring? Is it used routinely? Will the staff use the new technology of telemetry, or must you stay in bed while being monitored?
- Do the LDR rooms have comfortable labor tubs, so that you can use water to ease your labor discomfort?
- Are you allowed to drink and snack as you wish during labor?
- Is the baby placed on your abdomen immediately after birth?

- Must the baby spend time in the nursery for observation? Are nursing babies given supplemental feedings or encouraged to feed on demand? Are mothers encouraged to keep their babies with them and nurse during the night?
- What education is provided to assist you in getting the right start with your newborn? Infant-care classes? Consultations with lactation specialists or certified breastfeeding consultants?
- Are there any restrictions on taking photos and videos?
- What are the routines concerning mother-infant bonding? Is full rooming-in available? If baby needs to be transferred to a special-care nursery, are you allowed to visit as you wish?
- What are the hospital costs? What are the extra costs (for telephone and television, for example)? Be sure to find out what your insurance will cover and what it will not.
- What are the policies concerning visitors? Who can attend the birth? Who can visit afterward? When can siblings visit? Is there an age restriction?
- Does the hospital provide a visiting nurse or lactation consultant to check on you and baby at home?

America may make it an unsafe option for the majority of women. In European countries where home birth is common, obstetricians and midwives work together in a shared enterprise, obstetricians and hospitals provide backup for midwives attending home births, and there is an efficient transport system in case of emergencies. In the majority of areas in North America, there is currently no safe, established backup system for home birthing. For the majority of women in the majority of

communities, until this European model is set up in North America, home birthing is an unwise and risky decision.

Many obstetricians are philosophically very comfortable with the concept of home birth, but they do not choose either to perform home births or to provide backup home birth services. The problem with providing home delivery backup from an obstetrician's point of view is that he or she inherits another birth attendant's complications and is

Checking Out a Birth Center

If you are considering a birth center, evaluate the following:

- Is the birth center licensed and a member of The National Association of Childbearing Centers (NACC)?
- What are the credentials of the midwives? Are they licensed midwives? Are they certified nurse-midwives?
- Are there obstetricians affiliated with the center? Is there adequate obstetrical backup in case unanticipated complications occur during your pregnancy or your birth? Will you meet the backup physician ahead of time?
- Ask about the criteria for delivering in a particular birth center. Do you have an obstetrical history that meets these criteria, or do you have risk factors that might jeopardize the health and safety of yourself or your baby if you have an out-of-hospital birth?

- To which hospital does the birth center transfer mothers? Do they have a regular working relationship with this hospital? What is the transfer rate of the birth center (i.e., the percentage of mothers who begin their labor in the birth center but are transferred to the hospital for delivery)? What are the criteria for transfer? What are the transfer procedures?
- If you need to be transferred to the hospital, who will care for you there? The obstetrician who backs up the birth center? The midwife who attended you at the birth center? Will someone from the birth center stay with you at the hospital for your birth?

Browse around the birth center for a while. Ask for the names of parents who have recently labored in the center and talk to them. Do you feel safe and comfortable laboring and delivering in this facility?

then held responsible, as well as liable, for the outcome. Obstetricians believe safely performing a home birth requires an entire system to be set up, with standards applied to that system. In the United States, this system is not adequately organized for home birth.

During the writing of this book we had the opportunity to talk to many maternity health-care providers in various areas of the country, and even to visit some in Europe. Our conclusion is that it is not always the place of birth that determines the safety for mother and baby; rather, it is the overall system of maternity care. Organizations that discourage home birth claim that hospital birth is safer, even for low-risk women, in case an unforeseen complication occurs. Birth re-

formers argue that home birth is safer because with less intervention a complication is less likely to occur. Hospital birthing and home birthing have different risk factors that each couple and their health-care provider must consider.

Morbidity and mortality statistics are on the side of home birth, but those statistics may not apply to you or your community. If you dare to bring up the topic of home birth, choose your listeners wisely. Some may think you are foolish for even thinking of any option that they assume could jeopardize the health of you or your baby. Others may be more empathetic, considering you to be an informed consumer — wanting to do what is actually best for yourself and your baby.

During one of my childbirth classes, I overheard two women discussing their birth choices. "You are brave to have a home birth," said one concerned woman. "You are brave to have a hospital birth," replied the other. Why do some women rave about home birth while others feel it can be risky?

Women who fear a home birth because it is risky certainly should not have one. Women who rave about home birth probably entered the experience with a different mind-set. Here are the advantages of home birthing that women have reported to us:

• They feel more in control in their own homes than in a strange, new place, such as a birth center or hospital.

• They feel less anxious at home. For many women, birthing in their own home takes a lot of the fear factor out of birth. In the hospital, the machines and staff hovering around instill a fearful and constant reminder that something awful might happen.

• In their home, they set their own routines. The policies are those that they have worked out ahead of time with their family and birth attendants. They can invite those they wish; no strangers are allowed.

• In some cases, because they are less fearful and more relaxed at home than in the hospital, they can work with their body, helping their labor progress more efficiently and with less pain, even though they do not have access to medical pain relief.

• They can labor at their own pace, without being hurried by the system.

• If they want to have a midwife-attended birth, they usually have more options at home, since most hospitals are currently not set up to allow mother-chosen midwives to deliver babies.

• Family bonding is easier at home, and naturally baby rooms-in with mother. There are no trivial routine procedures, classes to interrupt mother and baby's postpartum peace, check-out procedures, and drives home. Many women enjoy having their birth be a family affair. Appropriate-age children (usually three years of age and up) can more readily bond with the new baby, and they can learn a lot about their mother and about birth. Carefully selected friends and relatives can be present, and they set the visiting hours.

I really want to have a home birth, but I don't want to do anything crazy to endanger the health of myself or my baby. What should I do to increase my chances of having a safe home birth?

First, interview yourself to be sure you really are a candidate for home birth. Do you really want a home birth for your own reasons and not because of pressure from friends? Do you really want to deliver at home, or are you just afraid of hospitals? It's better to have a home birth because you truly believe home is where you belong rather than because you don't like hospitals. Answer the following questions:

☐ Do you trust your body to work for you? While it's normal for all women to carry some fear into birth, regardless of the birth attendant or birth place, you need an especially positive attitude for a safe home birth. If you're afraid to have a home birth, you shouldn't have one.

☐ Are you truly convinced that your body will work better for you when birthing at home?

☐ Do you have a proven pelvis? Have you previously delivered safely at home or had an uncomplicated birth in a hospital or birth center? Knowing that in the past your body worked well for you helps you feel it's more likely to come through for you again. That feeling takes much of the fear and riskiness out of home birth. (Consider, however, that no two deliveries are the same, and unforeseen complications can occur with any pregnancy and delivery, even if there was no previous history or warning.)

☐ Do you and your mate agree on having your baby at home? Many men are more fearful of home birth than are women, perhaps because of the common male mindset of wanting to fix or control anything that could go wrong. Most men feel more secure in the hospital setting, with their wife and baby being monitored by machines and medical personnel and with equipment being instantly available should a complication arise. If you are seriously considering a home birth, you may have to do a lot of educating and even more marketing to convince your mate.

☐ What is your history of handling stress and pain? Remember that epidural anesthesia that your friend raved about so much in her near-painless childbirth? Epidurals are not an option at home, and in most instances no medications for pain relief will be available. For women strongly considering a home birth, this can be a blessing, since if medication is not available, they are more motivated to use natural and creative ways to ease the discomforts of labor. On the other hand, for many women, even those committed to the most natural of all childbirths, it's comforting to know that medical pain relief is available should they want it. That is not an option for most midwife-attended home births (though midwives do know much about nonmedical pain relief, such as positioning and relaxation, with the big plus of being able to fully use water for pain relief at home).

☐ Who is your primary birth attendant? Do you have a licensed and certified midwife in whom you have unquestionable confidence? Does she have obstetrical backup? (See pages 38 to 43.) Do what you can to lessen the birth surprises. Even though you plan for your primary birth attendant during pregnancy and delivery to be your chosen midwife, it's wise to cover all your bases by scheduling a couple of appointments with the backup physician. To lessen surprises at the time of delivery, this physician, in addition to performing a hands-on exam, may recommend an ultrasound or other tests that, if normal, can actually lessen your fear and increase your confidence in your choice to birth at home.

Above all, do whatever you can to lessen the chances of the following scene:

I believed in my body, my midwife, and my home. I took impeccable care of myself during my pregnancy and read every birth book. But through no one's fault, our baby's heartbeat started to go down during my home labor, and we rushed to the hospital. As soon as I got to the emergency room, I was quickly labeled "one of those irresponsible home birth fanatics." I was assigned an anonymous obstetrician, and the hospital staff were less than friendly — some even to the point of being punitive. I wished I had found a doctor beforehand who could have met me at the hospital and cleared my path.

In some ways having a home birth is simpler than a hospital birth, and when it works, it is a beautiful family experience. In other ways, choosing a home birth is more complicated: it requires more homework to decide if it is the right option for you and to learn what home-birthing attendants are available in your community and what backup facilities are available should your home birth not go according to plan. For expectant parents who want to be more informed about the options for out-of-hospital births, especially home births, try the following resources:

NAPSAC (National Association of Parents and Professionals for Safe Alternatives in Childbirth)
Route 1, PO Box 646, Marble Hill, MO 63764
(573-238-2010)

National Association of Childbearing Centers
3123 Gottschall Road, Perkiomenville, PA 18074 (215-234-8068)

American College of Home Obstetrics
PO Box 508, Oak Park, IL 60303
(708-383-1461)

Association for Childbirth at Home International
PO Box 430, Glendale, CA 91209
(213-667-0839)

California Association of Midwives (CAM)
PO Box 417854, Sacramento, CA 95841
(800-829-5791)
(Request their publication "Midwife Means 'With Woman,'" an informative fifty-six-page booklet about choosing and using a midwife.)

The American College of Nurse-Midwives (ACNM)
818 Connecticut Avenue NW, Suite 900, Washington, DC 20006 (202-728-9860)

Informed Homebirth and Parenting
PO Box 3675, Ann Arbor, MI 48106
(313-662-6857)

MANA (Midwives Alliance of North America)
600 Fifth Street, Monett, MO 65708

At home I felt more like a participant than a patient. If my midwife offered a suggestion, I could participate in the decision because I felt like the star of the show. In fact, I was the star of the show; everyone else was a member of my supporting cast.

I liked being able to feather my own nest and then crawl into it. As soon as labor began, I could tune into my own body without having to worry about packing bags, shuttling kids off to friends, driving to a hospital, and having my husband whisked off to do all that paperwork.

I liked the idea of being in my own home. Yes, no one in the hospital will ask you, "What should I do with the clothes that are in the dryer?" or "Which bedsheets?" just as a contraction is starting. But I did have the comfort of my own bed, my own bathroom, and as much privacy as I wanted. The midwife and her assistant were guests in my home and did things my way, so that I could concentrate on myself, my husband, my older son, and my new baby.

I could tune into my body, go with my instincts, move when I wanted to, and get into any position that helped me feel better. I could squat, kneel, moan, grunt, whatever I felt like doing without worrying about whether I was doing something wrong, unusual, or against hospital policy.

I had a long but steadily progressive labor. I loved laboring at the pace that was good for me — and I felt that what was good for me was good for my baby — without being compared to the "usual laboring woman" on a chart. Because my labor didn't fall within the usual "normals" in the hospital, I probably would have been offered many interventions to hurry my labor, along with the not-so-subtle implication that if I didn't go along I would be jeopardizing myself and my baby.

I made a pretend decision to deliver my baby at home. I then lived with that decision for a couple of months, making an agreement with myself that if I still felt as strongly about home birth later as I did then, I would go through with it. Living with this decision for some time gave me the peace of mind I needed that this was the right choice for me and my baby.

Unlike your choice of a birth attendant, a decision that should be made very early in your pregnancy, choice of birth place can, and often should, be made later in pregnancy, after you have had a chance to explore your options and formulate your own philosophy and plan of birth. While it's best to make your decisions early and stick with them, some women will change their chosen attendants and place of birth later in pregnancy, after they've explored all their options. Take your time. You owe it to yourself and your baby to have the best birth experience you can. Since there are so many choices to make during the first couple of months anyway, it's easy to get overwhelmed by all the child-birthing options. For many women, it's best to settle on a birth attendant early in the pregnancy and then ease into the rest of the decisions as their birth knowledge increases and their pregnancy progresses.

Be Flexible

You may have worked out your birth philosophy, negotiated your maternity leave, assembled your health-care-provider team, and mapped out your labor plan right down to the final push when, for no reason other than the quirks of biology, something happens and your pregnancy or delivery takes a more complicated course. If your pregnancy takes an unexpected turn, in the best interests of your baby and yourself, you just make mid-course adjustments. You may feel disappointed if you have to leave work earlier than you planned, or if your hoped-for natural birth becomes a high-tech one. Nevertheless, in the long run, the important issue is having a healthy baby. And remember that being flexible does not mean you skip all the planning; the more you prepare for birth and the more you know about what you want, the more likely you are to have a positive, fulfilling experience — even if it's not exactly the birth you originally envisioned.

THE SIXTH MONTH

❖   ❖   ❖

Emotionally I feel: _____
_____
_____
_____

Physically I feel: _____
_____
_____
_____

My thoughts about you: _____
_____
_____
_____

My dreams about you: _____
_____
_____

What I imagine you look like: _____
_____
_____
_____

My top concerns: _____
_____
_____
_____

My best joys: _____
_____
_____
_____

My worst problems: _____
_____
_____
_____

VISIT TO MY HEALTH-CARE PROVIDER

Questions I had; answers I got: _____

_____

_____

Tests and results; my reaction: _____

_____

Updated due date: _____

My weight: _____

My blood pressure: _____

Feeling my uterus; my reaction: _____

_____

How I feel when I feel you kick: _____

_____

_____

How Dad feels when he feels you kick: _____

_____

_____

What I bought when I went shopping: _____

_____

We started taking childbirth classes at: _____

_____

Our teacher is: _____

The method we chose is: _____

Because: _____

_____

We decided to deliver you at: _____

_____

Because: _____

_____

_____

The main person who will help me deliver you is: _____

_____

Other helpers I would like in the delivery room are: _____

_____

photo at six months

Comments: _____
_____
_____
_____
_____
_____
_____
_____
_____
_____
_____
_____
_____
_____

Seventh-Month Visit to Your
Health-Care Provider
(26–29 weeks)

During this month's visit you may have:

- examination of the size and height of the uterus
- examination of your skin for rashes, enlarging veins, and swelling
- weight and blood-pressure check
- urinalysis to test for infection, sugar, and protein
- hemoglobin and hematocrit, if indicated
- review of your diet, an opportunity to discuss your weight, if necessary
- an opportunity to hear your baby's heartbeat
- an opportunity to see your baby on ultrasound, if indicated
- an opportunity to discuss your feelings and concerns

If your health-care provider has extra concerns, he or she may want to check you twice a month during months seven and eight.

The Seventh Month — Big and Loving It

THE MIDDLE TRIMESTER is over, the final trimester begins, and your thoughts turn toward giving birth. During this month your baby gains at least 1 pound. You may gain anywhere from 3 to 5 pounds, and your uterus grows to midway between your navel and your rib cage. Naturally, your bigger baby makes herself felt in a bigger way. You may be awakened by a punch to the ribs, or find yourself staring in awe at the basketball-size hump that's sticking out of where your abdomen used to be. By the seventh month, your body demands you make lifestyle changes, whether you want to or not. You are simply too pregnant to go about your business at your previous pace. The waddle so characteristic of pregnant women creeps into your walk. Bending over to tie your shoes grows difficult, and putting on panty hose becomes an exercise in gymnastics.

HOW YOU MAY FEEL EMOTIONALLY

As you've undoubtedly figured out by now, there is no such thing as a "typical" emotional state during pregnancy. Every pregnant woman goes through unique emotional changes in the first two trimesters, experiencing feelings that are more intense, more interesting, more vivid, and more changeable than they were before she became pregnant. The third trimester is no exception, though in many ways it's an emotionally easier time. By now you have learned that pregnancy can be both unspeakably wonderful and incredibly challenging, and you have become used to handling these mixed emotions. Thus, many of the emotional and physical "growing pains" of pregnancy are now behind you, and the emotions that lie ahead are mainly those directly involved with delivering a baby. Here's how you may feel this month:

Euphoric. As you wander around town, waddling as much as walking, reveling in your pregnant state, you may experience a natural high quite unlike anything you've ever felt, a combination of feeling special and proud and wanting the whole world to acknowledge how important you are. After all, it's because of women like you that the human race continues. You may have moments, even days, when you forget the many discomforts you've been through and the intense work of labor that lies ahead.

I feel better emotionally than I ever have before. I'm in love with my husband, happy with life, and I adore being pregnant. I love the whole world right now. My mother keeps telling me not to get used to this euphoria, that being a mother is certainly not worry-free. But for right now, I'm enjoying going into parenthood wearing rose-colored glasses.

Savor every moment of these worry-free times. You deserve this emotional break. Sooner or later a thump in the ribs, a stitch in the side, an irritating itch somewhere, or an attack of heartburn will pull you out of pregnancy heaven down to earth-mother reality.

Forgetful. Preoccupation with pregnancy and the approaching birth causes many women to be a bit spacey and prone to day-dreaming. You may forget important events, such as birthdays and appointments. You may stop in the middle of a sentence, unable to remember the point you were trying to make, and, what's even more amazing, you don't care, because the point you were trying to make doesn't seem that important anyway. Everything pales compared to your pregnancy. While you now have nature's best excuse for your absentmindedness, life must go on. There are children to pick up at school, employers to satisfy, and other necessities of life that, though they seem less important than birthing a baby, still need your attention. You may have to consult your calendar hourly or post notes to yourself in places where you can't miss them, such as on the steering wheel of your car, the refrigerator, or the bathroom mirror. Perhaps the normal forgetfulness is a signal to focus on your baby

and realize that many other things were not worth remembering after all.

My husband called me "Spacey Gracie." Although I remembered my doctor's appointment, I forgot to pay the electric bill, left a quart of milk on the counter to spoil, left a friend dangling on the phone while I ran to the bathroom and forgot the call, and found the checkbook even more out of balance than I was. All this seemed funny until the other day, when I ran a stop sign and realized there are times when I have to keep my head together.

Needing to escape. It's not strange to fantasize about getting away from it all, especially if your pregnancy has visited you with every little irritation described in this book. You've been through a lot and still have a lot of work ahead of you. You are not a "bad" mother for having these thoughts. Think of them as rehearsal for the low points of parenthood, the days when you will feel like resigning, even though that's not an option (and one you wouldn't take even if it were offered).

Eager to get things done. You may be thinking, "I'd better get this done while I have the energy to do it." Many women feel a renewed desire this month to tie up loose ends at work, organize the photo albums, clean out closets, or catch up on social obligations. Often the nesting instinct, that desire to wallpaper the nursery or scrub the house for the baby, kicks in this month, though some women do not show this obsession with getting things in order until the eighth or ninth month. While it's true you have more energy now than you will have in the last two months, don't overdo it. Remember, your first priority is making sure you have the energy you need to take care of yourself and grow your baby. To do this, you will need to become good at delegating. You might as well begin delegating responsibilities to your mate now; in the first few weeks after the baby arrives, his help will be crucial to your survival.

Each day I feel more of an urgency to get things done. I've been making lists, trying to keep track of things I want to get done before the baby comes: get all those baby clothes out, get them all washed and put away, get the little bassinet ready. Then there are lots of things around the house I want to get done, and sewing projects, too. I know the end is coming very quickly, and I have a lot to do to prepare, not just for the baby, but so that I can devote time to the baby. I want so much to get things in order. I also have thoughts of, "Will I actually be able to do this? Will I be able to take care of the baby?" At times these thoughts seem a bit overwhelming.

Overwhelmed by birthing decisions. You may be halfway through your childbirth classes before you think seriously about your birth philosophy and begin to consider the many birthing options available to you. It's easy to be confused by all the choices and to feel burdened by the pressure to make them. Or you may find yourself thinking about changing your plans midstream. Second-guessing oneself as the time approaches is normal. (See "Working Out Your Own Birth Philosophy," page 256.)

HOW YOU MAY FEEL PHYSICALLY

Big! The little person who occupies so much of your middle takes up as much space as a basketball, and you are bound to feel the effects of carrying her around. You're beginning to find out that a big, hard belly can be a real impediment to your usual routine.

Heart-pounding sensations. Throughout your pregnancy, as you already know, blood volume steadily increases to accommodate your body's increasing need for oxygen and nourishment. By the third trimester you have 45 percent more blood than you started with. Your heart has to work harder to pump this extra fluid: your heart rate increases by around ten beats per minute and the heart pumps about 30 percent more blood with each beat. These changes peak during mid-pregnancy when you may be able to feel your heart working harder; many women feel heart-pounding sensations during the second half of pregnancy, especially when they exercise or change position suddenly.

The heart's occasional pounding is a normal response to the major circulatory changes that take place during pregnancy. But it is also a signal that your heart, at the moment, is working too hard. The more fit you are, the better your heart adjusts to the extra demands of pregnancy. If the pounding increases noticeably during exercise, slow down. Rise from lying to sitting (or from sitting to standing) more slowly. These heart-pounding sensations will disappear within a few weeks after birth, as your heart rate slows and your circulatory system returns to its prepregnant state.

Working Out Your Own Birth Philosophy

How you approach birth is intimately connected to how you approach life. Working out a birth philosophy and making adjustments along the way can be therapeutic for your labor — and for life. You may or may not have worked out your own personal philosophy of birth, and you may not yet even understand what that means or why you should. Like working out the philosophy of life, the philosophy of birth means the type of birth you want: What's important to you? What are your priorities? And how much are you willing to work for them? What are the things you have to do to get the birth you want? What should you read? Whom should you consult? Besides the end product of birth, the process of getting there is also important.

Having a birth philosophy implies participating in your baby's birth and the decisions accompanying it. It means valuing the process of pregnancy and birth, not just the end product. Birth is the fullest expression of your femininity, and the memories last a lifetime. Besides delivering a baby, you want a positive birth experience (which means different things to different women).

Pregnancy and birth are physiological, not pathological, processes. It is a normal process of life that millions of women have experienced, and most even choose to do it again. Working out your personal birth philosophy takes some of the scariness out of birth. The more you learn about labor, the more you realize that more is under your influence than you may have previously thought.

If you haven't developed a birth philosophy by now, perhaps these tips will help you to do so:

Imagine your dream birth. As an exercise, write down what you want your birth to be like (realizing that not all birth wishes usually come true). If you know the birth you want, you are more likely to get it. Make a list of "wants" and "don't wants." As your pregnancy progresses, you will undoubtedly update this list.

Empower yourself. As your pregnancy progresses, not only are your body and your baby growing; your mind is also filling with more and more information and

Shortness of breath. During pregnancy your respiratory system undergoes magnificent changes that enable it to take in extra oxygen as you breathe for two. Your lung capacity increases, and you may actually add a few inches to the size of your rib cage. While you may notice that you breathe slightly faster while pregnant, you may not know that you are breathing more efficiently, exhaling and inhaling more air during each breath. At times during your pregnancy you may feel short of breath. You may even have occasional moments when you feel as if you're not getting enough air. These feelings of breathlessness do not mean that you or your baby is lacking oxygen. They just mean there is less room for your lungs to expand, and your body is protesting. During pregnancy the circulatory system, like the respiratory system, is incredibly efficient, ensuring discernment about using all the information and options to get the birth you want.

Trust your body. As millions of women have proven, you can trust that your body is built to give birth. By understanding how your body labors to give birth and how you can work with it instead of against it, you are more likely to have a safe and satisfying birth.

Think positive. Surround yourself with positive birth consultants. Depending on what you read and to whom you listen, it's easy to get caught up in all the what-ifs and dwell on all the things that could go wrong with your birth, not realizing that most often birth goes right. The more you believe that your birth will go right, the more likely it will.

Choose birth attendants and a birth place that share your philosophy. If you want a high-touch, low-tech birth, be sure you seek out health-care providers that share these birth beliefs. If you prefer or need a medically managed birth, be sure you participate in your birthing decisions. Formulating your own philosophy of birth also affects how your health-care provider

formulates his or her philosophy about your care during pregnancy and his or her role in assisting your labor. Choose a childbirth class that helps you work out a birthing philosophy that's best for you and doesn't just sell its own philosophy. Not every woman wants the "full experience" of birth; many just want a baby.

Formulating a philosophy of birth gives you a head start in formulating a philosophy of motherhood. Many of the same mental exercises you will go through in achieving a healthy pregnancy and satisfying birth prepare you for similar mental processes you'll go through as you become a mother. You learn to trust yourself more and be more discerning about advice. You also appreciate that your body was not only marvelously designed to give birth but is also marvelously designed to be a mother.

Your labor and delivery day are precious moments to be remembered, and hopefully treasured for the rest of your life. You can influence the memories you keep.

that both you and your baby receive the extra oxygenated blood you need. Most of the time you are not even conscious that you are breathing more deeply, but sometimes you may catch yourself sighing, which is another way your body helps you take an extra deep breath.

During the third trimester, breathlessness increases in both frequency and intensity as your expanding uterus limits the ability of

your lungs to expand with each breath. To compensate for cramping your breathing space from below, pregnancy hormones stimulate you to breathe more often and more efficiently, just to make sure you and your baby are getting the oxygen you need.

Here are some ways to increase the efficiency and capacity of your breathing and to cope with feelings of breathlessness during the third trimester:

- Change position as soon as you feel breathless.

- Slow down when you feel short of breath. Listen to your body's signals that you are exceeding your limits.

- Try breathing exercises to raise your rib cage and promote more chest breathing (deep abdominal breathing obviously becomes more difficult as your uterus grows). Stand up (this will relieve some of the pressure on your diaphragm), then inhale deeply while raising your arms outward to the sides and upward. Exhale slowly as you bring your arms back down to your sides. Raise and lower your head as you inhale and exhale. To be sure you are breathing more into your chest than down into your abdomen, check for rib cage expansion by placing your hands on the sides of your rib cage. Make your ribs push out against your hands as you inhale deeply. Focus on how this deep chest breathing feels so that you can switch to it whenever the crowding of your uterus on your lungs makes abdominal breathing more difficult.

- Practice breathing for labor: slow, deep, relaxed breathing rather than shallow panting. (This is the type of breathing used throughout labor if you are using The Bradley Method®. If you are using the Lamaze method, this is the type of breathing you'll be doing throughout much of the active stage of labor.)

- Exercise regularly. Aerobic exercise begun early in your pregnancy improves the efficiency of both the respiratory and the circulatory systems.

- Experiment with sitting and sleeping positions that help you breathe more easily. Sitting in a straight chair using correct posture — chest lifted, shoulders back — is easier on the lungs than sitting slumped over in a recliner. Sleep semireclined, propped up on pillows. Or try elevating your head with an extra pillow while sleeping in the side-lying position shown on page 225.

As long as these normal episodes of breathlessness are few and far between, don't worry. During your ninth month, as your baby drops down into your pelvis and takes pressure off your diaphragm, you will be able to breathe more easily.

If you experience sudden, severe shortness of breath accompanied by chest pain, rapid breathing, or a much more rapid pulse, or severe chest pain while taking a deep breath, seek medical attention immediately. This could be a signal that a blood clot has dislodged and settled in your lungs — a rare but serious problem.

Facial puffiness. Don't worry if you wake up in the morning with a swollen face, especially the eyelids. The normal facial puffiness of pregnancy is due to the accumulation of extra fluid beneath thin tissue. During the day gravity usually drains the face of this extra fluid. If your puffy eyelids are accompanied by rapid weight gain and excessive swelling all over your body, call your doctor; otherwise, just accept the swelling as another of pregnancy's harmless changes in your body.

Swelling of hands, legs, and feet. Your body needs a lot of extra fluid to nourish a healthy pregnancy. The hormones of pregnancy naturally cause you to be thirsty and to drink more water. These same hormones make sure your body uses this extra fluid to refill baby's amniotic pool, increase the water level in your circulating blood (making it easier for your kidneys to wash away waste), and furnish baby's needs for fluid in his or her own growing body. The demand for fluid is so great that your body will take it as needed from the intestines, contributing to constipation. By the end of your pregnancy you are carrying around an extra 10 quarts, or 20 pounds, of fluid.

Most women with healthy pregnancies will notice some fluid accumulation, especially in the third trimester. Anytime from the fifth or sixth month onward, you can expect to lug around heavier hands, legs, and feet — the areas where gravity causes fluid to settle by the end of the day. Add to the effects of gravity the fact that a growing uterus slows the circulation in the legs, and it's no surprise many women gain a shoe size by the end of their pregnancy.

When swelling is normal. Some women retain more fluid during their pregnancy than others. These are signs that your swelling is within normal limits:

• The swelling shifts with gravity, with different areas of your body being swollen at different times of the day. (This is called "gravity edema.") The swelling in your legs and ankles lessens after elevating your feet for an hour.

• You are gaining weight normally. A sudden, unexplained weight gain may indicate a problem.

• Your diet is adequate and balanced.

• Your blood pressure is within normal limits.

• Urine checks at your health-care provider's office do not show protein in the urine.

Basically, if you are feeling fine and both your body and your baby are growing nor-

mally, your body is carrying just the right amount of extra fluid for you and your baby.

When swelling is not normal. At each of your prenatal checkups your health-care provider will check the amount of swelling your body displays. Talk to him or her if you are concerned about the fluid you are carrying. Fluid retention that is excessive and builds up rapidly may be a sign of a problem, such as preeclampsia, or toxemia (see the glossary, page 415), especially if it is accompanied by these signs:

• The swelling in your legs is excessive — pressing on the swollen areas with a finger leaves a noticeable dent. (This is called "pitting edema.") The swelling doesn't lessen after elevating your legs for an hour.

• You are gaining too much weight too fast.

• Your blood pressure is high.

• Your diet is inadequate.

• Urine checks show excessive protein in your urine.

• You are generally feeling unwell and/or your baby is not growing normally.

Lessening the discomforts of swelling. Normal swelling can be a nuisance and can contribute to fatigue at the end of the day, especially of legs and feet. Try these tips:

• Avoid standing or sitting for long periods of time. If you need to stand or sit for more than an hour at a stretch, exercise your legs and feet (see the exercises on page 181). Don't cross your legs when you sit, as this can restrict circulation in your legs.

• Elevate swollen feet for an hour, especially at the end of the day; the swelling should diminish a bit.

- Relax in a rocking chair while flexing your feet against a footstool. This movement promotes circulation in your legs. A rocking chair will be on your "must have" list for when the baby arrives, so you might as well get it now and start enjoying it.

- Walk, swim, or ride a stationary bike. All three are excellent for increasing circulation to your arms and legs.

- Avoid sleeping on your back. Sleeping on your side (see the best sleeping position, page 225) takes the pressure of your weighty uterus off the major blood vessels and promotes better blood return from your legs.

- Wear loose clothing. Avoid tight bands on pants, socks, or any other clothing, as they can restrict circulation.

- Elevate your feet on a stool during the day and on a pillow at night.

- Elevate your hands when sitting.

- Enjoy a healthy diet. Drink at least eight 8-ounce glasses of liquid daily, especially in hot, humid weather. Make sure that you have adequate amounts of protein in your diet (100 grams a day), and use salt to taste. Do not go on a fluid- or salt-restricted diet unless your health-care provider advises you to due to a specific medical indication. Drinking less fluid will not alleviate the swelling, and your body needs salt for a healthy pregnancy. The only self-help measures you should try are the exercises, position changes, and other tips mentioned above. Do not make any dietary changes without first consulting your practitioner. To check if you are drinking enough water each day, notice the color of your urine. If your urine is almost colorless or slightly yellow, chances are you are drinking enough fluid. If your urine is a darker color, like apple juice, this may be a sign of dehydration.

Backache. "Oh, my aching back!" is an almost daily complaint of nearly 50 percent of moms-to-be in the last half of pregnancy. Back muscles get a triple whammy during pregnancy: your ligaments, which are relaxing to allow for easier passage of the baby through the pelvis, are looser all over, putting more strain on your muscles, especially those supporting your spine; your overstretched abdominal muscles force you to rely more on your back to support your weight; and the change in your posture and the curvature of your spine as you compensate for your front-heavy body create still more work for the back muscles. In the third trimester especially, these overworked muscles and back ligaments will protest in pain.

I've now developed the "pregnancy sway." When I walk I swing my arms out from my side, and my belly gets its own momentum going separate from my body. If I don't catch myself and correct my posture, my back goes into an extreme sway and my shoulders slump forward. This posture causes my back and hips to ache, so I try to keep my pelvis tucked under and my shoulders square.

Preventing backache. The best treatment for backache is prevention. Practice the pregnancy posture tips on page 181 and do exercises to strengthen your lower back (e.g., the kneeling and back-lying pelvis tilt described on page 179) and your abdominal muscles. Simple aerobic exercises such as swimming and biking can also strengthen abdominal and lower back muscles. Also, take these precautions:

- Wear sensible shoes. Both high heels and totally flat shoes can strain back muscles. Try shoes with wide, medium-height heels (no higher than 2 inches) for dress, and walking shoes for casual wear.

- Instead of jogging on hard surfaces, such as concrete or asphalt, which can be jarring to the spine, try fast walking, and on natural surfaces like grass, earth, or sand, which are easier on the muscles and joints than a hard surface.

- Don't twist your spine. When you stand or recline in bed, be sure your shoulders and hips are aligned. Avoid awkward reaches, such as when getting a heavy box down from the top of a closet or lifting a sleeping toddler from a car seat. If you must undertake activities that call for awkward lifting, try to rethink the job. Consider unbuckling a toddler's car seat, for example, and turning the seat toward you before you lift your child out.

- Avoid sitting or standing for long periods of time. When you do sit, use a footstool to raise your knees a bit higher than your hips and take pressure off your lower back. If you must stand in one position for a while, put one foot forward and place most of your weight on it for a few minutes, then switch your weight to the other foot. Better yet, prop the forward foot up on a stool, telephone book, drawer, or cabinet ledge.

- Sleep on your side in the position shown on page 225 and shift sleeping positions whenever you awaken.

Treating backache. Usually, simply resting strained muscles will ease the pain. Also, try soaking in warm water or standing in the shower with a jet of warm water focused on the painful area. Many women swear by a hot or cold pack (or alternating both) placed on the painful area. If baby pressing against your spine seems to be the cause of pain, as is common during the final month, try the knee-chest position for a while (see illustration on page 181).

Ask your mate to give you a back massage. Practice these back massages now so he can later become a useful masseur to help ease the pain of back labor. Partners, try the "I Love U" technique:

- I   Massage down each side of her spine, using your thumbs to apply pressure along the way.
- Love Next, extend the massage along both sides of her lower back along the top of her pelvic bone.
- U   Finally, include the shoulders. Knead her neck and shoulder muscles. Then massage down her backbone and across her lower back.

Clumsiness. The combination of your unwieldy body, relaxed ligaments, and forgetful mind may cause you to stumble on curb corners, trip over toys, or drop your fork in the middle of a meal. Your ungraceful gait cannot be entirely attributed to the 20 or more pounds you have gained. Your waddle and your klutziness are also a result of the loose and water-logged ligaments in your hand, pelvic, and leg joints. Realize that you have temporarily lost your nimbleness in both feet and fingers, and be extra cautious. Pay more attention, for example, when on unfamiliar terrain and when using scissors, lifting a hot skillet, or carrying a toddler down steps.

I love to shop, but lately I've been bumping into counters and dropping things. My husband kidded me and said I shouldn't venture into a china shop. At least he didn't call me a bull.

Aching hips. During the last few months you may notice discomfort in your hips and pubic bone while walking. The ligaments in your hip and pelvic bones stretch and the cartilage softens, preparing these bones for the passage of baby. This stretching and softening is not only uncomfortable while walking, but can give you "loose hips," contributing to the "waddle walk."

More movements — new movements. The nightly "kick fest" continues. The baby's repertoire may now be more entertaining but also more uncomfortable. Studies show babies kick most frequently during the seventh month and kick more often in the night and early morning hours (from midnight to 6:00 A.M.). Of course, baby's limbs are longer and stronger now, so the punches are more powerful. Don't worry that those periodic, annoying jabs in the ribs might get worse in the months to come. The increasingly crowded living conditions in the womb will soon take some of the leverage out of baby's punches. Studies have shown that babies move less in the final two months than they do during this month.

We've been enjoying our baby's nightly gymnastics, the way he has of engaging our attention. But I'm beginning to feel his movements are more restricted, like he's going from an Olympic-size pool to a wading pool.

It really cracks me up when I'm in a business meeting and Stephanie is in there kicking and tumbling away. It's like our own private joke. It's kind of neat.

Fetal hiccups. Besides the kicks and shiftings you love to feel (though not necessarily at 3:00 A.M.), you may notice fetal hiccups early in the third trimester — short, spasmodic blips in your lower abdomen. Hiccups are usually short-lived, but they can last as long as twenty minutes. By the time you've hollered for your mate to "come feel this" and he finally gets there, they will probably have stopped. Hiccups often occur around the same time each day, so you may be able to catch another performance soon. These sudden new twitches may take you by surprise, but they don't bother baby, and most mothers just think they feel funny.

Some mothers have noticed that their babies who turned out to be sensitive to certain foods hiccuped a lot in utero. One mom actually figured this out because her baby got hiccups within an hour every time she drank milk. This helped her focus on milk as the offending food in her diet when her baby developed colic at two weeks of age.

Common annoyances. Many of the physical feelings you experienced in the first trimester return in the third, along with some new annoyances.

- *More frequent urination.* As your growing uterus increases pressure on your bladder, you will need to urinate more frequently. Be sure to urinate as often as you feel the urge, and empty your bladder completely at each urination. Do not hold your urine in, as this may increase your chances of developing a urinary tract infection or even trigger premature contractions.

- *More breast changes.* Your breasts continue to enlarge, and you may start leaking a thick, yellowish substance called "colostrum."

- *Vaginal pain.* An occasional sharp pain in your vaginal area is normal due to the pressure on your cervix.

- *Pelvic pains.* You may experience sharp pains and a feeling of pressure in your pelvic area, especially when you lift your leg up to get out of bed or put on your underwear. These pains are most likely due to the shifting of your pelvic bones and the loosening of the ligaments attached to these bones in preparation for the little passenger who will soon be coming through. The more pregnancies you have, the more you may experience these pelvic sensations.

- *Groin pain.* You may notice a sudden sharp pain when you laugh, cough, sneeze, twist, change position, or reach for something. This is caused by stretching of the ligaments that attach your uterus to your pelvis. Adjusting and changing position will ease this pain.

- *Increased thirst.* You are thirsty all the time. This is your body's signal that you need to drink a lot of water to keep up with your body's increased fluid demands this trimester. Drink to your thirst's content — and then some.

- *Faintness.* After you have been standing or active for a long time, or when you rise too quickly, you may experience a faint or dizzy feeling similar to what you felt in the second trimester. Sit or lie down immediately. Low blood sugar can contribute to this light-headed feeling, so be sure to snack frequently. Resting, eating nutritious food, and avoiding sudden moves to the upright position will lessen faintness.

- *Increased vaginal discharge.* Expect more whitish vaginal discharge, enough to necessitate the use of a panty liner.

- *Heartburn.* During the second trimester you may have had a reprieve from the heartburn of the first few months, but now that burning feeling reappears. This trimester it is due more to the upward pressure of the growing uterus than to pregnancy hormones. Propping yourself upright during sleep, eating small, frequent meals, and keeping yourself upright after a meal should help. (For more on treating heartburn, see page 71.)

- *Constipation.* Your enlarging uterus and its growing occupant push your intestines aside, contributing to constipation. Your increasing need for water elsewhere in your body may steal needed fluid from your intestines, also leading to constipation. Be sure you drink at least eight 8-ounce glasses of water a day and try the suggestions for easing constipation listed on page 70.

HOW YOUR BABY IS GROWING (26–29 WEEKS)

By the end of this month baby weighs 2 to 2½ pounds and measures around 14 inches long. During this month baby has a growth spurt, gaining around 1 pound. Fat deposits smooth out some of the previous wrinkles, giving baby a more filled-out appearance, but he is still much skinnier than he will be at birth. Baby's limbs are longer, stronger, and these delightful little kicks make more of an impression in your abdomen. Baby's eyelids open. Baby can now see, hear, smell, and

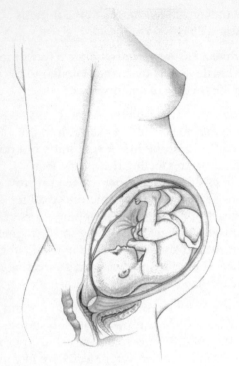

Baby at 26–29 weeks.

taste. Baby's bone marrow now takes over from the spleen as the major site of red blood cell production. At this stage, baby moves vigorously and responds to touch and sound. During this month, baby gets smarter as major changes occur throughout her nervous system. Nerve fibers are clothed in a fatty layer called "myelin" that allows nerve impulses to travel faster. The brain grows so rapidly that it folds on itself, accounting for the many indentations, called "gyri," that are characteristic of the human brain. Early in this month a major development occurs that begins to prepare baby to breathe outside the womb. Cells lining the rapidly budding alveoli (air sacs in baby's lungs) begin to secrete a soapy substance called "surfactant"

that keeps these air sacs from collapsing — similar to the substance that keeps the soap bubble expanded. Depending on how well developed the alveoli and surfactant secretion are, if baby were born now, she might be able to sustain air breathing and life outside the womb. Before the seventh month, most babies choose to lie in the breech position because it's easier for them to rest comfortably in the pear-shaped uterus, but most will flip to the head-down position by thirty-four weeks.

CONCERNS YOU MAY HAVE

Braxton Hicks Contractions or Premature Labor?

During the third trimester, normal Braxton Hicks contractions (see page 223 for explanation) increase in frequency and intensity. They may even become uncomfortable and cause you to worry that you are going into premature labor. True labor contractions show a definite pattern. To tell if it's really preterm labor, employ the 1–5–1 formula: if your contractions last at least 1 minute, are 5 minutes (or less) apart, and continue for at least 1 hour, you are, most likely, in labor. (This would mean you should alert your health-care provider immediately.) Braxton Hicks contractions come and go and don't settle into a regular pattern. (See also how to distinguish labor contractions from prelabor contractions, on page 354.) Don't forget to practice relaxing and breathing with these trial-run contractions.

I'm having plenty of little contractions, and I'm starting to expect them every day. I know the time is getting closer and they're just getting me warmed up for the final event. They don't last too long. If I'm walk-

Kick Counts

Feeling your baby kick can make you so happy you want to burst; not feeling your baby kick for long periods can make you worry. How often and how much a baby moves may be more a reflection of baby's personality than his or her well-being. And, of course, babies do rest and sleep. How many movements are "normal" has been the subject of many studies and much needless maternal anxiety. But because fetal movements are an easy way for mother to monitor fetal well-being, your doctor may ask you to do a daily kick count, especially if you have any risk factors (such as diabetes or high blood pressure) that could jeopardize your baby's health.

The kick-count theory is based on the simple idea that an active baby is a healthy baby. But that doesn't necessarily mean that a quiet baby is less healthy than an active one. Nevertheless, a sudden and sustained change in your baby's normal level of activity is an early sign to alert your practitioner to a possible problem; he or she will perform more definitive tests to tell if the change in kick count is significant or not. Here's how to do your baby's kick count:

- Choose a time that's convenient for you when you are most likely to notice baby's movements. Early evening, after a meal, or before bedtime is the best time for most women. Lie down on your left side and relax.
- Use the "count to ten" technique. Record how long it takes to feel ten movements. (Count only real jabs, not tiny twinges.) After a week or so of kick counts, you'll have your baby's personal average score. Studies show the average time to feel ten kicks is around twenty minutes.
- Since the kick count will vary from pregnancy to pregnancy, and your health-care provider may find a different kick-count method effective, ask him or her if and how you should record a kick count. Also, be sure to ask your practitioner what specific changes in kick count should concern you and when you should call. The usual recommendation is to call your practitioner if, during one of baby's favorite kick times, you haven't felt any movement for one or two hours.

Sample Kick Count Chart

Follow your practitioner's instructions on the method and frequency of doing a kick count. Your recording will be something like this:

Date/Time	Number of Movements/Time
May 21, 8:00 P.M.	10 kicks / 20 minutes
May 22, 8:15 P.M.	10 kicks / 22 minutes
May 23, 7:45 P.M.	10 kicks / 28 minutes
May 24, 8:00 P.M.	10 kicks / 18 minutes

ing and I have them, I sit and they go away. If I'm sitting and I get up and walk, they go away. That's just one more way that I know it's not really time yet, but getting closer.

Worries About Delivering a Premature Baby

Around 90 percent of mothers carry their babies to term (which means at least thirty-seven weeks), so your chances of delivering a mature baby are excellent. Most of the causes of premature delivery are beyond your control, quirks such as an incompetent cervix, placental abnormalities, or an irritable uterus. Your health-care provider will have already discussed with you any of the more obvious risk factors — structural abnormalities of the uterus, multiple babies, and chronic maternal illness, such as diabetes or high blood pressure.

However, mothers with no risk factors can go into premature labor without a known cause. Many times this premature labor can be stopped with medication. Even if you do deliver your baby prematurely, modern advances in newborn intensive care mean the chances are good that a baby of at least twenty-eight-weeks gestation will survive and thrive.

Here are some things you can do to reduce the risk of delivering a premature baby:

- Avail yourself of good prenatal care.
- Don't smoke. Quit before conception if you can.
- Avoid alcohol consumption.
- Eat nutritiously and gain the right amount of weight for you.
- Avoid illegal drug use and use of over-the-counter medications not okayed by your health-care provider.
- Avoid chronic unresolved stress throughout your pregnancy.

Here are the signs that you are in premature labor — *call your health-care provider immediately:*

- Your membranes rupture and amniotic fluid either trickles or gushes from your vagina.

- Contractions that you may have previously thought were Braxton Hicks contractions now become more intense and more regular (see page 264 for how to tell the difference).
- You experience the sudden onset of low back pain or crampy pressure in your pelvic area, a feeling that you have not felt before.

If any of these possible signs of premature labor occur, stop whatever you are doing and call your health-care provider. Sit or lie down while you wait to hear what he or she advises.

High-Risk Pregnancy

The label "high-risk" is unnecessarily scary. Hearing the term naturally makes you wonder, Risk of what? "High-risk" is just a medical term that obstetricians use to describe mothers who have a higher-than-average risk of experiencing health problems during their pregnancy or birth, or of delivering a baby with problems. Common risk factors are insulin-dependent diabetes, high blood pressure, or signs of premature labor. Remember, this term reflects only a statistical probability that a problem may occur in your pregnancy or with your baby; it is not an absolute prediction, and you, in fact, may have no problems at all.

My doctor sent me to a specialist, who told me my pregnancy is "high-risk." I'm not sure I like that term, but I want to do whatever I can during my pregnancy to stay healthy myself and deliver a healthy baby.

We prefer the term "high-responsibility" pregnancy. Our term goes beyond using specialized, more attentive medical care and a high-tech hospital; it implies that *you* must take greater responsibility for your own care and for your own birth decisions. Instead of resigning yourself to the high-risk label, becoming a passive patient, and leaving all the birth decisions up to your doctors, become a high-responsibility mother. Take an even more active part in the birth partnership. Cooperation between you and your care providers is essential if you have been labeled "high-risk." You need to be more informed, more responsible, and more involved in decision making than the average mother, and you need to take better care of yourself.

The first question you should ask your doctor after you are classified as high-risk is what specific things you should do to lower your risk.

Confined to Bed

At any time during pregnancy, complications can confine you to your bed for days, weeks, even months. While the occasional woman may welcome this doctor-mandated time off her feet, for most women all rest and no work or play is no vacation.

I looked so forward to showing off my pregnancy. Now my doctor says I have to stay in bed for six weeks.

Complications that banish a pregnant woman to bed in the first half of pregnancy are unexplained bleeding and the threat of an impending miscarriage; in the second half of pregnancy, the most common reason for bed rest is the threat of preterm labor. Other reasons for prescribed bed rest later in pregnancy include high blood pressure, preeclampsia, incompetent cervix, premature rupture of membranes, and chronic heart disease.

Doctors prescribe bed rest (medically called "therapeutic positioning") for problem pregnancies for a number of reasons. The less active mother is likely to have a less active uterus. Bed rest decreases the pressure of baby on the cervix, thus reducing the likelihood of premature cervical stretching and contractions. Rest increases blood flow to the placenta and thus improves the delivery of nutrients and oxygen to baby. Rest is also likely to reduce a mother's high blood pressure.

Around 20 percent of women are confined to a week or more in bed at some time during their pregnancy. In many cases, being ordered to bed comes as a complete shock to the woman — and to her employer. Following a visit or call to your doctor, your whole agenda is put on hold for days, weeks, or months. Even if you are in the middle of a household move or a big project at work, you go to bed because the stakes are so high.

It was easy to agree with the doctor's decision that I should go to bed, because there was no decision for me to make. When I considered the stakes at hand, I would have done anything to increase my chances of delivering a healthy baby.

I was put on bed rest at twelve weeks because of complications from amniocentesis. At this point, no one other than my trusted sister knew we were pregnant. Suddenly, I was inexplicably canceling social arrangements and mysteriously withdrawing from commitments at church. It was impossible for my husband to take time off work, and my sister has three children of her own, so we had to tell my mother and my other sister about the pregnancy because we needed their help with our kids. I went from being independent and healthy to being strangely dependent on everyone. It was necessary but tough, and very lonely. A week later, ultrasound showed that everything was okay, and bed rest was over. Two weeks after that, the amnio results showed a healthy baby boy, and I was joyfully, publicly pregnant at last.

Making the Best of Your Rest

While most women willingly abide by the doctors' orders for bed rest, for most it's an unwelcome inconvenience. There are always so many other things to do in addition to growing a baby. Yet when you consider that you will have plenty of other chances to do those things but have only one chance to complete this pregnancy, being in bed for nearly twenty-four hours a day can be managed. Here are some ways to cope with your confinement and actually enjoy it.

Know exactly what you may and may not do. Be sure you understand what your health-care provider means by bed rest. You can pretty much figure that bed rest means refraining from the more "active" activities that go on in bed — sex and orgasm. But check to be sure you know whether your doctor recommends total bed rest, which means sponge baths in bed and bedpans, or whether you get the luxury of bathroom privileges and an occasional walk to the kitchen. Ask if you can slowly walk up and down stairs or if you are confined to one floor. Bear in mind that most doctors overprescribe the degree of bed rest, realizing that most human beings do not easily adapt to such a drastic change in lifestyle and will occasionally cheat. Find out if your doctor thinks mental stress is a problem. Some women need to rest their mind in addition to their body. Can you deal with office work over the phone? While you won't want children using your bed as a trampoline, can they stay in the room with you for much of the day?

Set up a comfortable nest. If you have to stay in bed, you might as well create a bed you like to stay in. Have your bed placed near or facing a window so you have fresh air and a view. Put anything you'll need within arms' reach on a table next to your bed. Use a cordless phone or one with a long cord if the phone jack isn't near your bed. Keep address books, phone books, your journal, and all kinds of reading material on an adjacent table. Move the television or the sound system into the bedroom. Buy or rent a small refrigerator for your bedside snacks. Be kind to your recumbent body: place a foam egg crate–contoured pad on top of your mattress.

Think positive. Rather than dwell on what you're missing, think about what you are enjoying. Sure you are missing the strokes at work, the school play your child is starring in, or the simple pleasure of strolling through the park. True, a person can take only so much down time, especially if you have been used to being busy; you can read only so many novels, watch only so much TV, and meditate on your baby for only so long. Even if you find yourself feeling bored and depressed, these feelings will eventually subside, and you will have happy days again. Focus on what you are doing for your baby and on the benefits to you of resting and relaxing. The good thing about the emotions of pregnancy is that downs are usually followed by ups.

I lay there imagining what my life would be like if I didn't have to stay in bed. I had to stop thinking about that since it served no purpose and only made me more depressed.

Your feelings are normal. When you have so much time to just sit and think, your emotions are likely to run wild. You may worry about the baby's health and survival, fret about how your husband and kids are coping, be bored with too little to do, feel anxious about things you should be doing, and dislike feeling dependent. You may feel angry and disappointed about the course of your pregnancy. You may grow impatient as the days get longer. You'll probably feel tempted to cheat. Each day in bed will bring on new emotions to work through, yet continuing to focus on the goal of your pregnancy will help you overcome these feelings and keep you in bed as long as you need to stay there.

Seek your mate's help. This may be the first time in your life that your mate waits on you and seems to get very little in return — except, of course, that you are growing his baby. Prolonged bed rest during pregnancy can bring couples together or tear them apart. Abstaining from sex and curtailing the activities that you usually do together don't help a marriage that may already be stressed. Expect stress on your marriage for these reasons and because your husband is now holding down two jobs: taking care of you and bringing home the bacon. Yet, if you are creative, a lot of bedside romance can take place: candlelight dinners followed by a video; breakfast in bed; and daily massages that promote circulation and feel so good. Being cared for by a sensitive mate can add new depth to your relationship. And for a spouse turned waiter, masseur, entertainer, and cook, this could be the first time in his life that he has had to put someone else's needs ahead of his own — good preparation for becoming a father.

Now that my husband is being mom, shopper, and housekeeper, he realizes how tough my job is and has quit making cracks about how I have an easier job than he does. While I'm in bed, he has to cover all the bases.

Direct traffic. If you have older children, get used to issuing orders from your bed or couch. On the day you begin bed rest, call a family council and, together with your spouse, lay down the house rules, telling your children the importance of your resting in bed, being waited on, being served, and being loved. Your husband should take the lead and show your children how he expects them to behave toward you and that they should avoid disturbing you. Be sure they realize that they can't just run in and jump on your bed anytime they wish.

With children younger than four or five, you'll probably need some baby-sitting help if you are to get any rest. For times when you don't have another grown-up around, welcome your children around your bed, but on peaceful terms. You might even enjoy having a daily tea party there with your three-year-old. Have your bed or couch set up so that the VCR, snacks, and children's books are easy for you to reach. Make sure there are lots of toys around, too. But don't forget that even an eighteen-month-old toddler can follow simple instructions to get a tissue or turn off the TV. Expect cooperation and you will get it.

Work from your bed. While you can't be physically active, you can usually do mental work while lying in bed — balance the checkbook, work on a laptop computer, make appointments by phone, write shopping lists, or help with the children's homework. If the doctor permits, you can also keep up with your job by teleconferencing or doing paperwork. Or, if you need to go on "disability leave," be sure to apply for it.

Keep fit while in bed. With your doctor's okay, do some exercises in bed, such as leg lifts, calf stretches, and upper-arm exercises with light weights. Exercising helps promote circulation, as well as keeping your muscles (including your heart) in shape.

Pamper yourself. Staying in bed does not mean denying yourself all the pleasures of life. Hire a massage therapist (or ask a friend) to give you a head-to-toe massage at least once a week. See if your hairdresser will come to your bedside.

Bond with your baby. Many women on prolonged bed rest face a dilemma: though this would seem an ideal time to contemplate the miracle of pregnancy and to really bond with the baby, the usual reason for being on prolonged bed rest is the very real possibility of losing the baby. So some women find that even though they have plenty of time to think about and plan for the baby, they are afraid to invest any emotional energy because they might lose the baby. Without the usual distractions and tasks of daily life, it's easy to worry that every spot of blood is going to be the end of your baby, or that each contraction may be the one that sets off labor. Remember that the vast majority of women who are confined to bed go on to deliver healthy babies. And as for the few who don't, they never regret loving the little person who was briefly part of their lives.

Use your down time. This may be the only time in your whole adult life that you will have so much time to do just what you want to do, providing you stay in bed. There are many activities a bed-rester can enjoy. Read the classics you've been too busy for. Catch up on soaps. Write that article you've been meaning to write, or get on the Net. Write letters. Make plans. Study a language using audiocassettes. Learn about real estate, teaching, or some other field you've been too busy with your real job to explore. Hand-piece a quilt. Read to your kids. Laughter makes boring bed rest tolerable. Treat yourself to funny friends and video comedies. You get the idea.

I had to really work at it, but after a week or so I came to enjoy being waited on a little. It's been years since I've been on the receiving end of so much loving attention.

It dawned on me one day that I was learning more about patience and acceptance than most people ever did. It made parenting later a whole lot easier!

Choose your visitors carefully. Lying in bed for long periods of time can make you crave adult conversation. Invite over friends who are good listeners. It is likely that many of your friends will not understand your feelings about staying in bed. Be prepared to hear, "You are so lucky. I'd love to stay in bed for two months." Other friends may be more empathetic and realize that continued bed rest isn't all that natural or enjoyable. Pick out a friend who makes you laugh and invite him or her over frequently. Be sure it's someone who brings her own treats and doesn't expect you to play hostess.

Some people felt that I was so lucky to just sit there and watch TV and rest all day, but it's not that simple. I couldn't get up without feeling guilty and wondering if this was the trip to the bathroom that would push me into a miscarriage or a preterm delivery.

It really helped when my friend came by and did my hair and then just sat and listened.

Get support. Ask your practitioner to give you the phone numbers of other mothers similarly confined to bed. Sometimes you can talk each other through a particularly dull day. Or contact a support group called Sidelines (714-497-2265), which maintains a national hotline of volunteers who offer support and match you with other bedridden moms-to-be. This group is the brainchild of a California mother who was confined to bed during her high-risk pregnancies and figured out a way to use her free time for the good of other women in her circumstances. Ask these experienced bed-resters for practical suggestions on what helped them cope. Mothers who have lain in bed for six straight weeks or more will give you ideas on how to pass the time.

A volunteer at Sidelines suggested that since I had so much time on my hands to connect with my baby, I might want to find out its sex to help me connect better with him. Previously, I hadn't wanted to know the sex — I wanted to be surprised — but I took her advice. Using this time to bond more specifically with my son meant I wasn't just sitting there twiddling my thumbs. There was something special about calling our baby by the name we had chosen. This suggestion helped me a lot.

Don't overdo it when you come off bed rest. When you finally get out of bed, it's easy for your mate, kids, and anyone else around your house to feel that you are sud-

denly available to them again full-time. Serve notice that you are going to ease back into the household routine and will still be needing a lot of help and rest. When you do stand up after lying in bed for a long time, you may feel that parts of your insides aren't quite with you. The aches and pains from being in bed will gradually ease over the next few days, and your body will accustom itself to being active again.

When I did get the green light to get out of bed occasionally, I didn't push it. I didn't want to blow three months in bed in one day. I kept focusing on what my goal was: to bring my baby to term.

Children at Birth

We want to have our children, four and seven years old, present at the birth, and they want to be there. We believe it will be a good experience for them. Any problems with this decision?

Letting children share the birth experience is a wonderful way to begin family bonding. All our older children were present at our last three births, and we are all glad they were there. Two main issues to think about are, can your children handle the experience? and, can you handle their being there? Consider these factors:

• *The age of your child.* In our experience, children over three years of age can understand the emotions of labor and respect the dignity of birth. For some children under three, the intensity of birth may be more than they can understand or cope with. Children are usually more comfortable at a home birth than at a hospital birth because they are in their familiar environment and can more freely come and go.

• *The temperament of your child.* Only you know how much raw emotion your child can take. Will your child be frightened by the normal theatrics of labor — your groans, your red face, your bleeding, and the fact that mommy appears to be unhappy and in distress? How will your child cope with the restrictions of the hospital or other birth place?

• *Your ability to tune out your child and focus on your birth.* You must be allowed to concentrate on delivering a baby and not be distracted by the demands of other children. Will you be able to ignore the distractions of having your child there and focus on your labor? (If your child is attending your birth and is diverting some of your energy away from the work you need to do, by all means have him escorted out of the delivery room.)

• *The availability of familiar caregivers for your children.* Make sure that there are enough familiar adults present (other than your partner), so that each child is someone else's only responsibility.

Tell your children ahead of time what the birthing-room rules will be and what behavior you expect of them. Impress upon them that you want them there but also that you need them to behave so that "mommy can do her hard work to push our baby out."

Prepare your children for being bored during periods in labor when nothing seems to be happening. You may want to bring them in only toward the end of labor. If you choose to bring them in just before you're ready to deliver, you'll need a plan for where your child will be cared for throughout labor,

which could be quite a long time by three-year-old standards. One way to solve this dilemma is to stay home for most of your labor. Once things are moving along, you go ahead to the hospital. Then have your child and the child's caregiver come after you've been assessed and are settled.

Prepare your children for what they can expect to see and in terms they can understand: "Mommy may yell or cry, and you may hear some groaning noises that you've never heard before [demonstrate some of these noises]. It's okay, the noise just means mommy's working real hard to push our baby out."

A valuable resource for further reading is *Children at Birth,* by Marjie Hathaway and Jay Hathaway (Academy Publications, 1978). Write to PO Box 5224, Sherman Oaks, CA 91413, or call 818-788-6662 (also available on video).

Enjoying Late-Pregnancy Sex

Your sex life changes again in late pregnancy. In the third trimester a woman is often preoccupied with her imminent birthing and mothering roles. Her husband may find that his own feelings are undergoing a metamorphosis; his wife's body is not just exciting and different — it is the harbinger of imminent change. As the abdomen reaches its full shape, couples come to the realization that they are no longer just a twosome, and they begin to look ahead realistically. Women focus on birthing and nurturing the baby; men focus on their new roles as father and (at least temporarily) sole breadwinner. Your mate may be worried that he's losing you to motherhood. Both of you may experience ambivalence about the changes ahead. All these anxieties can get both your minds temporarily off sex.

Nevertheless, most couples do engage in sex late in pregnancy. As you grow, your sexual relations will out of physical necessity become more creative. Desire can be the mother (or perhaps, in this case, the father) of invention. You will have to experiment with workable and comfortable positions for intercourse. The man-on-top position is usually the most awkward — it is difficult, literally, to get over the hump — and least comfortable; penetration is deepest in this position, and the man's weight on the woman's abdomen and breasts, while not harmful for baby, is uncomfortable for the woman. Besides, in the last few months, women are often uncomfortable lying on their backs for anything. Experiment with these alternatives that allow the woman to control the depth of penetration and the amount of weight she bears:

- woman on top
- man on top, but with his weight supported on his arms
- couple side-lying front-to-front or back-to-front (woman raises her upper leg and supports it with pillows)
- rear entry (woman on hands and knees with partner behind her)

Use whatever position gives you the most pleasure. Expect sex in the last months to be less passionate, less frequent, less athletic, but more inventive. If the desire for sex overrides your physical discomforts and your mental distractions, you will discover new ways of being together.

Choosing a Labor Support Person

Soon after fathers were finally admitted to the delivery room, women began whispering

"Natural" Childbirth

I am not a martyr, nor do I feel I will be less of a woman if I ask for a shot of pain reliever or an epidural during delivery. I just don't handle pain well. For me, "natural childbirth" means going to the hospital without my makeup on. Is a medically assisted birth really all that unnatural?

"Natural birthing" means different things to different mothers. To childbirth educators, however, it means delivering a baby without drugs. Birth reformers have recently added a new term to childbirth chat, "pure birth," which means no drugs or technological interventions. What you call your birth means little; it's what the birth experience means to you that matters the most. A medically assisted birth may be perfectly natural for you; and if medical assistance helps you avoid a surgical birth, you will have achieved the natural phenomenon of vaginal birth.

We prefer the term "responsible childbirth." This is a birth every woman can have. Responsible childbirth means you have done your homework — studied the options, worked out a birthing philosophy that suits you, assembled the right team, chosen the appropriate birth place, and educated your mind and trained your body to have a safe and satisfying birth. Regardless of whether or not your birth goes according to your plans or your wishes, enter the delivery room with these tools, and you can call your birth anything you wish — and feel good about it.

a little secret to each other, one they'd never tell their husbands or their doctors (who might throw the men back into the waiting room): many dads aren't cut out to be labor coaches. So who provides the missing link?

Enter the labor support person. A woman, and probably a mother herself, a labor support person brings the relaxed, natural approach of the midwife to a traditional hospital birth. Her presence means a mother does not have to rely solely on her husband for help in dealing with pain. She can instead enjoy his emotional support and love at a time that is special, but stressful, for them both.

Though a friend can certainly be a labor support person, mothers typically have the best results when they hire a professional labor assistant (or PLA, also called a "labor support doula" or a "monitrice"), who, in addition to providing comfort and companionship to the laboring mother, has special obstetrical training as a midwife, obstetrical nurse, or educated laywoman. Her knowledge of and experience with birthing, and her sole focus on the mother's needs, make her a unique and, to our minds, indispensable part of a hospital birth. She coaches, counsels, supports, and anchors a laboring woman, helping the process move more quickly and comfortably. With the hospital staff she acts as an advocate for the parents, conveying their wishes and freeing mom and dad up to focus on the labor and impending birth.

Studies show that woman-supported labors are shorter (by as much as 50 percent) and involve less medical intervention than non-woman-supported hospital labors. (In one study, 18 percent of non-woman-supported but only 8 percent of woman-supported mothers had cesareans; fewer women-supported mothers had epidurals,

episiotomies, and perineal tears.) PLAs are new players in the birthing game, and few hospitals and insurance companies yet recognize the benefits gained from using professional labor support. For that reason, you may end up paying for a PLA yourself — fees ranging from $250 to $550. Negotiate with your insurance carrier if you can, but don't hesitate to take the money out of savings if you have to. PLAs are often instrumental if mothers choose to avoid medical interventions (e.g., IV, epidural, and internal fetal monitoring); they are especially valuable in high-risk pregnancies where the necessary use of such technology makes natural methods of pain control much harder to use. Most important, they aid immeasurably in getting a mother to relax and work with her birthing body.

I had a previous cesarean section, and with this pregnancy I wanted to do everything possible to have a VBAC. I read that having a professional labor support person would increase my chance of having the birth I wanted. So I negotiated with my insurance company. I told them about the studies showing less chance of a repeat cesarean delivery in births that are attended by professional labor assistants. I asked them to pay for the labor assistant if I didn't end up with a cesarean birth, and they agreed. This not only eased my mind during my pregnancy, but it was also good business for the insurance company: paying my labor support person a few hundred dollars was better than paying $5000 for a C-section. I used a wonderful labor support person, got my vaginal birth, and my insurance company willingly paid her fee.

If you're lucky enough to live in a part of the country where the use of PLAs is becoming standard practice, your hospital or obstetrician may have a list of them for you to call. Most mothers, however, find their PLA through childbirth educators, local La Leche League groups, or the recommendations of friends. For information on PLAs, contact Doulas of North America (DONA), 1100 23rd Avenue, Seattle, WA 98112 (206-324-5440; fax 206-325-0472; E-mail http:\\www.dona.com\).

Be sure to interview PLAs as you would any other professional (see the questions for doctors and midwives on pages 36 and 41). Remember that you must be able to trust this woman in order to get the most out of her services. Once you've chosen your PLA, she will schedule a meeting or two during your third trimester to help you work out a realistic birth plan. Most PLAs will then meet you at the hospital once you are in labor, but some will come to your home and help you labor there until it is time to leave for the hospital.

Questions You May Have About PLAs

Would a PLA cause my husband to feel displaced in the birthing room?

Not likely. In our experience, fathers welcome this experienced woman with open arms. The PLA does not displace the father at birth; instead she takes the pressure off him to perform as coach and frees him up to do what a man does best — love his mate.

Neither should your obstetrician or obstetrical nurses feel displaced by a PLA. She fills in the gaps in the health-care team and frees these professionals to do what they do best.

I'm categorized as high-risk because of high blood pressure, and my doctor is worried about toxemia. Could a PLA help in my situation?

Absolutely! As we mentioned previously, both studies and common sense show that the probability of having a satisfying birth and a healthy baby is increased by the presence of someone who provides accurate information and support and empowers a woman to work with her body and make wise birthing choices. PLAs really shine in crisis moments during delivery when, due to an unanticipated complication, there is a sudden change in birth plans, requiring decisions to be made about technology or surgery for the best interests of mother and baby. During these situations, you often do not have a clear enough mind to understand your options completely. The PLA acts as an advocate or a go-between, often interpreting the medical information for you so that you can more easily understand and be part of the decision.

Dr. Linda notes: As an obstetrician, I love professional labor assistants. They can help relax both the woman and her spouse. If things don't go well, professional labor assistants can really help with interventions and with lending acceptance to the physician's recommendations.

I chose to employ a PLA because, after doing my homework, I realized there was a missing person in the current maternity system. Due to economic pressures, obstetrical nurses are often overworked, and obstetricians are overloaded. I wanted more than just my next-door-neighbor friend holding my hand during delivery, and I feared my husband would panic at my first pain. After talking to other mothers about their deliveries, I realized that many first-time mothers are left alone a lot during delivery and don't really know how to interpret what's going on in their bodies. My PLA was the missing link that I needed to keep me cen-

tered on my body to make it work more efficiently, and I think she saved me a lot of pain — literally.

My husband and I feel getting a PLA was one of the best decisions we've ever made. My husband was freed from the primary role of guiding me through labor; he and I were able to labor lovingly together. I didn't rely on him to somehow save me from the pain of labor, so there was no tension between us from expectations. He said he was glad to be part of the experience rather than carrying the burden of the experience.

When One Becomes Two

A new life begins —
   a fresh heartbeat,
   a flutter of feet,
   a new soul.

Little miracle placed in my womb —
    I feed you, I nurture you
    and the string between our hearts grows
      strong.

Little one growing in my womb —
    Daddy and I lay our hands upon my
      growing belly
    and wait for you to flutter a reply.

Little person living in my womb —
    I welcome and cherish your consuming
      presence
    and long to gaze into your deep, warm
      eyes.

Little babe curled up in my womb —
    I anxiously prepare for your arrival
    and dream of touching your soft new skin.

Little child born of my womb —
    I embrace your tiny self
    and dream of holding you forever.

Oh baby, sweet baby —
   a fresh heartbeat,
   a flutter of feet,
   a new soul.

— JACQUELYN deLAVEAGA

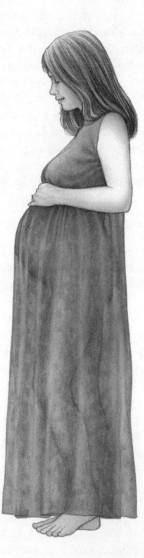

THE SEVENTH MONTH

❖ ❖ ❖

Emotionally I feel: _____
_____
_____
_____

Physically I feel: _____
_____
_____
_____

My thoughts about you: _____
_____
_____
_____

My dreams about you: _____
_____
_____

What I imagine you look like: _____
_____
_____
_____

My top concerns: _____
_____
_____
_____

My best joys: _____
_____
_____
_____

My worst problems: _____
_____
_____

VISIT TO MY HEALTH-CARE PROVIDER

Questions I had; answers I got: _____
_____
_____
_____
_____

Tests and results; my reaction: _____
_____
_____
_____
_____
_____

Updated due date: _____
My weight: _____
My blood pressure: _____
Feeling my uterus; my reaction: _____
_____
_____

How I feel when I feel you kick: _____
_____
_____
_____

How Dad feels when he feels you kick: _____
_____
_____
_____

Reactions of your brothers or sisters when they feel you move: _____
_____
_____
_____

What I bought when I went shopping: _____
_____
_____

photo at seven months

Comments: _____
_____
_____
_____
_____
_____
_____
_____
_____
_____
_____
_____
_____
_____
_____
_____

Eighth-Month Visit to Your Health-Care Provider (30–33 weeks)

During this month's visit you may have:

- examination of the size and height of the uterus
- examination of your skin for rashes, enlarging veins, and swelling
- weight and blood-pressure check
- urinalysis to test for infection, sugar, and protein
- hemoglobin and hematocrit, if indicated
- review of your diet, an opportunity to discuss your weight, if necessary
- an opportunity to hear your baby's heartbeat
- an opportunity to see your baby on ultrasound, if indicated
- an opportunity to discuss your feelings and concerns

If your health-care provider has extra concerns, he or she may want to check you twice a month during months seven and eight.

The Eighth Month —
Almost There

A S YOU ENTER MONTH EIGHT, your mind and your body will likely turn toward birth. Your uterus has grown to reach your breastbone and rib cage. You are now so big you can't imagine getting bigger, but you and baby still have some growing to do. Baby, who begins this month 16 inches long and around 3½ pounds, will probably gain ½ pound and ½ inch each week from now until delivery day.

HOW YOU MAY FEEL EMOTIONALLY

Anticipating baby's arrival is bound to stimulate your imagination to work overtime. There may even be periods when you daydream so often you may feel your brain is going soft on you. It isn't; you've just filled it with baby stuff. Here are some typical emotions of the eighth month:

Wanting your pregnancy to be over. Even though you've come a long way, two more months to D day (i.e., delivery day) seems like an eternity. If you are like many women, you are growing tired of being pregnant and feeling like you can't wait to hold your baby. This normal impatience is likely to get worse, especially since there are so many questions that will be answered only on delivery day: Is baby (really) a he or she? What does she look like? What color are his hair and eyes? How will she act? What will I feel when I meet him? How will her father react? Waiting for baby to come can be as frustrating as watching a flower grow — time seems to stand still. As much as you want to see your little one, as much as you want your body back, you still have a lot of baby-growing to do — two more months of adding the finishing touches to this little person. Remind yourself that this is the last chance you'll have for a while to sleep in, go to a movie without paying a sitter, make love without possible interruption. Make the most of this special time.

Imagining your baby. As your pregnancy progresses, the things you've imagined all along seem more real. What once seemed a fantasy is almost a reality. You may imagine your baby, or picture the baby and your other children playing together. You probably think about baby's personality now as much as you do his or her looks.

Feeling baby kick is usually the trigger for

these imaginings. Sometimes they really run wild and you start fast-forwarding your imaginary tape, picturing what your child will be like in school, as a teenager, even as a grown person. You'll likely begin to formulate ideas about the kind of person you want your child to be. Fantasizing about your child's life will also trigger vivid replays of your own childhood. As they reflect, many women begin to feel closer to their mothers, feeling anew the love that was behind typical childhood scenes, such as eating breakfast together each morning or being told to wear a coat.

In this month you will probably start giving some serious thought to how other family members will take to your baby. Most mothers-to-be begin to imagine what kind of father their husband will be. If your mate has not been as attentive to you and as enthusiastic about becoming a father as you might have hoped, you may fear that he'll be a distant dad. Don't worry. Many times men who seem inattentive and uninvolved in their wives' pregnancies become very caring and involved dads once they hold their baby and the reality of fatherhood sinks in. You may also imagine how your parents and your in-laws will interact with your baby. It's normal if one of your parents is deceased to reflect on how much you miss your mother or father, and to feel sad that he or she will miss the joy of loving this grandchild. You may even begin to imagine how your deceased parent would look holding your baby. Many mothers enjoy thinking about the love an older sibling will have for the baby, imagining sweet scenes of sister's kisses or of big brother helping to change a diaper.

Driven to replay a previous birth. If you've given birth before, you may begin to think a lot about your previous birth, recall-

ing both pleasant and unpleasant events. How will this labor and delivery be different? Will it hurt more or less? Will it be shorter or longer? This is also a good time to mull over the lessons you learned from your previous labor and delivery. What do you want to do the same this time? What do you want to do differently? Will you use the same pain-relieving techniques? The same labor and birthing positions? You are much wiser this time around. Put your experience and your wisdom to work for you over the next month. Though you have probably been working out your feelings about earlier births all during your pregnancy, it is normal to replay them a lot. Channel any worry you have into more practice of relaxation skills, and talk to a few friends who can encourage you. If you can't stop worrying about this birth, see a professional to help you reduce your fear.

Superstitious. Even if you've never been a superstitious person, you may start looking for omens. A black cat crosses your path and you worry about what that means. Then all those baby catalogs start coming — your name is already on multiple mailing lists, and your baby isn't even born yet. You can't bring yourself to buy baby's layette because something bad may happen to baby. Guard against letting this form of worry disturb your peace.

Worried about your baby's health. By now you have undoubtedly been on the receiving end of many comments from well-meaning mothers who simply must tell you what could go wrong. Your practitioner may unintentionally magnify these health worries by explaining what could go wrong. That's part of the job of a good doctor or midwife — to inform you about all the possibilities. Consider those worst-case scenarios just that: rare happenings that are unlikely to happen to you or your baby. If negative conversation like this disturbs your peace during your prenatal visits, tell your practitioner.

Don't allow health worries to rob you of the joys of pregnancy and motherhood. While it's normal to be concerned — you are, after all, thinking like a mother — the fact is, most births go right. Chances are great that the two of you will celebrate birth day as a healthy mother and healthy baby.

I loved every part of my prenatal visit — even weighing in — except when my doctor started talking about the tests to be sure my baby didn't have those awful things. I know she's obligated to tell me these things, but it put a damper on the joy of my visits. At least she saved all the bad stuff till the end of the office visit.

Worried about your weight gain. If you are obsessed with weight and get depressed after every monthly weigh-in, just stop looking at the scale. Ask the doctor and the nurses not to tell you how much you weigh unless there is a medical reason to do so. As long as you are feeling well and your baby is growing normally, don't worry about your weight. And certainly don't think about going on a diet now. If your doctor doesn't say anything to you, you can assume you're at the right weight for you. Focus on nutritious eating habits rather than on the scale. The number on the scale is not an absolute anyway, since your body undergoes rapid fluid shifts. Fluid retention can be higher on the day (or hour) of your checkup. (See "Preeclampsia," page 415.)

I worried if I gained too much, I worried if I gained too little. Once the midwife assured me that every woman (and baby) has a different growth pattern, I relaxed, ate well, and didn't worry.

I worried so much about my weight gain that I resented my monthly weigh-ins. I made a deal with my doctor that she would not tell me unless there was a problem. If she was mum, then my weight was OK and I didn't need to worry.

Relieved. If you were preoccupied about going into premature labor, you can take comfort knowing that your baby would, with a lot of medical help, probably survive if born now. In fact, by the end of the eighth month, most babies have achieved sufficient lung development to enable them to breathe on their own. And many premature babies born at this stage experience very few complications. (Babies born earlier than thirty-six weeks often need a few days to a week or so of assistance with their breathing while their lungs mature.)

Curious about your dreams. When delivery is looming on the horizon, you tend to dream in themes — usually birth themes. You may dream about your labor and delivery or about taking care of your baby. These dreams are often a bit bizarre.

I dreamt the other night I went into labor and was at the hospital when I looked down at my tummy and could see the baby's head emerging through my skin. It was a scary sight. He looked like an alien. I also dreamt the same night that my husband got abducted by aliens. I guess you could say there was an alien theme running through my head that night.

I dreamt my baby suddenly wasn't there, and when I woke up, I rushed to the doctor's office begging for an ultrasound. It was only when I saw a healthy baby on the screen that I realized that my dream was just a nightmare.

I dreamt I left my baby at the house while I went shopping, and when I got home the police were waiting to arrest me. I wondered if this dream was from a subconscious fear that I won't be a fit mother or able to take care of my children.

I dreamt I forgot the baby and left him in the trunk of the car in the broiling heat of the Arizona desert. I dreamt I forgot to feed him for a couple of days and he was starving. I guess those mean I am just nervous about having responsibility for a child.

I dreamt that my daughter was born able to walk!

The new baby does feel like an alien, a strange being. All moms are nervous about being responsible for such a helpless little person, and thoughts about the future are inevitable. Your dreams may be as easy to interpret as these ones were, or they may be bizarre, frightening, or jumbled, with very strong feelings attached. Write down the ones you remember. They will help you identify your unconscious fears and concerns.

Worried about being a good mother. Many mothers report serious ambivalence about parenthood during this month. One day you may feel excited about the big event soon to happen. Another day you may feel incredibly nervous about the tremendous changes the birth of your baby will bring to your family. All these feelings are normal and not unlike the emotional highs and lows of motherhood: there will be times when you love being a parent, and there will be times when you wonder what you've gotten yourself into. One very common, but unnecessary, concern that nearly all mothers have throughout pregnancy, but most strongly near the end, is whether they will be good mothers. They hear about this mysterious "mother's intuition" that is somehow supposed to be in the hospital gift pack along with the baby oil and diapers. Be assured that you will develop this mother's intuition. Your hormones helped you grow this baby and they will also prepare your mind to have clear insight into your baby's needs after birth.

Pregnancy brings out a lot of soul-searching in a woman. You may wish you were more patient, less selfish, more giving, less obsessed about your weight, less impulsive about cleaning the house. The desire to perfect yourself is a byproduct of wanting to be a perfect mother — a goal your child won't expect of you, so you needn't expect it of yourself.

HOW YOU MAY FEEL PHYSICALLY

In month eight you're probably feeling mostly, well, BIG. Your belly is big. Your baby is getting big. You're beginning to have problems getting around. Chances are you're taking these problems in stride because you know you have only another month or two more to deal with them. Your Braxton Hicks contractions may become more intense this month, too. They may feel like strong bands tightening across your uterus. You may feel your uterus itself harden. A couple of these Braxton Hicks contractions may occur every hour this month, and many will make you wonder, "Could this be it?" Probably not. Your uterus is still just warming up for the real contractions at the end of next month. (See page 354 for the difference between prelabor and labor contractions.) Use these prelabor contractions to practice your relaxation and natural pain-relieving techniques. Condition yourself to relax, not tense up, with each contraction.

Stronger kicks. In the final two months it's usual to feel fewer kicks, but stronger ones. Studies show that women often feel half the number of kicks in the eighth month compared to the seventh. You can expect your reaction toward these precious jabs to change. Previously you enjoyed each little nudge as a reminder of the miracle happening inside you. In the final month or two, each kick may be a downright pain in the ribs, gut, bladder, groin, back, or wherever else your growing baby feels like stretching out. And you begin to feel movement at both ends of baby — feet kicking up against your ribs, for example, while the head is pushing down on your pelvis. You may even begin to feel that baby is kicking purposely, as if she's trying to tell you to please change position because she needs more room. Some women notice that baby moves when they start to talk and are certain this is baby's way of responding to their voice. In month eight, it's especially fun to place a piece of paper on your abdomen and watch baby kick it off. (Is it on purpose?) We loved playing "Guess the Body Parts." ("Is it the heel of his foot, or a bony little elbow?") It's fun to map out the profile of your baby's body beneath your abdomen. Ask your practitioner if you've mapped it out right.

I'm woken up by a kicking spell at night, and I even get a kick out of it. I can tell that baby is much bigger, and oftentimes it makes me uncomfortable when baby

moves. I can sometimes see an elbow move from side to side or feel its little bottom pooch out on my tummy. It must be getting pretty cramped for space in there because it's trying to stretch its little nest a bit bigger. It can be sort of uncomfortable, but overall it's really enjoyable. These kicks will wake me up, but if I change sides or just walk a little bit, the discomfort goes away, and I settle back down.

The baby moves most right after I eat. It seems like the baby says, "Yeah, some food, yum, yum."

I encouraged him to kick by talking and patting him whenever I felt it. I believe that when he heard me talk to him and say, "Hi, whatcha doing in there?" he would kick in response.

Feeling bigger. You will feel bigger because you are bigger. The good news is this is about as big as you're going to get, or at least your baby is as high under your ribs as she is going to be. Next month baby will begin to drop lower into your pelvis, and if you don't look any smaller, you will at least look different as you view your profile in the mirror.

Being bigger brings plenty to complain about. It's harder to move around; your joints ache and your feet swell. It may even be more of a chore to walk and bend over to tend to a toddler.

I love how my bigness gets responses from my three-year-old. She reaches over and pats my tummy and says, "Baby, baby." She's also getting more excited, wanting to know where the new baby is going to sleep and asking, "Is the new baby going to sit in the high chair to eat?" When she was helping me get out some little baby clothes and baby shoes, she said, "These little shoes are so cute."

Needing to rest. Even when your body is not tired, your brain may tell you to take it easy. Having your mental signals anticipate your physical needs may take you by surprise. Your legs may not hurt, nor are you out of breath, yet something inside says, "Sit down." Listen to your mind, even when your body says to keep going. Your energy reserves are just about tapped out, and in this case, your body can benefit from listening to your perceptive mind. If you keep going until you crash physically, it will take a lot longer to recharge.

Frequent night waking. Guess what? Babies don't sleep through the night and neither do pregnant women. Welcome to the world of nighttime parenting. There are several reasons for night waking in the final months. One is that your sleep cycles change, and you may experience more REM sleep — a sleep state in which you dream more and awaken more easily (see page 119). Also, your enlarging uterus makes it difficult to sleep. It presses upward on your stomach, causing heartburn, and downward on your bladder, necessitating frequent nighttime trips to the bathroom. And if your enlarging uterus doesn't wake you up, its occupant will. Babies in the womb seem to have their days and nights mixed up. Daytime motion lulls baby to sleep. Then when you rest, baby awakens, stretches, and wakes you up by knocking on your insides. You may also wake up just to roll over, as you squirm to find a comfortable sleeping position. Most mothers find sleeping on their side supported by pillows to be the most comfortable. If heartburn is a problem, try sleeping propped up slightly on several

pillows. Be sure to steal several catnaps during the day to make up for the sleep you miss at night. Keep a bottle of juice or water handy at bedside to quench night thirsts.

You certainly want to be as well rested as possible for D day and beyond. Here's how you can get more sleep:

- Reread the advice beginning on page 73.
- Try catnapping during the day.
- Go to bed earlier. You may crave time for yourself after a hectic day, but make yourself retire at least an hour earlier than usual. The energy payoff will be worth the lost reading or TV time.
- If leg cramps awaken you, try a before-bed massage and the leg-cramp exercises described on page 218.
- If indigestion or shortness of breath keeps you awake, try sleeping slightly upright, propped up on pillows.
- Try the position illustrated on page 225.
- Change sleeping positions whenever you are awakened by discomfort, especially if you experience pelvic pains from the stretching of the uterus, or pressure of the uterus on the pelvic nerves (see relief for round-ligament pain, page 182, and sciatica, page 222).
- If itchy skin wakes you up, use soothing lotion to massage the sensitive spots before bed.
- To help yourself fall asleep, practice the relaxation techniques you are learning in childbirth class. Try mental imagery (see page 307); imagine yourself floating in water, or moving back and forth on a swing. Practicing relaxation techniques to get to sleep quickly will make it easier for you to relax when your labor begins. The ability to rest or sleep even momentarily between

contractions is an important energy-saving aid during early labor.

HOW YOUR BABY IS GROWING (30–33 WEEKS)

By the end of this month, baby weighs from 3 to 4 pounds and is 16 to 18 inches long. During this month fat deposits double, giving baby a more filled-out appearance. Her skin begins to shed the silky, lanugo hair that covered the skin, while the hair on her eyelids and eyebrows grows longer, and some babies sprout a full head of hair. She can blink her eyes in reaction to outside light. During this month of rapid brain growth, your baby experiences definite REM and non-REM sleep stages. Hiccups, which a mother may experi-

ence as sudden jerks, are common now. Baby becomes more aware of her outside world and can react to its stimuli. If she is born now, your baby may be able to breathe outside the womb on her own without medical assistance.

CONCERNS YOU MAY HAVE

Worried About a Cesarean Birth — What You Can Do

The rate of cesarean deliveries in American hospitals, which was on the rise for decades, has now finally begun to level off. Yet, the

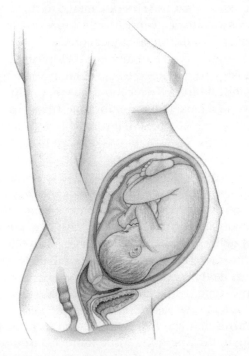

Baby at 30–33 weeks.

One of our other books, *The Birth Book,* is a useful companion to *The Pregnancy Book.* In it we delve deeper into helping you work out a philosophy of birth, the options of various birthing environments, the wise use of tests and technology, and relaxation tips that will help your labor progress more efficiently and less painfully. Much of *The Birth Book* focuses on labor and delivery. We share our own birth experiences and devote an entire chapter to other mothers' birth stories. The process of labor and delivery is explained in depth in *The Birth Book,* and each stage of labor is illustrated. Reading *The Birth Book* will empower you to get the birth you want and equip you to enter your labor knowing your body, reading its signals, and trusting your responses. It will help you make informed choices to increase your chances of having a safe and satisfying birth.

rate is still very high. From 1970 to 1990 the percentage of women being delivered surgically rose from 5 to 25 percent. Why does one in four mothers in the United States have a surgical birth? Only 5 to 10 percent of women in European countries have cesarean births. Do American women have smaller pelvises and grow bigger babies than European mothers? Not likely. What's going on here?

Vaginal birth has worked beautifully for most babies and mothers since the beginning of time. So who's to blame for this new propensity for delivering babies by abdominal incision? The doctors? The hospitals? The mothers? None of these groups is to blame. Despite claims in birth-reform newsletters, doctors don't do surgical births to make more money; the slightly higher obstetrical fees earned attending a surgical versus a vaginal birth are not proportionate to the vastly increased time and energy involved in performing major surgery and doing postoperative patient care. And hospitals do not make judgment calls on what is the safest way for baby to be born. And certainly mothers are not to blame.

The truth is that the high cesarean rate is a side effect of changes in the obstetrical system, and, for that matter, of a changing America. As obstetrical care grew more sophisticated and used more technology, its side effects increased. Consider these factors influencing the high rate of surgical births. More women with chronic diseases (such as diabetes and heart disease) are now able to conceive healthy babies, and these "high-risk pregnancies" are more likely to need a surgical delivery to ensure the health of both baby and mother. Modern fertility drugs increase the number of multiple births, and many of these require a surgical delivery. A surgical

birth is now safer in some instances than a potentially problematic vaginal delivery. For example, some tiny preemies who previously would not have survived a vaginal birth can now be safely delivered by cesarean section and have a good chance of survival. Decades ago abdominal and uterine surgery and the accompanying anesthesia carried higher risks, so much so that doctors had no choice but to deliver all but the most endangered babies vaginally. For example, if a baby was having trouble getting through the birth canal, high or mid-forceps were used to bring the stuck baby down through the vagina — but not without risk to the baby. Now that surgical birth is much safer, the risk-benefit analysis favors a cesarean over forceps. Another example of the changing balance of risks is the current recommendation that most breech babies be delivered by cesarean. Studies show that the risk of damage to these babies is statistically greater during a vaginal birth than during a surgical one.

Some features of modern childbirth technology have helped to raise the incidence of surgical births. The same drugs that help women have more comfortable labors can increase the chances that they will need surgical births. The epidural — that godsend that many women tout as the obstetrical advancement of the century — may also in some situations increase a woman's chance of having a surgical birth. (In some instances, though, epidural anesthesia may increase her chances of delivering vaginally; see page 326.) Electronic fetal monitoring, the tool that can detect fetal problems and alert the doctor to intervene before damage to the baby occurs, is not always easy to interpret, and false alarms may send the whole birth team rushing to the operating room unnecessarily.

Finally, and significantly, the increasing cesarean rate is a side effect of our litigious times. Despite many claims to the contrary, the fear of malpractice suits is a powerful force that has driven up the rate of surgical birth and the cost of medical care. For most of human history, birth was understood to have risks, and parents were prepared to take those risks. Until there is malpractice reform (a promise on which the government is unlikely to deliver), obstetricians aren't going to do any risky vaginal deliveries. Today, for better or for worse, a take-no-chances, "when-in-doubt-get-baby-out" mind-set prevails in most delivery rooms, and this is a mind-set that both parents-to-be and their doctors seem to be able to live and labor with. Given this scenario, doctors aren't motivated to lower the cesarean rate.

Though having a baby has never been safer, even for women with problem pregnancies, both doctors and parents believe the time has come to start chipping away at the rising rate of surgical births — without compromising the health of mother or baby. While there are medical situations beyond your control that require a cesarean section, the good news is that there are many things you can do during your pregnancy and labor to influence whether or not you will need a cesarean.

Modern advances in surgical techniques and anesthesia have made the cesarean a much safer operation than in previous decades; the lives of many babies and mothers have been saved by this procedure. Yet it is major surgery, from which it takes time to recover; a cesarean should be avoided unless it is absolutely necessary.

The five most common reasons for a cesarean are: failure to progress, a repeat cesarean section, fetal distress, cephalopelvic disproportion, and active maternal herpes.

You can influence all five of these situations.

Failure to progress. Labor that doesn't progress according to the usual timetable accounts for around 30 percent of cesarean deliveries. For various reasons the cervix does not open enough and/or the baby does not descend. Some cases of failure to progress cannot be avoided, such as a very short cord. Most cases, though, are due to inadequate support for the laboring woman and violation of the basic physiology of labor. Of all the reasons for a cesarean, "failure to progress" is the most under your control. Think about it. No other system in your body "fails" 10 percent of the time. Why should your "delivery" system? Of course, you must use the system the way it was designed to work. Emotional and physical support for the mother, walking during labor, upright pushing, along with the prudent use of medication and technology, will help labor progress by increasing the efficiency of uterine contractions rather than interfering with them.

Repeat cesarean. This is the most common reason for a surgical birth, and it is under your influence as well. (See "Questions You May Have About Cesarean Births," page 291.)

Fetal distress. The third-most-common situation leading to a cesarean delivery is fetal distress. Fetal heart patterns on the electronic fetal monitor may suggest that baby's well-being is in jeopardy unless he or she is delivered quickly. A fetal heart rate that is higher or lower than average is a sign that baby may not be getting enough oxygen or recovering well from the decreased heart rate that is normal during contractions. While some of the reasons babies receive insufficient oxygen are beyond your control, the choices you make in labor do help determine your baby's well-being.

Cephalopelvic disproportion (CPD). Another reason for surgical births is CPD — baby is too big to pass through the pelvic outlet. Laboring and delivering in a more upright position, namely squatting, can enlarge the pelvic outlet, often allowing even a small mommy to deliver a big baby. (See also FPI, page 411, and Pelvimetry, page 414.)

Active genital herpes. If you have active genital herpes at the time of labor, your doctor will probably recommend a cesarean birth, so that you don't transmit the infection to your baby during passage through the birth canal. If you had a previous history of genital herpes but during this pregnancy do not have any visible sores, the American College of Obstetricians and Gynecologists currently recommends that weekly vaginal cultures for herpes are not routinely necessary and the baby could safely be delivered vaginally. If you have a new outbreak or a recurrence of a previous herpes infection during your pregnancy, your doctor will monitor these lesions and sometimes treat them with antiviral medicine throughout your pregnancy.

Other possible reasons for cesareans are multiple babies, breech and other unusual presentations, and structural abnormalities of the uterus and pelvis. Now that you understand why cesarean sections are done, here's what you can do to increase your chances of delivering your baby vaginally:

• *Inform yourself.* Read, read, read; study, study, study. There are support groups (see page 292) for mothers who are grieving

about a previous cesarean and are adamant about doing everything within their power to avoid another. Attend these meetings, and talk to mothers who have delivered vaginally after a previous cesarean. Besides providing you with practical suggestions during your pregnancy and labor that will increase your chances of delivering vaginally, the information you obtain from this group can empower you to have an easier and more efficient labor.

• *Eat right.* Overeating may cause you to gain too much weight and your blood sugar to be too high. Both of these factors increase your chances of having a baby too large to be delivered vaginally.

• *Exercise regularly.* In-shape women typically have easier labors and healthier weight gains than couch potatoes.

• *Employ a professional labor assistant.* Studies show that mothers who use a professional labor assistant are much less likely to have a surgical birth. (See "Choosing a Labor Support Person," page 273.)

• *Be upright.* Back-lying is the position for surgical birth; the more time you spend on your back, the more likely you are to have one. (See "Working Out Your Best Birthing Positions," page 347.)

• *Get moving.* Avoid spending most of your time lying in bed wired to monitors like a surgical patient. When you get moving, your labor will, too.

• *Trust your body.* Believe that your delivery system will work. Believe that your pelvic passages are designed to birth your baby. The fear that you can't go through with the delivery can be a self-fulfilling prophecy, since fear frightens the uterus into not working efficiently (see page 302). Surround yourself with positive advisers. Even if your family tree or circle of friends is full of cesarean deliveries, know that you can beat these statistics.

- *"What's good for mother is good for baby."* Keep this truth in mind during your pregnancy and labor. Choices you make during your labor that help it progress more efficiently and less painfully are also likely to contribute to the well-being of your baby and lower the chance of fetal distress. (See "Working Out Your Own Personal Pain-Management System," page 302; "Helping Your Labor Progress — What You Should Know," page 340; and suggestions for increasing your chances of having a vaginal birth after a previous cesarean, page 292. Following the suggestions in these sections will lower your chances of needing a surgical birth.)

Questions You May Have About Cesarean Births

I had a cesarean with our last baby, and I'm worried I might need to have one again. Am I at higher risk for having another cesarean?

Chances are greatly in your favor that you can deliver your next baby vaginally. As with so many other medical myths, the rule "once a cesarean always a cesarean" no longer applies. The main reason for sentencing a first-time cesarean mother to lifelong birthing in the operating room was the fear of uterine rupture. Years ago, cesarean incisions were made vertically, in the upper part of the uterus — the area most prone to rupture. Nowadays, most cesarean incisions are made horizontally, in the lower part of the uterus (even in emergencies). This cut, a low-transverse incision or "bikini cut," is unlikely

to rupture. With a low-transverse incision, authorities now estimate the risk of uterine rupture in subsequent labors to be around 0.2 percent, which means there is a 99.8 percent chance of mother going through a labor without rupturing her uterus. In a survey of thirty-six thousand women attempting VBAC (vaginal birth after cesarean; pronounced "Vee-back"), no mother died of uterine rupture, regardless of the type of prior uterine incision. In a study of seventeen thousand women attempting VBAC, no infants died as a result of uterine rupture. (Don't let the term "rupture" scare you — it does not mean that your uterus will suddenly explode. Instead, the previous cesarean scar gradually pulls apart. Fortunately, the threat of uterine rupture can be detected by electronic fetal monitoring.) So the numbers are greatly in your favor — having a VBAC poses only a small risk for most women and is less risky than a surgical birth.

Whether you are a candidate for a VBAC may depend upon the reason for your previous cesarean. If you needed a surgical birth because your baby was in a breech position, you had an active herpes infection, you had toxemia, or the baby was experiencing true fetal distress, there is no reason to expect you will need a cesarean again. These factors were unique to the earlier pregnancy and may not recur. If the diagnosis leading to your previous cesarean was cephalopelvic disproportion (CPD) — your baby's head was thought to be too big to pass through your pelvis — there's still no reason to worry. New studies show that this diagnosis does not lessen your chances of having a VBAC. True CPD is very uncommon, and in most instances the births could just as easily have been labeled "failure to progress." Studies report a 65 to 70 percent chance of successful VBAC despite a previous diagnosis of CPD. A woman's pelvic outlet often becomes more flexible with each delivery, and various changes of position during labor can make it easier for baby to find the way out.

However, don't count on the positive statistics alone to carry you through a VBAC. Do your job, too:

Select birth attendants and a birth place friendly to VBACs. Your doctor's mind-set and your hospital's policies about a vaginal birth after a previous cesarean will make a difference to your outcome. Be sure both your practitioner and your hospital are up on the latest studies. And consider these fascinating statistics: The nationwide VBAC success rate is around 20 percent, but if a mother is under the care of a practitioner who regards VBAC as no riskier than any other delivery, the mother delivers in a hospital that does not consider VBAC women high-risk, and the mother uses the suggestions for helping the labor progress that are mentioned below, the VBAC success rate is 75 to 90 percent. This means that a woman choosing a VBAC may, in fact, have an even smaller chance of having a cesarean than the general population because she is now more motivated than most mothers to use a variety of tools to help her labor progress. Perhaps the obstacles to VBAC lie in the birthing policies of some obstetrical systems rather than in the pelvises of mothers. Find out what your prospective birth attendant's VBAC success rate is. For normal low-risk pregnancies, it should be at least 70 percent. Shun practitioners and hospitals who try to label you high-risk even if you have no risk factors besides a previous cesarean. Studies show that even mothers with two or three previous cesarean births have a 70 percent success rate with VBAC if they deliver in a birth place supportive of VBACs. Obstetrical centers that specialize in VBACs

do not consider most VBAC candidates high-risk and treat them no differently from any other obstetrical client. In fact, they consider it counterproductive to attach the "high-risk" label to VBAC mothers. Most women wishing a VBAC should be treated like any other woman delivering a baby. They require no more or less technology, intervention, or monitoring. Beware especially of birth attendants who have a "pelvic prejudice" against small-hipped mothers wanting a VBAC. Many petite women have successfully pushed out big babies.

Employ a professional labor assistant. If you're serious about delivering your next baby vaginally, a PLA is a must. In our experience, mothers using a PLA were much more likely to have the birth they wanted. (See "Choosing a Labor Support Person," page 273.)

Don't let technology or the measurements it produces scare you. VBAC studies fail to show any correlation between the size of the baby and the chances of uterine rupture. Also, estimates of fetal size and weight by ultrasound are not always accurate, especially in the final month.

Join a support group. There are support groups for mothers who need help grieving about their previous cesarean or avoiding another one. ICAN (International Cesarean Awareness Network, 310-542-6400) is one of the best and has chapters nationwide. This support group will help you deal with feelings of regret from your previous cesarean while arming you with information on how to avoid another one. You will hear helpful suggestions from mothers who have gone the surgical route once and were highly motivated to try a VBAC the next time. One great piece of advice from this and other support groups is to keep your mind in your present labor and not allow yourself to have flashbacks from the labor that led to the cesarean. Otherwise, you may panic at the first monitor alarm and undo all the good work of a previously efficient labor. If you want to feel fully empowered for a VBAC, a support group is your best bet.

I had a previous cesarean and I haven't yet gotten over feeling that I was a failure. I'm afraid this will affect my next birth and I'll have another cesarean.

You are no less a woman if you had a cesarean. After all, you nourished this baby through pregnancy, and your baby grew in your womb, even though the exit was not the one you planned on. Medical circumstances beyond your control may have led to your previous surgical birth. In all likelihood, you were doing the best you could at the time.

This time around you can avoid feelings of regret by being more informed and better prepared, and by following the suggestions we have given throughout this book on having a healthy pregnancy and efficient delivery. In our experience, women who begin studying up for a VBAC often realize that there were things they could have done to lessen their chances of having the cesarean. Mothers who can satisfy themselves that they did all they could to influence a positive birth outcome typically do not experience feelings of guilt and failure, because they realize they had a truly necessary cesarean.

So why feel guilty? Truthfully, you are not guilty for what happened to cause a cesarean. This is easy to see when you know you didn't "bring on" a breech position, a cord tightly wrapped around your baby's neck, a multiple pregnancy, or even an active case of herpes. In these cases your most likely reaction would be, "Thank God for modern obstetrics." But if the situation is less clear-cut, with no obvious physical reason you can point to, it's easier to look for someone to blame. If there is some doubt as to your performance ("I didn't walk enough," "I took the drug too soon," "I didn't relax enough," and on and on the list could go), the easiest person to blame might be yourself, and you would feel loaded with guilt. But that is hardly realistic. In many ways you are the victim in the scenario. You must never blame the victim. Resolve in your mind that you did the best you knew how, and blame the system if you need to blame someone. (Be careful not to shift blame onto your mate or you'll set up long-lasting conflict that will damage your relationship. He is no more to blame than you.) But don't get stuck in the blaming mode. Move on from there to forgiveness and the resolve to learn from the past — perhaps the greatest gift of all next to your precious baby. Rejoice in your motherhood and the prize of your delivery, and don't dwell on the way in which your baby came out.

Could my baby be less healthy if delivered by cesarean rather than vaginally?

Your baby should not be any less healthy if delivered by cesarean. In fact, depending on why the cesarean is done, he could turn out to be healthier. If a baby is found to be in distress during labor, waiting for a vaginal birth could compromise his health. As an obstetrician and a pediatrician, we can say with authority that how a baby gets out seems to make little difference to her health. Cesarean-birthed babies do often display the picture-perfect round newborn head, compared to the typical "cone head" of a baby who worked his way through the narrow vaginal passage. Surgically birthed babies do sometimes require more suctioning right after birth. They tend to be a bit more mucousy, probably because fluid was not squeezed out of the lungs as it would have been in a vaginal birth. Cesarean-birthed babies are sometimes slower to breastfeed, but that may be the result of mother and baby being separated and the drugs used in labor.

One possible health complication from a cesarean arises when a baby is delivered too early. This may happen when a C-section is performed before the mother goes into labor, perhaps because she is diabetic or has a heart problem. The due date may suggest that the baby is mature enough to be born, when in fact he isn't ready. If there is uncertainty about your dates or the maturity of your baby and you need a prescheduled cesarean, your doctor may elect to do an ultrasound and perform tests on the maturity of the baby's lungs to be sure she is ready for life outside the womb. If there is any doubt and there is no reason to suspect baby would be in jeopardy by being in the womb a week or so longer, it is best to wait.

There are benefits and risks to not doing a cesarean until mother begins labor. But, you may think, why should I go through any labor if I'm going to have a cesarean anyway? Besides indicating the baby is ready to be born, contractions give baby and mother the benefit of the natural hormones of labor, endorphins (see page 306). Studies show that babies delivered by cesarean after mother has labored for a while have fewer breathing problems in the first few days after birth than those whose mothers never entered labor. On the other hand, the surgical complication rate for mother may be slightly less for a scheduled cesarean than when the surgery has to be done because of a complication during labor. When in doubt, it's best not to hurry baby out.

Last time I tried a VBAC, but I ended up having a cesarean anyway. I feel I went through all that pain for nothing. I'm not sure I want to try again.

You didn't go through labor for nothing. If your newborn could talk, he would thank you for your labor of love. The natural hormones released during labor prepare a baby to adapt more easily to life outside the womb. Studies show that babies delivered by cesarean after mother labors awhile have fewer breathing problems in the first few days after birth than babies whose mothers were not in labor. (For additional information on this subject, see "Is Labor Good for Baby?" page 369.)

So many women are having cesareans nowadays. It seems to be no big deal. What complications might happen?

True, with modern surgical techniques and better anesthesia, cesarean sections have never been safer. Yet a surgical birth is a big deal. Cutting through all the layers of your abdomen and into your uterus is major surgery. Though minimal, there are risks of complication, such as hypersensitivity to the anesthetic, excessive bleeding, postoperative infection, and pain. Also, you are required to do double duty: healing yourself while learning to care for a newborn — not the most joyful way to enter motherhood. It's best to do whatever you can to lessen your chances of needing a surgical birth.

My due date is almost here and my baby is still butt down in a breech position. My doctor says it's safest for my baby to be delivered by cesarean. Is a cesarean necessary, or are there alternatives that are just as safe?

Studies show that breech babies have a lower risk of birth injury and newborn complications if delivered surgically rather than vaginally. Hence, the trend toward cesareans for babies in a breech position. Some specialists wonder whether the statistical increase in vaginal birth complications could be related to the breech position itself rather than to the mode of delivery, but currently in most hospitals, from 80 to 90 percent of breech babies are delivered by cesarean.

The main concern with a vaginal delivery of a breech newborn is that, with the feet or buttocks presenting first, the head will not have enough time to mold itself to the pelvic canal and may get stuck once the rest of the body is out. Also, a breech delivery can cause damage to the major nerves leading to the arms and hands. Both of these complications are less likely when baby presents buttocks first ("frank breech") rather than feet first. Prolapse of the umbilical cord (the cord slips through the cervix before baby's body and gets pinched), an emergency requiring an immediate cesarean delivery, is more common in breech deliveries.

Baby's being in a breech position does not mean you absolutely must have a cesarean birth. The American College of Obstetricians and Gynecologists officially sanctions vaginal births for breech babies as safe in *selective* situations. Your doctor will weigh the risks of a surgical versus a vaginal birth and recommend the course of action that is best in your situation. Here are some of the alternatives to explore with your doctor that may make it possible to deliver your breech baby vaginally.

Consider the possibility that your baby might turn. Around half of all babies start out bottom down early in pregnancy. Most turn head down by thirty-two to thirty-four weeks. If baby hasn't turned by thirty-six weeks, he or she is likely to remain in a breech position. For some unknown reason, 3 to 4 percent of babies never turn head down.

If your baby hasn't turned on her own by thirty-six to thirty-seven weeks, your doctor (or a specialist to whom you have been referred) can attempt a maneuver called "external version," in which he or she manipulates your abdomen to turn baby into the head-down position. External version is successful 60 to 70 percent of the time (40 to 50 percent for first pregnancies), but some babies turn back and require a second attempt. A few stubborn babies keep reverting to the breech position and remain there. A version is generally a safe and only mildly uncomfortable procedure, but sometimes it can be painful to mother and can cause distress to baby.

Another alternative is to search out a doctor who has experience in vaginal delivery of breech babies. He or she will most likely be affiliated with a hospital that has the technology and support staff to care for the baby properly should a complication occur. We have found that in most cases, doctors experienced in vaginal delivery of breech babies either practice at a university hospital obstetrical center or have gray hair and began delivering babies at least twenty years ago, when more than 90 percent of breech babies were delivered vaginally. You may get discouraged looking for one, since many of the doctors who have this kind of experience are now retired. Since in the past ten years, most breech babies have been delivered surgically, newly trained obstetricians may have delivered only a few breech babies vaginally. Also, if the obstetrical standard in your community is that breech babies are to be delivered surgically, don't be surprised if your doctor is forced to comply with this standard.

Obstetricians and hospital centers with a lot of experience in vaginal breech deliveries usually follow the American College of Obstetricians and Gynecologists guidelines for breech delivery. The criteria you need for a safe vaginal delivery of a breech baby include the following:

- Baby is in the frank breech position — bottom down instead of feet first or legs crossed in tailor sit.
- Baby weighs between 5.5 and 8 pounds (baby's head getting stuck during delivery is more likely to occur in small and premature babies, probably because the head is proportionally larger than the rest of baby's body).
- Baby is mature or at least older than thirty-six weeks.
- Baby's head is tucked down, chin on chest, prior to delivery.
- Mother is judged to have an adequate pelvis as determined by a technique called the "fetal-pelvic index" (see page 411).
- Mother's labor progresses normally.
- The hospital facility and staff are equipped for an emergency cesarean within thirty minutes.
- Mother's having delivered a previous baby vaginally adds another plus to the OK list.

If your baby is a footling or a complete breech, weighs more than 9 pounds, or is premature, your doctor will probably choose to deliver your baby surgically. Be aware that each specialist is likely to have his or her own variations on these criteria. Also, remember that an X-ray diagnosis of "inadequate pelvis" may be inaccurate, since your pelvic outlet will enlarge during delivery, especially in the squatting position (see explanation, page 349).

If you wish to have a vaginal delivery of your breech baby, and your doctor feels that you meet the criteria, expect that your labor will be monitored more closely than most. Even though you will experience careful surveillance during labor, take special care not to let the fear factor interfere with your labor. This is a good example of where a professional labor assistant can help, making sure that birth attendants are not hovering over you "waiting for something to happen."

By being informed of all the options for delivering your breech baby and by consulting a doctor experienced in vaginal delivery of breech babies, you and your doctor are likely to make a wise choice.

I had a vaginal herpes outbreak early in my pregnancy, but seem to be OK now. Will I need a cesarean section because of herpes?

A newborn baby can contract herpes during passage through an infected birth canal, so it is considered prudent obstetrical medicine to deliver via cesarean section all babies whose mothers have active herpes at the time of delivery. Herpes infections are life-threatening in newborns. If you have herpes, your doctor may do monthly or weekly vaginal cultures throughout your pregnancy to monitor your body's response to the stress of pregnancy (stress can cause genital herpes to flare up). Women with prior herpes outbreaks actually pass some immunity to their newborns. Women who acquire herpes for the first time during their pregnancy and have active sores at the time of delivery pose the greatest risk of infecting their babies. When you begin labor, your doctor may judge that it is safe for you to deliver vaginally if he or she sees no new herpes sores. If, however, your vaginal cultures continue to show herpes throughout your pregnancy, or if you have herpes sores when you begin labor, you may need a surgical delivery.

I'm scheduled to have a cesarean section. I know that in my situation it's best for my baby, but I'm disappointed. I wanted so much to have a natural birth. Besides, I'm scared of surgery.

It's normal to feel disappointed when the birth you hoped for will not be the birth you get, but the end result will be the same: you'll have a baby! A healthy baby is your main goal, even if you will need some technological help. You have grown this baby inside you. He or she will be your most important accomplishment, regardless of what route this special little person takes to get here.

All the natural childbirth information that is now available to women is a great thing, but it does set women up to feel like failures if they have to have surgery. Remember that a hundred years ago surgical birth was not a safe option, and be thankful that your cesarean will help ensure your baby's health. It's nice that you know about the surgery ahead of time so you can cope with the change of plans and not fight disappointment at the time of birth. You can also plan ahead and make the birth a positive experience for yourself and your baby. It takes maturity and a willingness to set aside your own desires to make the best of this situation. Having your baby surgically will be no less of an accomplishment than having a natural birth.

Because cesarean births are so common nowadays, one of your childbirth classes may be devoted entirely to cesarean deliveries. At least you won't enter the labor room unprepared. Remember, a cesarean section is primarily a birth, and there are things you can do to make this surgical birth a wonderful experience for yourself and your baby:

- Ask your doctor for a spinal or epidural anesthetic so you can be awake for the birth.

- Have your partner sit next to you at the head of the operating table. If he's hesitant, remind him that the actual procedure takes place behind a sterile curtain. He won't see anything unsettling.

- Ask your obstetrician to lift baby high enough so you can see him or her right after delivery. It is a beautiful sight to see your newborn lifted "up and out" during a cesarean birth.

- Immediately after your baby is delivered and quickly checked over (for temperature, breathing and pulse, and heart rate), ask that baby be brought to you to be held and hugged. You may need some help since you may be a bit groggy and one arm may be immobilized by an IV. This mother-father-baby bonding time, though brief, is an ideal time for pictures, and in many cases, the anesthesiologist or attending pediatrician will act as photographer for you.

- While your uterus and abdomen are being stitched closed (this takes about thirty minutes) and the operation is completed, your husband should accompany baby to the nursery so he or she will not be alone with strangers. This extra father-baby bonding time will have a deep impact on both of them.

- To decrease postoperative pain, ask your anesthesiologist about using a long-acting analgesic given in the anesthetic tubing. This do-it-yourself analgesia, called "patient-controlled analgesia" (PCA), is set up so you can administer your own medication through your intravenous. Just turn the pump on and off as you need relief. This medication is safe for your breastfeeding baby.

• In most cases baby can be brought to your bedside within an hour or two of surgery. If your husband or a nurse is present in the room and baby is healthy, it's even possible for a cesarean-birthed baby to room-in with mother. The best postoperative pain reliever is an injection of baby in your arms.

• Be planning ahead for some good long-term help, one thing you'll need more of since you'll be recovering from major surgery.

Recovery from abdominal surgery and the anesthetics used is rarely complicated. Remember, this event is a birth. You will feel just as elated when you first see your little one, and you will long to put baby to your breast. You will have the same need to gaze at your baby for hours on end, delighted with each yawn, burp, and wiggle. You'll be a proud mom, having given life to a precious new human being.

When I walked into the delivery area, I felt like my doctor was already sharpening his knife. I had barely gotten my shoes off and I was hooked up to continuous fetal monitoring and an intravenous line, and I, or at least my uterus, was viewed by the nursing staff as a disaster waiting to happen. As a final blow to my confidence, the lab technician came in to blood-type me "in case I needed blood" during an emergency operation. I was made to feel I was doing something unnatural to myself and too risky to my baby for wanting a VBAC — a feeling that did nothing to help my labor progress. Nevertheless, I went on to push out a healthy 10-pound baby. He was a full pound

larger than my previous baby who was delivered by cesarean because of "CPD."

Most of the women in my family "had" to have cesareans because, they were told, their pelvic bones were too small. With our first child I lived up to the family history and had a cesarean. With this baby I did my homework. I chose the right birth attendant, the right birth place, and I was not a patient but a participant in my delivery. I pushed out a healthy 9-pound baby. I let my body birth the way it was intended.

My cesarean birth and my vaginal birth left me with completely different feelings. With the cesarean I felt defeated. I thought everyone and everything had betrayed me. We have pictures of me right after the surgery. I look like I am dead. Someone even folded my hands over my stomach! With my VBAC I felt elated. All I can say is, "I did it! I did it!" One positive thing about having a C-section is that it taught me to become responsible for my birth. It helped me to grow up.

Dr. Linda notes: *There is now enormous pressure on doctors and patients to have VBACs. This is overall a good thing, and I think it improves women's well-being. But be sure you are having a VBAC because you and your caregiver think it is appropriate, not because your insurer thinks it will be cheaper. I see women who literally have Post-Traumatic Stress Disorder (PTSD) from a difficult labor and surgical delivery; it is wrong to force those women to go into a VBAC without appropriate counseling for the PTSD. While our practice has a 90 percent VBAC trial rate and an 80 percent success rate, the other 20 percent are very important women. They include the 10 per-*

cent who after careful consideration decide along with their caregivers that this particular pregnancy may best be served by a repeat cesarean. The final 10 percent are the women who end up with a cesarean despite doing all the right things. The morbidity (complication) rate of cesarean section in laboring patients is greater than the morbidity rate of a cesarean scheduled electively. This fact is often ignored in the VBAC literature, but I think it is an important issue for women who want to be informed consumers. Therefore, important questions to ask your caregiver include, How many of your prior C-section patients attempted a VBAC? What is your success rate? If either the trial rate is under 80 percent or success rate is under 50 percent without a good explanation, then you may want to find a group with more experience and expertise in this area.

What matters to me more than the way he got here is having a healthy baby. I know my cesarean was necessary, and I don't regret having it or feel less of a woman because of it. Recovery was certainly no picnic, but at least I could enjoy sex more comfortably than my vaginally delivering friends!

MANAGING PAIN IN CHILDBIRTH

Today's woman has more options for pain relief in childbirth than ever before. Not only is there much more the laboring woman can do for natural pain relief, but medical pain relievers are also getting better and safer. Because there are so many analgesic options, today's mother needs to be well informed. It's best to learn about natural and medical pain relief a couple of months before labor day. It's no fun getting a crash course in pain management when the first contraction hits. Of course, safe and effective pain relief in childbirth depends on the partnership between you and your practitioner. But learning how you can use your mind and body to enhance the progress and ease the pain of labor is more important than knowing what shot of analgesic or whiff of gas your doctor will offer. Here's what you should know and what you can do to ease the discomfort of labor.

Why Childbirth Hurts

It takes a lot of pushing and stretching to move a baby the size of a melon through a cervical opening that starts out the size of a kidney bean. Muscles don't flex and tissues don't stretch without letting your body know it. Your uterus will be working very hard to accomplish the feat of childbirth.

Contrary to popular belief, it's usually not the contracting uterine muscles that produce the pain. Most childbirth pain originates in the stretching of the cervix, vagina, and surrounding tissues as baby passes through. During labor the uterus doesn't squeeze baby out; what really happens is that uterine contractions work to pull the cervical muscle up out of the way so that the baby's head can then be pushed through. (Think of a turtleneck sweater being slowly stretched as you pull it over your head.) The muscles and ligaments in the pelvis are richly supplied with pressure receptors and pain receptors in the nerves, so the stretching produces powerful sensations that may be interpreted as pain, especially if there is tension in the surrounding muscles.

Like any muscle, uterine muscles don't hurt unless they are forced to work in a way

The Purpose of Pain

Why does childbirth have to hurt so much? The "curse of Eve" concept — the idea that childbirth pain is every woman's punishment for Eve's having eaten the apple — is neither sound biblical theology nor acceptable postfeminist philosophy. That childbirth pain is a rite of passage that prepares a woman for the hard work of motherhood is not a bestselling concept either. Even the wisest obstetrical researchers have not yet come up with a good scientific statement as to the purpose of pain in childbirth. So we are back to the drawing board of common sense.

It's no wonder many women sign up for epidurals when they preregister at the hospital. Movies and television often portray pregnancy as an illness to be endured and labor as a crisis event in this illness, one that must be treated with drugs while a woman lies on her back in bed. Childbirth educators, on the other hand, try not to even mention the *P* word, substituting the more technical term "contractions" for "pains."

Could it be that pain serves some useful purpose in childbirth? After experiencing birth and watching thousands of women manage (or not manage) their labor pains, we have two theories about pain and birth:

1. Pain does serve a useful purpose.
2. Unmanageable pain is not normal, necessary, or healthy in childbirth.

Overwhelming pain is the body's signal that a muscle group is not working the way in which they were not designed to work. Yet tired, tense, and strained muscles do hurt, which is why you need to learn how to help your birthing muscles work efficiently for you. When a muscle is overly tired, the natural chemistry and electrical activity within the muscle tissues get out of balance. These physiological changes produce pain.

How You Feel Pain

In order to manage childbirth pain well you need to understand how your body processes pain and how your mind perceives it. If you follow a typical labor contraction from stretched pelvic tissue to verbal "ouch!" you will see how you can influence the amount of pain produced in your pelvis versus the amount of it you feel in your brain.

The contraction begins, tissues stretch, and the tiny pressure receptors in the nerves are stimulated, sending lightning-fast impulses along the nerves to the spinal cord. Pain receptors are stimulated as well if the surrounding muscles are tense. In the spinal cord these impulses must pass through a sort of gate that can stop some impulses and allow others to pass through into the brain, where they can be registered as pain. So you can influence pain at three sites: where it's produced in the first place; at the gate in the spinal cord; and in the brain, where the pain is perceived. In working out your own techniques for pain management, you will want to employ pain-relief measures that can control pain at all three of these sites.

Another way to understand this pain pathway is to picture pain impulses as miniature it is designed to, or that something is going wrong in the body and needs attention. If you are running a marathon and find you are becoming painfully exhausted, you take this as a cue that you need some nourishment or liquid, or that you need to change your breathing technique or style of running. You make whatever changes are necessary to increase your energy and ease your pain, while still progressing toward your goal.

The same is true of birthing a baby. If a mother feels excruciating pain in her back, she interprets this as a signal to keep changing her position until she feels relief. What's good for mother is good for baby: by changing her position, she allows baby to shift and find an easier — and less painful — way out. Pain, properly understood and wisely managed, is a valuable labor assistant. Listen to its signals. This is why in some cultures childbirth pain is referred to as "good pain."

"Pain for a purpose" is not some weird, New Age concept developed by males, a few stoic women, or some ivory tower researcher who has never felt the sensations of birth. Nor does it mean that childbirth is just another endurance contest; the "no-pain, no-gain" concept has little merit. (Sports medicine specialists don't even believe in it.) Think of pain as the birth communicator: manageable pain means your cervix is doing its job, opening so you can push baby out; unmanageable pain means you need to change what you're doing.

race cars. They speed from the stimulus site in the pelvis to parking spaces, or microscopic pain receptors, located on the nerve cells of the spinal cord and brain. The more cars that park, the more sensation you perceive. You can influence the activity of these pain cars. First, you can limit the number of cars getting started in the first place. To do this, you can practice relaxation techniques (described on page 305) to keep your muscles from getting tired and tense. And you can use efficient positions for labor (see page 347) that keep your muscles working in the way in which they were designed to work. Next, you can close the gate in the spinal cord so the cars can't get through. A pleasant touch stimulus, such as massage, sends positive impulses that can block the transmission of pain impulses through the spinal cord. You can also cause gridlock at the gate by sending through a lot of competing vehicles, such as impulses from music (see page 307), specific mental imagery (see page 307) or counter-pressure (see pages 310 and 312). Finally, you can fill up the receptor sites in the brain so that the pain cars have no place to park. Blocking access to this third pain-perception site is how pain-relieving drugs work. You can achieve the same effect naturally by manufacturing your body's own painkillers, called "endorphins" (see page 306).

Also, distraction techniques can be used to fill up pain receptor sites in the brain and thus block the perception of pain. With the distraction method, you endeavor to fill your brain with alternative images, the idea being that your focus on them will overshadow your perception of pain. These techniques sound good in childbirth classes, and even seem to work when you are practicing in the living room, but they often fail when the real labor begins. Concentrating on an image requires great mental discipline, the kind that takes years to acquire. For most mothers, the effort soon becomes mental strain, which tends to put the body on edge. In our experience, neither mind nor muscles relax when a mother tries to concentrate on something else to escape from her labor. Managing pain during labor requires attention to both mind and muscles.

Martha notes: With my first few labors I tried distraction techniques, such as fixing my eyes trancelike on a focal point, breathing in patterns, and tapping out a tune with my fingers. But when my labors became so demanding that these techniques no longer worked, I intuitively began to do what did *work: I let my body take over and do what it had to do. When I learned to release my body during labor rather than try to control it, I was more relaxed, as were my muscles.*

Working Out Your Own Personal Pain-Management System

Every person perceives pain differently: one person's "sensation" is another person's "hurt." For this reason, every woman must come to the labor room armed with her own personal pain-management system and a backup plan. The responsibility for pain management during labor is primarily yours. Your birth attendants are there as consultants. Even though no amount of reading and preparation will totally prepare you for what this particular labor is going to feel like, odds are, the more informed and prepared you are,

the less fearful you will be — and the less your labor will hurt. In showing you how to work out the right pain-management system for yourself, we will focus on ways to lessen both pain production and pain perception.

Forget your fears. There is a connection between fear and pain. The efficiency of the magnificent uterine muscle depends upon your hormonal, circulatory, and nervous systems all working together. Fear upsets these three systems. Fear and anxiety cause your body to produce excess stress hormones, which counteract the helpful hormones your body produces to enhance the labor process and relieve discomfort. This results in increased pain and a longer labor. Fear also causes physiological reactions that reduce blood flow and thus oxygen supply to the uterus. An oxygen-deprived muscle tires quickly, and a tired muscle is a hurting muscle. Fear produces muscle tension, and the last thing you want during labor is tight muscles. Tense and tight muscles not only hurt, but they also have a harder time working in harmony to open the cervix enough to allow you to push baby out. Normally, the muscles in the upper part of the uterus contract and pull up while the lower ones relax and open. The contractions of the upper muscles and the relaxation of the lower ones open the cervix and pull the uterus over baby's head during contractions. Fear affects primarily the lower muscles, causing them to tighten instead of relax. As a result, the strong muscles of the upper uterus contract against the tight lower uterine muscles and cervix, producing much pain and little progress.

British obstetrician Grantly Dick-Read, author of *Childbirth Without Fear,* was the first to describe this fear-tension-pain cycle. While examining women in labor he noticed that a woman's cervix was softened and dilating when she was relaxed, but harder and tightened when she reacted to a contraction with fear. Fear produces tension in the muscles, which produces pain, which produces more fear, which increases the tension, which intensifies the pain, and the cycle continues. By teaching women how to work *with* rather than against their bodies, breaking the fear-tension-pain cycle, Dr. Dick-Read proved that women do not have to suffer or be heavily drugged to give birth. Most of the pain-management systems taught in today's childbirth classes are based upon Dr. Dick-Read's observation of the way in which the mind can influence the body during labor.

Work out your fears before your birth. Some fear of labor is perfectly normal, springing from anxiety about the unknown and individual experience with pain. However, unresolved fears can impede your labor. Even though a fearless labor is as rare as a painless birth, you should try to resolve your fears before birth day. Here's how:

- *Address your fears.* What specifically do you fear about birth? Do you fear the pain, for example, having had negative experiences with pain in the past? Do you fear having a cesarean or needing an episiotomy? Are you afraid that you will lose control midway through labor? Do you have fears about problems with the baby? List all your fears and alongside each one, write what you can do to avoid having the fear come true. Realize, too, that some events and outcomes are beyond your power to change, and resolve not to worry about things you cannot change.

- *Be informed.* The more you know, the less afraid you will be. While no two mothers' labors are alike, and each birth a woman

experiences is different from another, childbirth does follow a general outline. There are sensations ("pains") that will always occur between the first contraction and the final delivery of a baby. If you understand what happens and why and what it will probably feel like, you will not be taken by surprise. Having a sense of what to expect — and when it will end — helps most mothers feel confident that they can handle labor and delivery. A good childbirth class can help you understand what happens and why. There is no class that can tell you what it will feel like specifically for you, because this will depend on your particular situation and your ability to cooperate with the forces of labor. Women can easily be taken by surprise at the intensity of labor. Some decide they do not like it one bit and wind up resisting the forces when fear takes hold.

- *Employ a professional labor support person.* An experienced woman who has gone through labor herself and who has made a profession of studying the normal sensations of labor and what to do about them will be a valuable person to have at your side. This special woman, a PLA, will help you interpret your sensations during labor, offer suggestions for managing your pain, and help you understand and participate in any medical decisions. (See "Choosing a Labor Support Person," page 273.)

- *Surround yourself with fearless helpers.* Try to bring as little extraneous fear as possible into your birthing room. By now you've probably learned who among your friends and family see birth as a horror story and who do not. Fear is contagious. Be sure you do not allow any of these horrified helpers to be in the labor room. Don't think that this is the time to finally prove something to your mother; if she has a fearful attitude about labor, it is better for her to watch your birth on video afterward than to be in the birthing room infecting you with her fears.

• *Avoid fearful replays.* Don't carry scary baggage from your past into the delivery room. Birth has a way of stirring up uncomfortable memories of previous traumatic labors or even of a past sexual assault. You may, at the height of an overwhelming contraction, automatically push "tense-up" buttons in response to events long past. Deal with the emotional fallout of traumatic experiences before labor day. Get professional counseling if necessary.

Dr. Bill notes: Many men, including fathers-to-be, are afraid of birth. They don't understand childbirth pain, and they find it very upsetting when their mate hurts and they can't "fix" it. Even Mr. Sensitive-and-Fearless may become Mr. Frightened at the height of a particularly hard series of contractions, or in response to a sudden change in birth plan. It helps to inoculate your mate against fear so that he won't pass the bug on to you. Prepare your partner for the normal sights and sounds of labor. Tell him what may happen if events don't go as planned. And try not to share your own fear. If he sees that you are not afraid, he is less likely to be so himself. A calm birth attendant can give your mate a much-needed break and help him keep focused on his job, which is to support you and share in the birth experience, not to protect you from this perfectly normal process.

Take Responsibility for Your Birth Decisions

While a painless childbirth is rarer than a sleep-through-the-night newborn, most pain in childbirth is under your influence — if you are ready for it. Check yourself against this list of the major factors that affect how painful a birth will be:

☐ Have you chosen your practitioner wisely? Does your doctor or midwife take an active role in teaching you about the birth process and helping you to trust your body to give birth? After each visit do you leave believing your birth will go right? Or does this person create a fearful mind-set about birth, filling your mind with all the possibilities of what could go wrong?

☐ Do you understand the labor and birth process? Do you know what happens during contractions, what it is those "pains" do? Do you understand how being upright and changing positions during labor can influence how you experience contractions?

☐ Are you armed with a variety of relaxation techniques? (See below.)

☐ Have you employed a professional labor support person, especially if there is a possibility that the doctor or midwife you are counting on for support will not be available when you go into labor?

☐ Are you certain that everyone you have invited to your birth (friends, relatives, and mate) is going to help you labor confidently and not undermine your confidence with a fearful attitude?

□ Do you understand which technological tools (e.g., electronic fetal monitoring) are likely to be used during your labor? Are you confident that you are knowledgeable enough to participate in decisions about the use of technology in your labor?

□ Are you aware of the options available for medical pain relief, such as narcotics and epidural anesthesia? Do you understand their benefits and risks?

□ Do you realize how important it is to release and surrender to your body during labor? Are you determined to assume whatever position works for you rather than tensing up, resisting the labor process, or becoming a passive patient and spending a lot of time in the horizontal position?

You need to enter the delivery room with each of these questions thoroughly answered. Women who enter the delivery room armed with their own answers are the ones most likely to have a satisfying birth.

Learn to Relax Your Birthing Muscles

"Relax? Are you kidding? These contractions feel like a Mack truck plowing through my belly!" So said a mother we know to her coach midway through labor. "Relax" is more than just an empty word for helpless bystanders to throw at a mother who is experiencing the most intense physical work of her life. It is exactly what she must do in order to help the work progress. Relaxing will help her cooperate with what her uterus is doing rather than resist it. Being able to relax makes the difference between a happy birth experience you want to treasure in your memory and a "war story" you would just as soon forget.

Why relax? Relaxing all of your other muscles while only your uterus contracts eases the discomfort and speeds the progress of labor. If there is tension anywhere in your body, especially in your face and neck, this tension will spread to the pelvic muscles that need to stay loose during a contraction. Tense muscles hurt more than relaxed ones, and they tire sooner. Chemical changes within an exhausted, tense muscle actually lower the muscle's pain threshold, and you hurt more than if the muscle were working unopposed. When tight muscles resist the relentless, involuntary contractions of your uterus, the result is pain. Exhausted muscles soon lead to an exhausted mind, increasing your awareness of pain and decreasing your ability to cope with it. You lose your ability to explore options and make changes that would lessen your misery.

Running a marathon is hard and constant work. Laboring a baby out takes even longer (usually), but the hard work is done in spurts with periods of rest in between, a sort of charge and recharge. Once a contraction is finished, you need to let go of it so you can totally rest. If you don't relax between contractions, you will not be able to recharge and welcome the next contraction with its good work. Labor becomes steadily more intense and energy-consuming as it progresses, so relaxation is important for conserving energy for what's ahead — the active phase of labor and the pushing stage, when enormous energy will be needed for the hardest work you will ever do.

Relaxation also helps balance your hormones for birth. As we mentioned earlier, two sets of hormones help you labor efficiently. Adrenal hormones (also called "stress hormones") give your body the extra power it needs in situations that call for tremendous effort, like labor and birth. These hormones are often referred to as the "fight or flight" hormones, and they are there for the body's protection. The adrenal hormone, epinephrine, exerts a synergistic effect on the natural narcotics your body produces, adding more natural pain relief. During labor your body needs enough of these stress hormones to help you work hard, but not so many that your body becomes anxious and distressed, causing your mind and muscles to work inefficiently. Stress hormones may even divert blood from the hardworking uterus to the vital organs of the brain, heart, and kidney.

Another kind of hormone also works for you during labor — natural pain-relieving hormones, known as "endorphins." (The word comes from *end*ogenous, meaning "produced in the body," and m*orphine,* a chemical that blocks pain.) These are your body's natural narcotics, helping to relax you when you're stressed, and relieving pain when you're hurt. These physiological labor assistants are produced in the nerve cells. They attach themselves to pain receptor sites on the nerve cell, where they blunt the sensation of pain. Strenuous exercise increases endorphin levels, and endorphins enter your system automatically during the strenuous exercise of labor, as long as you don't do anything to block them. Tensing up blocks endorphin release. Levels are highest in the second stage of labor (pushing), when contractions are most intense. Like artificial narcotics, endorphins can work differently on different women, which may explain why some women seem to feel more pain than others. Unimpeded endorphins are better for you

than artificial narcotics. Instead of the periodic "blast" and subsequent groggy feeling you get with drugs, endorphins provide steady pain relief during labor and a feeling of mental well-being that laboring mothers often describe as "naturally drugged." Relaxing will allow these natural pain relievers to work for you. Fear and anxiety can increase your level of stress hormones and counteract the relaxing effects of endorphins. If your mind is less anxious, your body is less likely to hurt.

Endorphins also help you in the transition from birthing to mothering. Levels are actually highest just after birth and don't return to prelabor levels until two weeks postpartum. Endorphins stimulate the secretion of prolactin, the relaxing and "mothering" hormone that regulates milk production and gives you a psychological boost toward enjoyment of mothering. Endorphins also help you stay relaxed during pregnancy. Studies have shown that endorphin levels are increased by laughter, perhaps accounting for the verse from Proverbs, "A cheerful spirit is health to the body and strength to the soul."

When you labor the way your mind and body are designed to, your body produces just the right balance of stress hormones and endorphins. Fear and exhaustion drive these hormones out of balance so that the stress hormones override the pain-relieving hormones, resulting in a labor that hurts more and progresses less. When you relax during labor, you'll be amazed how your body is under the control of your mind. You'll feel better and your baby will be born more easily.

How to relax. When you are choosing a childbirth class, one of your criteria should be how much time is spent teaching you to understand the level of relaxation needed for birth. Realistically, your ability to relax is governed by your subconscious. Reading books and listening to lectures will not help you relax. You must spend as much time as possible practicing relaxation. Ask for extra help if you need it. Some one-on-one counseling and instruction may help you break the "relaxation barrier." Here are some time-tested relaxation helpers Martha and mothers we have counseled have found most helpful in their labors:

• *Relax and release.* "Relax and release" is the basis of all the exercises that follow: relax *between* contractions, release *during* contractions. You must keep these two words in mind during your labor.

Condition yourself to think muscle-relaxing thoughts that help you surrender to the normal workings of your body. When you feel a contraction beginning, instead of tensing your muscles and bracing yourself for what's to come, take a deep breath, relax, and release. Practicing "R&R" exercises conditions you to say to yourself, "Contraction coming, release" instead of "Oh, no, not another contraction!"

Practice relaxation with your partner. Get comfortable. Collect a bunch of pillows and teach the chief pillow-placer (your partner) where you like them. Do these exercises in various positions: standing and leaning against your partner, a wall, or a piece of furniture; sitting down; lying on your side; and even on all fours.

EXERCISE #1: Check your whole body for muscle tension: a furrowed forehead, clenched fists, and a tight mouth are the easiest ones to spot. Then practice releasing each group of muscles from head to toe systematically. Tense, then relax, each muscle group to help you identify the two different states. When your partner cues you with "contraction," think "relax and release." Then feel these tight muscles loosen.

EXERCISE #2: Practice touch-relaxation frequently throughout your final month of pregnancy. Touch-relaxation conditions you to expect pleasure rather than pain to follow tension. Find out which touches and what kinds of massage relax you best (see page 312). Do the head-to-toe progression described above. Tense each muscle group, then have your partner apply a warm, relaxed touch to that area as your cue to release the tension. This way you won't have to keep hearing the verbal cue "relax," which eventually becomes irritating. Another goal is to be able to relax a tense muscle when your partner puts just the right touch on that spot just as it begins to hurt. Practice: "I hurt here — you press hard [or stroke or touch] here."

• *Music to birth by.* Music can be a wonderful relaxation aid. Carefully choose a medley to fit your taste and help you relax. Play this music during your practice relaxation sessions at home so you are conditioned to relax when you hear these soothing sounds on labor day. (For favorite lullabies of labor, see page 314.)

• *Mental imagery.* A clear mind filled with soothing scenes relaxes a laboring body — at least between contractions. It also encourages the production of labor-enhancing endorphins. Sports psychologists use mental imagery to help athletes perform.

Determine now what thoughts and scenes you find most relaxing and practice meditating on them frequently throughout the day, especially in the final month of pregnancy. In this way you'll bring to your birth a mental library of short features that you can click on for a few minutes' relaxation between contractions. Most laboring mothers find these birth-related images

helpful: rolling waves, waterfalls, meandering streams, walking along the beach with their mate. You may also want to file away half a dozen mental flash cards of your

Childbirth Pain in Perspective

One day, after speaking at the 1996 International Childbirth Education Association (ICEA) convention, we had the opportunity to listen to a group of veteran mothers who were also childbirth educators discuss the topic of pain in childbirth.* We realized that they had a whole different perspective on pain from that of first-time pregnant women who are influenced by the war stories they hear from friends. A first-timer is programmed to expect that the pain she will experience at childbirth is the most awful pain in her whole life. She enters labor with fear. She has no idea what it will be like; she just knows it's going to feel awful. The experienced childbirth educator has often experienced several births and has a different perspective on pain. It's not that labor is worse than any pain you've ever felt in your whole life, it's just that it is different. Realizing how childbirth pain differs is what gets the experienced woman through labor in a much less painful way than a novice.

Ponder for a moment the worst pain you have ever suffered in your whole life, say, a bad toothache. It caught you by surprise; it went on for days. It started out severe and was unrelenting no matter what you did. It just wouldn't go away. You would have given anything for a few minutes of relief. Childbirth pain is different:

- You know it's going to happen, you just don't know how it's going to feel.
- It's not unrelenting. There are blissful pauses between the pains, and the pauses may last a lot longer than the pains, at least early in labor. Put the pain in perspective. Each one is only sixty to ninety seconds long.
- It's predictable. You know that within a minute or more another pain is going to come.
- After a while you begin to know what the next pain is going to feel like. It may be a bit more or less intense than the previous one, but it's going to feel similar.
- Childbirth pain builds slowly, giving you a chance to get accustomed to it and to cope with it.
- It has an ongoing purpose, signaling you to make adjustments for the benefit of baby.
- You know that it will end.
- When it ends, you get the world's most magnificent reward.

When you put these pains in perspective, it's clear that Mother Nature designed labor pains to be manageable. If they weren't, why would women go on having babies?

---

* *Many thanks to Jan Mallak and other childbirth educators for this perspective on childbirth pain.*

most pleasant memories: how you met your mate, a favorite date, lovemaking, a special vacation.

Visualize what's happening during your labor. When a contraction begins, picture your uterus "hugging" your baby and pulling itself up over his or her adorable little head. During the dilating stage, imagine your cervix getting thinner and more open with each contraction. Some mothers who have used visual imagery successfully during the pushing stage have visualized their vaginas opening up like a flower.

Change scenes from painful to pleasant. Try the strategy called "packaging the pain." Grab the pain as if it were a big glob of modeling clay, massage it into a tiny ball, wrap it up, put it in a helium balloon, and imagine it leaving your body and floating up into the sky. Do the same with distressing thoughts: wrap them up and picture them floating away. This exercise is especially helpful in conjunction with a cleansing breath during a contraction: breathe deeply, exhale, and blow the pain away.

Between and during the more painful contractions, imagine the prize rather than the pain you have to go through to get it. Picture yourself reaching down as your baby comes out, assisting your birth attendant in placing your baby on your abdomen, and nestling your child against your breasts.

Mental imagery is not a mind-over-body technique — it's mind helping body work more efficiently. Be sure to use mental imagery as a relaxing tool, not as a distraction gimmick. If you believe that you can put your mind on another planet to help you escape from what's going on in your body, you're probably in for a big surprise; contractions can be so overwhelming that efforts at mental escape will have little effect. It's more realistic to expect your mind to work with your labor rather than escape from it.

I found it helpful to completely erase the word "pain" from my thoughts. When my contractions began, instead of anticipating a pain, I imagined, "Here comes a pleasant."

Visualizing my favorite dessert helped me relax. My childbirth educator reminded me that "stressed" spelled backward is "desserts."

Consider Laboring in Water

Oftentimes the simple things in life — and labor — work the best. One of the most effective labor pain relievers also happens to be the least expensive. It is also without side effects. The miracle? Water — not to drink, but to float in.

Martha notes: *I personally experienced the benefits of water labor with the birth of our*

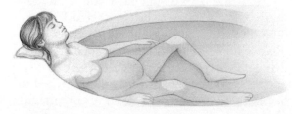
Water labor.

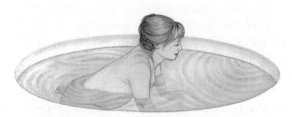

seventh baby, Stephen. After four hours of labor I began to feel an intense pain low in front. This was a strong signal to my body that something needed attention. If it had been pain in my back, the all-fours position would have helped. I tried that position anyway, but it only hurt more. Then I got into a large tub filled with warm water. I felt my entire body relax, just like that. I experimented with different positions and finally found one that allowed me just to let go and float from my shoulders down so that my whole torso and pelvis could remain totally relaxed. At that point, the pain literally melted away — better than Demerol! The buoyancy did for me what I was not able to achieve by myself.

The experience of total release accompanied by total relief was amazing. I stayed in the water for about an hour until I reached the pushing stage. Then I got out and delivered Stephen on the bed in a side-lying position. As the baby emerged, we discovered the reason I'd felt such pain; his little hand presented alongside his head, so two parts of him were coming through the cervix at once. My body needed total relaxation to allow my muscles to give way to the larger-than-usual presentation. Too bad it took me seven labors to discover how wonderfully water works.

Why water works. Remember your high school physics? Place an object in water, and the force of buoyancy equal to its weight lifts it up. To simplify Archimedes' principle, put it this way: water gives a pregnant mother a lift. Buoyancy feels like weightlessness. With less weight to support and less muscle tension, your body feels less pain and saves energy for where it is needed — your hardworking uterus.

Water relieves. Muscles that weigh less tire less and hurt less. Also, the counterpressure of water can ease the pain of sore muscles, especially during back labor. Recall our earlier discussion about relieving pain by filling the nervous system with pleasant sensations so there's less room left over for painful ones. Being in water is like a continuous body massage, stimulating all the touch receptors in the skin. It would take thousands of gentle fingertips to touch as many skin receptors as the water does when you soak in a nice warm bath.

Water relaxes. Immersing most of your body in a warm tub soothes your mind and body, reduces stress hormones, and allows your body's natural relaxing and pain-relieving hormones to take over.

Water releases. Changing positions and going with the flow of labor are the most important natural pain relievers and labor enhancers a woman can use. Being in water lets this happen more naturally and easily. Many women laboring on terra firma describe feeling rooted to one spot, afraid to move at all, lest it hurt more. A woman in water is free to float with her body supported until she finds the position that best eases her discomfort. Being in water also seems to free her mind, so she can tap into her deepest instincts and let tension float away. Next time you're in a swimming pool, see if this doesn't ring true. Notice how you are free to move your body and clear your mind.

Water labor has been used in Russia and France for the past thirty years, but it's relatively new to North America. A recent study of eighteen hundred women who labored in Jacuzzi-type pools showed these encouraging results:

- The women had shorter labors.
- Cervical dilatation was more efficient — 2.5 centimeters per hour compared with 1.25 centimeters per hour for mothers who did not take advantage of water during their labors.
- The descent of the babies was twice as fast.
- The women reported less pain.
- The cesarean section rate was one-third that of traditional hospital births.
- Mothers labeled "high-risk" because of high blood pressure showed a dramatic reduction in their blood pressure within minutes of immersion in the pool.

More gain with less pain — bring out the labor tubs!

Using water for labor. Some hospital maternity suites and birth centers have Jacuzzi-size labor tubs. If the hospital of your choice does not offer one, ask for it. This is just one more way in which women can influence how birth business is done. An alternative is to rent one; check with local midwives or childbirth organizations for information. (Of course, you will have to convince your birth practitioner and the hospital to go along with this.) The tub should be large enough to bring out the mermaid in you — at least five and a half feet wide. It's not only being in water that eases the discomforts of labor; it's the freedom to move that gives you the greatest benefit. Here are some ways to use water to your advantage during labor:

- Have the water at bath-water temperature, which is usually around your body temperature.

- Try lounging on your back or side or kneeling forward on all fours, so that the water covers your uterus, at least up to your nipple line.

- Enter the tub when the intensity of your contractions tells you you need some relief. For most women the best time to take the plunge is between 5 and 8 centimeters dilatation, when active labor is in full swing. You may also find water labor especially comforting during transition — the most intense stage of labor. The freestyle movements of mother help baby to find the path of least resistance (and least pain). Lying in a labor tub can also be used to accelerate a slow labor. The splashing of the water on your nipples can trigger the release of contraction-stimulating hormones. And water is also very effective in easing a fast-and-heavy labor, where the contractions threaten to overwhelm you.

- If your labor stalls while you are comfortably floating in the water, get out and walk or squat on land to get your labor going again; reenter your "womb" once labor gets going.

- When you enter and exit the water, be sure to do so between contractions and with assistance, so you don't slip.

- When you feel the urge to push, it's time to get dry. (Babies have been born in the water when there was suddenly no time to exit or when a mother was so comfortable she could not bring herself to leave the water. Babies do just fine, as long as they are lifted up out of the water and placed in mother's arms without delay. Baby simply goes from water to water and doesn't take a breath until his face meets the air.)

Unless your birth attendant advises you otherwise, it's safe to use water labor even after your membranes have ruptured. That's when contractions usually get more intense and you really need the relief of water. Maternity centers with much experience in water labor (and water birth) report no increased rate of infection in women using water after their membranes have ruptured, as long as the mothers are in active labor and proper infection-control hygiene is followed.

It is rarely necessary to leave the water for routine tests. If you need an IV, a heparin lock can be used in the veins of your hand, covered with a waterproof plastic bag, and sealed with a rubber band. If intermittent fetal monitoring is necessary, let it be done on a part of your abdomen that you can lift above the water; place a plastic bag over the handheld monitor if you aren't using a monitor designed for underwater use.

If your hospital or birth center does not offer a labor tub or you're unable to rent one, at least try sitting in a regular tub or taking a shower. A jet of warm water is often especially effective in easing back labor. And, in addition to the feel of water, the soothing sounds of the shower running or the tub filling are welcome during labor.

Don't expect all the pain of labor to float away into the water. Our personal experience, however, and that of other women who have used labor pools suggest that water is one of the most wonderful labor-saving devices available.

Use the Right Touches

A soothing massage, a caring caress, a passionate kiss, even a simple foot rub can be blissful relief to a laboring mother. The power of touch to relieve pain is based on the pain-control theory described on page 300. By stroking the receptor-rich skin and kneading the pressure receptors beneath the skin, you bombard the brain with pleasant stimuli, leaving less room for painful ones.

You won't really know where or how to ask your partner to rub or press till labor day is under way. But in the final months some practice rubdowns to relieve backache or to help you relax during Braxton Hicks contractions will prepare both of you for labor, when the right touch really counts. Tell your partner that a lot of prenatal practice will condition his hand muscles so they won't tire so easily on the big day.

Using pure vegetable oil or massage lotion, try different strokes in different areas of the body. Firm caressing with the fingertips is preferred on the face and scalp. Deep pressure and kneading is welcome for large muscles, such as the shoulders, thighs, buttocks, calves, and feet. Try counterpressure with the heel of your hand for easing the pain in lower back muscles.

The last couple of months not only provide an opportunity to work out massage strokes that you like but also give you a chance to weed out those you don't. For example, stroking down in the direction of body hair growth is pleasant, whereas light stroking upward, against the hair shaft, may irritate a laboring woman. Help your partner learn the intensity and rhythm of the pressure you enjoy. When you massage him, show him what you like so he'll learn by being on the receiving end.

My first labor was slow and I got the best, most relaxing, foot rubs. My second was fast and furious and my husband rubbed my legs hard and fast, up and down. Somehow he knew instinctively that only something intense could compete with the pain of passing a cannonball!

A tip for the masseur: don't take criticism of your massages personally. Expect your mate to be touchy during late pregnancy and irritable during labor. Rubs that she used to love may get you a curt "Stop that!" or "Don't touch!" on labor day, as you discover the "hot spots" that annoy rather than relax her. During your childbirth class you may practice with massage tools such as tennis balls or paint rollers, but be prepared to improvise. Experiment with many different touches in different places throughout different stages of labor. Just be quick to switch gears if your partner doesn't like what you're doing, and be patient. She'll try to let you know what she wants, but she'll be too preoccupied for politeness. Rest assured, she'll appreciate your efforts immensely.

During labor, I went ballistic when my husband tried to move my bangs in the opposite way from how I comb them. I used to love him to massage my abdomen as we talked to the baby while lying in bed, but during labor I couldn't stand to have anybody touch my tummy.

Breathe Right for Birthing

Breathing is so automatic you probably wonder why you have to practice it in childbirth classes. You may never even have considered how taking the right breath could relax your body and relieve your pain during labor, but it's important to breathe properly; every exercise has its optimal breathing pattern, and this is especially true of labor.

Forget those old birth videos that show laboring women panting robotically at the first uterine twitch. Even if mothers were able to remember the canned breathing techniques they learned in class, they usually found that this unnatural respiration pattern did little to relieve pain. Instead, it sometimes left them feeling a bit light-headed and often caused

them to become tense, the very thing you don't want.

My husband and I practiced our patterned breathing every night, but once I was in the grip of an overwhelming contraction, I would forget how I was supposed to breathe.

When breathing patterns are intended as a distraction, the true purpose and role of breathing in the body's physiology can be sabotaged. Breathing that is slow and deep has a relaxing effect and supplies the blood with plenty of oxygen. Fast, shallow breathing can easily do the opposite. If you find yourself breathing fast during a contraction, it's probably because you are in panic mode. Slow your breathing down, and you will automatically feel calmer.

As a labor and delivery nurse for ten years and now a professional labor assistant, I have observed and been involved in a thousand-plus births and rarely have I seen couples use patterned-breathing techniques successfully throughout labor. Most women become so frustrated with the concentration it takes that they find "the breathing" confuses and stresses them rather than relaxes them. Patterned breathing simply isn't sufficient to distract them from the intensity of the contractions, especially during later labor and transition. I have noticed that at this point most mothers switch intuitively to an internal focus, and to consistent, deeper, slower breathing that relaxes and tunes them in to the workings of their own bodies.

The right breathing technique is the one that works for you, the style of breathing that delivers the most oxygen to you and your baby with the least amount of effort. Try these dos and don'ts.

DO:

- Breathe naturally between contractions, as you do when you are falling asleep.

- When a contraction begins, inhale deeply and slowly through your nose, then slowly exhale through your mouth in a long, steady stream. As you breathe out, let your facial muscles relax and your limbs go limp as you imagine the tension leaving your body. Think of this exhalation as a long sigh of release.

- As the contraction peaks, remind yourself to continue to breathe at a relaxed, comfortable rate.

- Ask your partner to remind you to slow down if you start breathing too fast in response to an intense contraction. Have him take slow, relaxed breaths along with you.

- If you still find yourself breathing too fast, stop for a minute and take a deep breath, followed by a long, drawn-out blow, as if you are blowing off steam. Do this periodically to remind yourself to slow down.

- Partners should watch the mother's breathing patterns for cues as to how she is coping. Slow, deep, rhythmic breathing shows that she is handling her contractions well. Fast, spasmodic breathing communicates tension and anxiety. Use massage, model proper breathing, or suggest a change of position.

DON'T:

- Don't pant. Panting is not natural for humans. (Dogs and cats in labor pant because they don't sweat. It's their way of releasing body heat.) Panting not only exhausts you, it lessens your oxygen intake and may lead to hyperventilation.

- Don't hyperventilate. Breathing too fast and too heavily blows off too much carbon dioxide, causing you to feel light-headed and to have tingling sensations in your fingers, toes, and face. Some women tend to hyperventilate during the height of intense contractions and need caring reminders to relax their breathing. If you start to hyperventilate, breathe in through your nose and out through your mouth, as slowly as you can.

- Don't hold your breath. Even during the strain of pushing, the blue-in-the-face, blood-vessel-popping breath-holding you see in movies is not only exhausting but also deprives you and your baby of much-needed oxygen. (See page 363.)

- Don't worry too much about how you will breathe during labor. If you keep your wits about you, you will naturally breathe in a way that's best for yourself and your baby.

Prepare a Labor-Friendly Nest

The environment in which you birth affects the pain you feel. Mother cats search out the quietest, softest place in the house, one where they will not be disturbed. Even though designers outdo themselves in their efforts to beautify birthing rooms, you must bring to your place of labor some finishing touches. Take a tip from mother cat and create a peaceful nest in which to birth your baby.

Bring music to birth by. Why do you think dentists pipe in music for their patients? To occupy the mind while they work on the teeth. Music can actually ease bodily discomforts by a phenomenon called "audioanalgesia." Studies show that mothers using music during labor require fewer pain-relieving drugs than mothers who do not listen to music, because music stimulates a mother's body to release endorphins, the natural pain-relieving and relaxing hormones. Music also fills the mind with pleasant sensations, leaving less room for painful ones. And music has a mellowing effect on birth attendants, too, reminding them to respect the peacefulness of this event.

Play a medley of already tested favorites, taking care to choose songs whose rhythms relax rather than rev up your system. Many mothers make their own tapes using pieces that have previously helped them in times of stress. Music that triggers flashbacks of particularly pleasant events, such as the first time you danced with your mate, is particularly appealing. Some moms report that environmental sounds (such as waterfalls, wind, and ocean waves) and soft instrumentals that ebb and flow (New Age music or quiet jazz) are more soothing than vocal music. Along with your favorite tapes or CDs, bring along a player and fresh batteries.

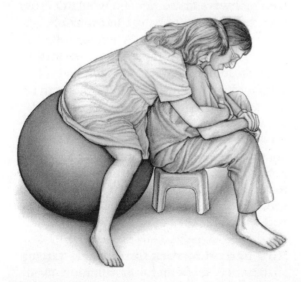

Birth ball.

Dr. Bill notes: Martha and I listened to harp concertos during her labor. Each time Boieldieu's "Première Concerto" came on, it recalled for her the scene where we first heard this piece: sitting by the fire in a friend's ski chalet and watching snow fall in the light from the porch.

Sit on a birth ball. In our living room sits a 28-inch "physioball" (a sturdily made inflatable ball available in physical therapy and birthing supply catalogs, see resource list page 401) that our children play on. Each time a pregnant woman visits our home, she gravitates toward it. "My, how relaxing to just squat on this ball" is a common response. Our daughter-in-law loved this ball so much during the final few months of her pregnancy that she asked to borrow it for labor. Cheryl spent more time sitting on this ball (see illustration) than in her bed during labor, which makes sense because sitting on the ball naturally relaxes the pelvic muscles.

Try a beanbag chair. When you shop, try out various beanbag chairs until you find a squishy nest that you can imagine yourself sinking into during early labor. Be sure to get an oval or rectangular bag large enough to allow you to sprawl. Practice relaxation with these nesting tools!

Bring along pillows and foam wedges. You cannot count on the hospital to provide you with plenty of pillows — you will need at least four. Thick, tapered foam wedges, available as leftovers at upholstery shops, make relaxing back supports for sitting; a thinner one can be used as a cushion between the bed and your abdomen when side-lying. Don't count on your birth place to supply these either. Buy beanbags and wedges early enough in your pregnancy to enjoy relaxing with them even before labor begins.

Try heat and cold packs. Heat packs improve blood flow to tissues; cold packs lessen pain perception in these tissues. You will need both kinds. A hot water bottle or a rubber surgical glove filled with warm water is a fine heat pack to nestle against your lower abdomen, groin, or thigh to relieve achy muscles or just to relax you. Packs of frozen veggies, covered with a cloth, work well as cold packs to soothe a hot forehead or numb an aching back. Try both heat and cold packs to see which one eases the pain; sometimes alternating them works best. Also, warm compresses on your perineum can help relax these muscles just before pushing to allow baby's head to pass through more easily and comfortably.

Consult the experts. Talk to other women about what pain-relieving tools they brought to their labors. Be sure to experiment with your bag of tricks at home to see what you think will work. Once you're in labor, try all sorts of combinations — cold pack, counterpressure, and all-fours position; side-lying, heat pack, and massage; cold pack here, heat pack there, and support with a wedge. You never know what will work until you try it. Here is where a professional labor assistant pays off. She can help plan and direct how you employ these tools and keep track of what's helping and what's not.

Pain and progress in labor are interrelated. Many of the things that help your labor progress also ease your pain. For additional pain relievers to put in your bag of labor tools, see "Helping Your Labor Progress — What You Should Know," page 340.

Medical Pain Relievers

Complete pain relief without risk is a promise on which no doctor can deliver. While today's analgesics and anesthetics are better and safer than ever, there is no such thing as a perfect pain reliever, that is, one that works yet is perfectly safe for mother and baby. By understanding what obstetrical drugs are available, what benefits and risks they carry, and how to use them wisely, you will best be able to decide which of them, if any, you want to use. Medical pain relief can be a welcome addition to — but not a substitute for — the natural self-help remedies we previously listed. Remember, studies show that mothers who take natural childbirth classes and study ways they can manage their own pain relief require less pain-relieving medication during their labors than uninformed mothers do.

Narcotic Pain Relievers

If only there were a perfect analgesic (meaning "painkiller") that would act on only the pain pathways in mother and wouldn't cross over the placenta to baby. Unfortunately, there is no such panacea. When narcotics relieve mother's body of pain, they also affect baby. An additional concern about narcotics is their effect on the mind, since they can impair one's ability to focus. When combined with natural pain relievers, however, properly used narcotic pain relievers can get a laboring woman back on track by providing temporary relief, which allows her to rest and recharge. Here is what every mother-to-be should know about choosing and using narcotic pain relievers.

How narcotics work for mother. Narcotic analgesics (e.g., Demerol, morphine, Nubain,

Stadol, and Fentanyl) relieve pain by blocking the pain receptors in the brain (see our parking-space analogy on page 301; narcotics fill up the parking places on the pain receptors). Analgesics affect different persons differently. Not only does the degree of pain relief narcotics provide vary from woman to woman, but so do the mental and emotional side effects. Some mothers feel a lot of relief within twenty minutes of the shot, while some report only slight relief ("It took the edge off the pain so I could manage it better"). Others report little pain relief, claiming the foggy mind was worse than a hurting body. Some women enjoy the euphoria narcotics can cause, a floaty feeling that helps them take their mind off their labor. Other mothers find narcotics compromise their ability to make decisions that benefit their labor progress. If a mother's mind is too muddled to participate in managing her labor with movement and changes of position, her labor may be prolonged, along with her pain. Narcotics can also make you feel very sleepy, so much so that you sleep between contractions and wake only as each one peaks, unable to focus and stay "on top of" the contractions. If this is your first pregnancy or your first use of a narcotic analgesic, you don't know how you may react. While you may tolerate these drugs well and experience pain relief without a lot of undesirable side effects, be prepared for the possibility of nausea, vomiting, dizziness, and the above-mentioned spaced out feeling. If you used narcotic analgesics to your advantage in a previous labor, chances are great that they will work for you again, though there is no guarantee.

How narcotics affect baby. When mother gets a drug, baby gets it, too. Let's follow a typical narcotic from the time it's injected into mother to delivery and postpartum, to see how it can affect baby. Within thirty seconds after a narcotic is injected into mother intravenously, it enters baby's circulatory system at around 70 percent of its concentration in mother's blood. Since babies can't talk and tell us how these drugs make them feel, we can only guess from studying external effects. Electronic fetal monitor tracings of babies whose mothers received narcotics during labor show heart rate patterns that differ from normal. Babies' brain-wave tracing (electroencephalogram, or EEG) changes, as do their respiratory movements. Depending on the type, dose, and timing of the drug, babies born under the influence of narcotics sometimes show respiratory depression and require temporary assistance to stimulate their breathing. They may also be a bit groggy as they first enter the world. Bonding may be affected; a drugged mother and a drugged baby don't make a good first impression on each other. These newborns are also slower at learning how to breastfeed. Narcotics given during labor have been detected in babies' bloodstreams up to eight weeks after birth.

How to use narcotics wisely during your labor. You may enter the delivery room studied up on drugs, armed with all the natural alternatives, and still conclude, with your birth attendants, that it would be in the best interest of you, your baby, and the progress of your labor to get some medical pain relief. Here are the safest and most effective ways to use analgesics during your labor:

• *Select the right drug.* With the assistance of your mate and your labor support person, discuss with your doctor or anesthesiologist which drug is best for your particular labor situation. Which one is likely to give you the quickest, most effective pain relief with minimal effects on your baby? In our experience, Nubain is the most effective in taking the edge off the pain and has the fewest number of side effects. We have also found that it is not as readily available in some hospitals because of cost.

It's important to avoid becoming exhausted during your labor. Sometimes it's sleep a mother needs more than pain relief. Instead of suggesting a narcotic during early labor, your doctor may advise taking a sedative to help you sleep so that you can enter active labor with more energy reserves.

• *Select the right time.* Analgesics given too early can slow the progress of labor. In the early stages of labor, narcotics are known to decrease the strength of contractions and slow dilatation of the cervix. If given too late, they can depress baby's breathing. The best time to administer narcotics is when your labor is very active (6–8 centimeters), just before you enter transition, or if your contractions become so overwhelming that you are losing control (see "A Balanced Mind-set About Pain Relief," page 322). Because the effect of narcotics on a newborn's nervous and respiratory system peaks around two hours after they are given, doctors prefer not to give these drugs within two hours of when they expect you to deliver. They want to give the drug time to wear off, at least to the point that it does not compromise baby's ability to breathe after birth. Thus, physicians do not feel it is safe to give narcotics to the mother once the pushing stage has begun. Fortunately, once you have the urge to push, your need for medical pain relief will

be greatly diminished. Don't worry, however, if a situation arises in which you *must* have a narcotic pain reliever during the pushing stage; baby can be given an injection of a narcotic blocker (Narcan) immediately after birth, which at least reverses the effect of the drug on baby's ability to breathe.

• *Select the right route.* Getting the drug intravenously gives you relief more quickly than an intramuscular injection. Intravenous drugs also wear off faster. After an intravenous injection a mother usually feels some relief within five to ten minutes; this relief may last for around an hour. Intramuscular injections, on the other hand, typically take half an hour to an hour to reach full effect, but the relief may last three to four hours. In either case, some mothers notice that the second dose is not as effective as the first. Most women choose the intravenous route; if labor pain is overwhelming enough to require medical relief, you want it to happen fast, and you probably also need intravenous fluids. Request a heparin lock, which allows you to move from your bed and to adjust positions more easily, rather than being tethered to a bedside intravenous bottle.

As in so many aspects of pregnancy, delivery, and parenthood, using medical pain relief is a judgment call of both mother and doctor. Make these decisions carefully. The progress of your labor and the health of your baby depend on it.

Epidurals

Many women want to hug their doctors for giving them an epidural during labor. In many hospitals, more than 60 percent of laboring women opt for this "gift from heaven." The epidural has made most other methods of pain relief obsolete — and has even done away with the belief that you must experience pain to birth a baby. Yet before you grab for this magic medicine, inform yourself about its benefits and risks. There are different types of epidurals, different times during labor to get one, and trade-offs you should know about.

Here are some medical terms to help you understand how epidurals are given and what they do:

- "Epi" is a Greek word meaning "around" (or ("outside") and "dura" is the membrane that covers the spinal cord. "Spinal" refers to the space enclosed within the dura. This space contains the spinal cord, spinal nerves, and cerebral spinal fluids. In an epidural, the pain-relieving drugs are injected into the space outside the dura. In a spinal, they are injected into the spinal space.

- "Analgesia" means "a lessening of pain without loss of movement." Pain relievers are therefore known as "analgesics."

- "Anesthesia" refers to "a loss of sensation and less movement in the affected area." Epidurals contain an anesthetic medicine, so they are termed "epidural anesthesia." Some of the newer procedures (see page 322) inject painkillers into the epidural or spinal space only and are called "epidural analgesics" or "spinal analgesics."

How epidurals are given — what you may feel. Before you receive an epidural, you will get a liter of intravenous fluids to build up your blood volume and prevent the decrease in blood pressure that sometimes accompanies an epidural. Your doctor or anesthesiologist will then ask you to sit or lie on your side and curl into the knee-chest po-

sition to round your lower back. This widens the space between the vertebrae, making it easier to find the right area for injection. As your doctor or nurse scrubs your lower back with an antiseptic solution, it may feel cold. Next, you will feel a slight stinging sensation as the doctor injects some local anesthetic under your skin to numb the area. When the area is sufficiently numb, he or she will insert a larger needle into the epidural space and inject a test dose to determine if the needle is in the right place. Once the needle is properly inserted, the anesthesiologist threads a plastic catheter through the needle into the epidural space and removes the needle, leaving the flexible catheter in place. The pain re-

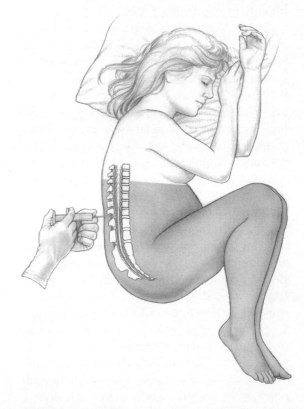

Epidural anesthesia.

liever you and your doctor have decided on will then be fed into the catheter. A few minutes later you may feel a shooting sensation, like an electric shock, down one leg. Within five minutes you are likely to begin to feel numb from your navel down, or you may notice that your legs are feeling warm and/or tingly. Within ten to twenty minutes the lower half of your body may feel sleepy, heavy, or numb, depending on the type of medicine used, and the pain of contractions will subside. The exact level of decreased sensation cannot be predicted precisely. Most mothers experience numbness from the navel down, some experience decreased sensation as high as the nipples. A few mothers notice some patchy areas on their skin where they can still feel sensations. You should still be able to wiggle your toes.

This is the point where most women sing the praises of the epidural, but this is also the instant at which a woman becomes more of a patient than a participant. Yes, once the pain is relieved, you can rest and recoup your energy. But because the lower half of your body feels heavy, you will need assistance changing positions. Since the sensation to empty your bladder is impaired, a nurse will insert a urinary catheter to take away urine. Because of the possibility of the epidural lowering your blood pressure, the nurse may monitor your blood pressure every two to five minutes until it is stable, and every fifteen minutes thereafter. To keep the pain relief even on both sides of your body, the nurse may turn you from side to side. To be sure baby is handling the epidural well, you will be hooked up to an electronic fetal monitor. You will also notice that the doctor or nurse periodically rubs the skin of your abdomen, checking to be sure the drug is giving you sufficient pain relief but not ascending high enough to interfere with your breathing. Now comes the juggling act of getting you just enough anesthetic to give you pain relief and help you manage your labor but not so much that it interferes with your labor.

I had a horrendous labor with my first baby and, quite honestly, wasn't sure I ever wanted to go through that again. But labor memories do fade and I got pregnant again. This time I opted for an epidural, and I'm glad I did. Even before my labor started, the fact that I knew I was going to have an epidural took a lot of the fear and dread out of labor. I actually loved the experience of birthing a baby without excruciating pain. I don't feel guilty or less of a woman because I opted for an epidural. For me, this decision was right. My epidural was marvelous. I can't wait to have another baby.

I felt like a beached whale. My legs felt like a sack of potatoes. I couldn't move. Everyone had to help me, and the nurse even had to tell me when I was having a contraction. Sure it didn't hurt, but I felt out of touch with what was going on in my body. For my next birth I may rethink the whole epidural question.

Types of epidurals. Not only are epidurals getting better and safer each year, but there are more kinds of them available, allowing laboring women and their doctors to choose which one best fits an individual labor. Here is the menu of epidurals that may be available at your hospital:

• A *continuous epidural* means that a bedside pump continuously infuses your epidural space with pain-relieving medication. The continuous epidural is the most common epidural used because it offers constant pain relief. Unlike with an intermittent epidural (see next option), blood pressure is more stable, and, overall, a lower dose of medication is needed.

- With an *intermittent epidural* the medicine is injected periodically as needed, al-

lowing mothers to juggle the level of pain they can tolerate with the degree of movement they desire. Some mothers do not like the roller-coaster effect of intermittent injections.

Epi-lite

The newest pain reliever in the anesthesiologist's medicine bag is a low dose of narcotics or a combination of narcotic and anesthetic medicines in the epidural. This lower dose allows a woman to maintain sensation and movement without unbearable pain, thus allowing her to manage her labor without fear of pain. Critics of epidurals fear that it is unsafe to obliterate all of the sensations during childbirth because pain can be a valuable signal that something is not going right and it can prompt mother to make adjustments. Critics also believe that some epidurals diminish a mother's awareness of what's going on in her body and detach her from her labor. Mother is less involved and unaware of what's happening in her body; father becomes equally uninvolved because he doesn't have to be involved. Epi-lite may be the answer to these concerns and a compromise that is both more beneficial and safer for mother.

With a lower dose, the mother can be more involved in her labor. With an epi-lite, mother can still feel when she's having a contraction. While the dose is high enough to relieve unbearable pain, it does not mask excruciating pain that could be the body's signal a problem exists that needs attention — from mother and doctor. A low-dose epidural can relieve just enough pain of labor so that an exhausted mother

can relax and get a second wind for pushing. A low-dose epidural allows mother to at least sit upright in a rocking chair — a "rocking epidural." If she can't walk, at least she can rock. In a further improvement, the anesthesiologist uses a combined spinal and epidural technique. A small dose injected into the spinal space takes effect immediately and lasts only two hours, but the epidural remains in place, allowing longer pain relief.

Not feeling anything going on in her body during labor is not healthy for mother or baby. Neither is excruciating pain, which may release stress hormones that diminish uterine blood flow. Somewhere in between is the safe sensation. For some women, epi-lite may be this compromise.

While no anesthesiologists can guarantee the amount of pain relief you will receive and the amount of movement you will have, the more homework you do and the more questions you ask, the more likely you are to get the pain relief that is best for you and your baby. If the anesthesiologist knows that you're willing to compromise, he or she may be willing to try a lower dose.

Epi-lite allows a woman to maintain sensation without unbearable pain, giving her the best of both worlds — feeling without hurting.

- *Mix and match.* The anesthesiologist can mix medicines (anesthetics and analgesics) to match the degree of sensation and movement you want, but there is no guarantee you will get the exact pain relief or movement you desire. Women react differently to pain-relieving medications.

- *Patient-controlled epidural anesthesia* (PCEA) allows the woman to self-regulate the amount of relief she receives by pressing a button that allows a preset computer-controlled amount of medication to be injected into the epidural tubing. With PCEA, some women use less medicine, some more, but at least you have a choice.

- *New epidurals.* Both mothers and doctors have long dreamed of an anesthetic that would allow women to enjoy sensation and movement during labor, but without the pain. With newer epidurals this dream has almost come true. Anesthesiologists are experimenting with combinations of narcotic analgesics and anesthetics, or with analgesics only, in hopes of blocking the pain nerves while sparing the motor nerves. Dubbed "walking epidurals," these types of analgesia allow the mother to stand, kneel, squat, and maybe even walk with support. Studies show that epidurals that allow mothers to walk or at least be upright during labor are associated with fewer interferences with labor and healthier babies than epidurals that take away a mother's mobility.

  The "walking epidural" is actually a spinal and epidural administered together. A small amount of narcotic is injected directly into the spinal space (not the surrounding dura) in a small enough dose to ease the pain of labor but still allow movement. Mothers can walk with assistance, shower, sit, stand, or squat. This type of anesthesia is particularly useful in cases where mother is experiencing unbearable contractions in early labor, and her pain and exhaustion are preventing her labor from progressing. If it is too early in labor to call upon the help of an epidural (before 5 or 6 centimeters), which could further delay the progress of labor, spinal analgesia may be just enough pain relief to allow mother to rest and recharge before she enters the next, more strenuous, stage of labor.

A Balanced Mind-set About Pain Relief

Some women enter birth absolutely opposed to taking medicines and willing to push their minds and bodies to the max; they regard anything less than a pure birth as failure. Other mothers ask their doctors to "give me everything you've got" in their quest for a pain-free childbirth. Somewhere between these two extremes is the right balance. For most mothers, it's wisest to enter labor armed with all the natural pain-relieving tactics we describe *and* with an open mind regarding the options available for medical relief should your labor or your individual obstetrical situation demand it. Birth is not a contest of who can cross the finish line in the fastest time with the least medical assistance. It is, first and foremost, your baby's entry into the world, and it is also a landmark in your life. The memories of this birth will last a lifetime. Whatever it takes to deliver a healthy baby and help you feel good about the process is the right pain package for you.

Some of these pain-relief options are still experimental, and many are not available in all hospitals. Nevertheless, you should be aware that "epidural" can mean many things. Ask what your options are. Discuss them ahead of time with your doctor and have some idea of what you plan on doing. Discuss your options again with the anesthesiologist, whom you may not meet until you are in active labor. Be sure to tell your practitioners that you are open to change should your labor situation change. A realistic fact of laboring life is that you will not know before labor day what your contractions are going to feel like and how you are going to manage them. Being informed about your options will at least help you make a healthier choice.

When deciding which, if any, epidural to choose, remember that there is a trade-off between how much pain relief you need or desire and how much movement you need and want. Complete pain relief and complete loss of movement interfere with your body's ability to help baby find the easiest path out and set you up for other medical interventions, possibly even a surgical birth. If complete freedom of movement with only minimal pain relief is not the best option for you, by all means look in the epidural medicine bag, keeping in mind that analgesics and anesthetics work differently in different women and that a doctor cannot guarantee how much pain relief you will receive or how much movement you will enjoy.

Composing Your Birth Plan

While birth, like life, is full of surprises, the more convincingly you state your birth wishes, the more likely you are to get them. The purpose of a birth plan is not only to increase your chances of getting the birth you want but also to alert your birth attendants to your personal needs. Obstetricians and obstetrical nurses attend mothers with a variety of birth wishes. Some mothers prefer a high-touch, low-tech, more "natural" style of birth. Others want or need more high-tech management and intervention during their labors. Your labor attendants may not know the style of birth you want, unless you tell them.

I've read your birth plan and know you don't want to have drugs. It would be easy for me to ask the doctor to prescribe some pain relievers, but you won't like me later. Before getting a shot of Nubain, let's try changing your positions. (A portion of a conversation between an obstetrical nurse and one of the Searses' daughters-in-law during her first birth)

In your birth plan you stated that you wanted the epidural turned off after transition so you could participate in and experience pushing. So I decided to use a lower dose of analgesics that wear off more quickly when you seemed not to need them anymore. (A portion of a conversation between one of the Searses' daughters-in-law and her obstetrician)

Personalize your plan. Don't copy it from a book or class. This is your birth, so it must be your plan. You will learn how to compose a birth plan during your childbirth classes. Also, there is a full chapter on how to compose a personal birth plan in *The Birth Book* (Little, Brown, 1994).

The timing of epidurals. When to get an epidural is as important a decision as which type to have. Getting an epidural too early in labor can stall your progress; getting one too late can impede your ability to push. (A continuous epidural can just be turned off when you are completely dilated and ready to push.) How epidurals affect a mother's labor is highly individual, so it is difficult to come up with absolute "shoulds" and "should nots" in obstetrical anesthesia. But there are some general guidelines. Your obstetrician and anesthesiologist are likely to recommend waiting to administer an epidural until they are satisfied that your labor is active, you are having regular contractions, and your cervix is dilating progressively. Different women reach this point at different times, but typically this will be when your cervix is dilated around 5 centimeters and you're just beginning the active phase of labor. Because you have to get "halfway there" before you are at the stage of labor where an epidural is safest and most effective, it is important to develop a pain-management system (as previously discussed) even if you know ahead of time you will want an epidural.

Some mothers and their birth attendants adopt a "wait and see" attitude about epidurals. If your own pain-management system is working, you are not overly tired, and your contractions are bearable, you may want to delay the magic stick in the back. But remember that the decision-to-effect time (the time between deciding on an epidural and its being in place and relieving pain) can be at least thirty minutes. Waiting too long may mean you cannot get the relief you need.

I was coping just fine until the contractions came on like gangbusters and I begged for an epidural. The doctor checked me and said I was already beginning transition. It

Managed Care

Sometime during your pregnancy, you may hear the term "managed labor" or "active management of labor" (AML). This means that if a mother's labor is not progressing at a predetermined rate (usually 1–2 centimeters dilatation per hour), rather than allowing the mother to set her own pace and risk exhaustion and failure to progress, the obstetrician intervenes by artificially rupturing the membranes, augmenting the labor with pitocin, and offering the mother an epidural anesthesia. The goal of AML is to lower the cesarean-section rate, and the rationale behind it is to intervene before the mother and her uterus become so fatigued they can't work efficiently. Maternity centers in which this type of "organized labor" is popular report shorter labors and fewer surgical births. AML does not mean either a doctor-directed or a mother-managed labor, but rather is a team approach in which all members do what they're trained to do to help labor progress most efficiently. AML offers the benefits of intervention before irreversible fatigue sets in, mother waits too long, and the intervention procedures don't work as well. Mother is then left no alternative but to have a surgical birth. The key to the wise use of AML is to select mothers whose labors truly are stalling and need medical assistance and those whose labors are normally "poky." If your labor seems to be stalling, your doctor may discuss the option of active management with you before exhaustion sets in or your particular obstetrical needs warrant this approach.

*would have been difficult for both the doc-
tor and me to try to do an epidural during
the height of these contractions, and besides, by the time the epidural took effect
the worst would be over, and I probably
wouldn't need it. So I toughed it out. But the
next time I won't wait so long to cry uncle.*

When to ask for the continuous epidural
to be turned down or off is an important decision. It's best to think about this one hour
ahead of time, too. Many mothers and physicians prefer to stop the infusion early enough
to allow the effects of the epidural to wear
off just as the pushing stage begins. This enables mother to move around and adjust her
body to the most comfortable position for
pushing. If you wait until your cervix is completely dilated to turn off the epidural, you
won't have the urge to push and won't be
able to push effectively for about an hour.
The pushing stage could last as long as three
hours — one hour of ineffective (fake) pushing, followed by two hours of real pushing —
once you can feel what you need to do. Of
course, these times depend on the mix of
medications you have. Remember, during labor as in life, what's good for mother is usually good for baby. If you're able to enjoy
freedom of movement, your baby will be better able to find the path of least resistance,
making the pushing stage easier and shorter.

*With my epidural I felt my body and I were
out of sync. My urge to push was obliter-
ated, so I couldn't tell when I was supposed
to push. I needed the nurse to put her hand
on my uterus and tell me when to push. I
felt like a bystander at my baby's birth.*

Questions You May Have About the Safety of Epidurals

Is an epidural safe for our baby?

Yes, probably. The truth is doctors do not
know for sure whether epidurals are completely safe for babies. Even the U.S. Food and
Drug Administration labels epidural anesthesia "generally regarded as safe" (GRAS). This is
a hedge, meaning the FDA is not certain either. There is no such thing as a risk-free pain
reliever. Small amounts of the narcotics and
anesthetics used in epidurals do cross the
placenta into baby's bloodstream within minutes. Some babies show changes in fetal heart
patterns following an epidural, though these
changes have been judged not to be harmful.
Some observers have noted that newborns
whose mothers had epidurals are more likely
to show feeding difficulties in the weeks after birth. When compared with newborns of
unmedicated mothers, some newborns of
medicated mothers do not search for the
breast as vigorously when placed on their
mother's abdomen immediately after birth.
For an unknown reason, a few mothers develop a fever following an epidural, and as
many as 5 percent of babies of mothers receiving epidurals may also have fevers. Deciding whether this fever is simply a side effect
of the drug or whether it signals a newborn
infection is difficult for the doctor caring for
the baby. Sometimes, to be on the safe side,
the doctor must order a lot of tests to rule
out infant infection, even though the fever
may have been caused by the epidural.

When we were investigating the various
obstetrical anesthetics, we found it very difficult to evaluate them in terms of efficacy and
safety. The field of obstetrical anesthesia is
improving so fast that on one occasion, when
we asked an anesthesiologist to comment on

a study, his reply was, "Oh, we don't use that drug anymore." Much of what you do read and hear about the potential problems associated with epidural anesthesia is indeed out of date. With improved needles and better drugs used in lower doses, today's epidurals are safer for baby and have fewer annoying side effects on mother. This is why it's important to discuss the safety issue with your anesthesiologist. Sometimes a mother's epidural actually benefits the baby; it's not good for baby if mother suffers through a prolonged, exhausting labor in which the blood flow to the uterus is compromised. In this situation, an epidural is good for both mother and baby.

Is having an epidural safe for me?

The problem with evaluating the safety of epidural anesthesia is that everyone so badly wants it to be safe that it's easy to lose objectivity. For the great majority of women, epidurals are safe and effective, and if you ask women who have had one, most would say they would gladly choose an epidural again. For other mothers, particularly those who don't like the technology and monitors that are part of the whole epidural package, being demoted to the role of "patient" and being unable to take as active a role in the birth as they would like is a disappointment. As with any drug, a few women may experience unpleasant side effects: a drop in blood pressure, shivering, nausea and vomiting, generalized itching, difficulty urinating, spinal headaches, and even seizures if the epidural "goes spinal," that is, enters the spinal cord and travels up the spinal canal. Some women who receive epidurals also report long-term backaches. While these side effects are merely uncomfortable and temporary, they are nevertheless enough to make you stop and think about whether or not you want

an epidural. In the main, most women breeze through their epidurals with few unpleasant side effects and carry home a healthy baby and pleasant memories of their birth.

Might an epidural interfere with my progress in labor?

An epidural can help or hinder the progress of labor. We have been present at births where a well-timed epidural actually increased the progress of labor, and we have observed births where a poorly timed or poorly chosen epidural interfered with labor. Like the studies on the safety of epidurals, the studies on their labor-prolonging effects reveal mixed results. In general, epidurals do seem to have a tendency to prolong the second stage of labor, especially for first-time mothers. The newer low-dose epidurals, however, do not generally prolong labor. Here are two examples of how epidurals can affect labor:

Jan and Tony were first-time parents who wanted to birth their baby "right." They attended two separate series of childbirth classes, took great care in choosing their birth attendants, hired a labor support person, and did all their homework, as befitting the importance of this event. They entered the delivery room well informed about all their options and well practiced in all the natural pain-relieving tools that they had learned about.

Jan's personal pain-management system seemed to be working for her until midway through her labor, when contractions got increasingly intense. Jan and Tony realized the natural way wasn't working anymore. Even though Jan walked, knelt, soaked, and squatted, even though Tony rubbed, supported, and coached, even though the obstetrician and labor support person did everything they were supposed to do, Jan's progress was slowing. She had used up all of her resources to cope with the pain and was now becoming increasingly exhausted. Her labor stalled: lots of pain, no gain. Together with her husband and her birth attendants, Jan made the decision to avail herself of whatever medical intervention was appropriate so that she could achieve her goal of a gratifying birth experience. She opted for an epidural, which allowed her to rest, regain her strength, and go on with the labor. Jan felt a twinge of "I couldn't do it naturally" remorse, but she knew when to say when, and she felt good about her decision. After about three hours of relief from the epidural, Jan asked that the epidural be stopped and allowed to wear off. Most of its effects had indeed worn off by the time she entered the pushing stage, and she was able to squat to push out her 9-pound baby.

In this case, the wise use of an epidural helped restart Jan's labor by allowing her time to get her energy back. Jan and Tony viewed the use of epidural anesthesia not as a failure of their resources, but as one more tool available to them in their quest for a safe and satisfying birth.

First-time parents John and Susan had a crowd of friends who praised the virtues of epidurals and wondered why any woman would want to go through the ordeal of labor without this "godsend." John and Susan attended the childbirth class at their hospital but concluded that, since Susan was going to have an epidural anyway, there was no reason to take time to practice relaxation, breathing, and position changes that they wouldn't need to use. Susan got her epidural as soon as the contractions began to intensify. After it was administered, however, and she was confined to bed, her labor slowed. To get her la-

bor going again, her doctor used pitocin, a synthetic oxytocin that stimulates contractions. The nurse who was caring for Susan couldn't help thinking, "First, she had a drug that weakened her contractions, then another one to make them stronger. Can two wrongs make a right?" Even with the pitocin, Susan's contractions stalled, and her labor soon fell into a growing diagnostic category, one that seems to be associated with modern managed labors: "failure to progress." She gave birth by cesarean section.

It's important to understand how any medication in childbirth, especially an epidural, can affect a mother's natural birthing hormones. Levels of oxytocin, the body's natural contraction-stimulating hormone, have been found to be higher during the second stage of labor in mothers who do not have epidurals. Studies also show that mothers having epidural anesthesia tend to have lower endorphin levels. In unmedicated labors, mothers get some degree of natural pain relief from endorphins (see page 306); these endorphins are also thought to be responsible for the "high" of childbirth most unmedicated women report. Thus, epidurals take away some of the pleasure of birth, as well as the pain. Of course, sometimes epidurals are the best thing for a mother's hormones, as in cases where a mother who is overwhelmed by the intensity of contractions is becoming increasingly exhausted. As her stress hormones go up, uterine contractions become weaker and blood flow to the placenta decreases — neither of which is good for mother or baby. For these mothers, epidural anesthesia helps reduce the level of stress hormones, enabling uterine contractions to become stronger and more productive.

Am I more likely to have a cesarean section if I choose to have an epidural?

Because there are so many reasons that a woman may need a cesarean, it is difficult to answer this question. Studies are inconclusive and based on older anesthetics and higher doses than are commonly used today. The newer lower-dose epidurals do not seem to increase the cesarean rate. For a moment, though, forget the studies and employ common sense. In order for a baby to progress down the birth passage, baby must be able to move and find the path of least resistance. A regular epidural prevents mother from moving, so she cannot take advantage of a valuable labor assistant — gravity. When she has no sensation, there are no cues telling her when or how to move or change position. If baby is coming down the birth canal in an awkward way, an unanesthetized mother will feel this and intuitively adjust her position. In effect, baby is looking to mother for help, and mother is asking baby to let her know what's working. If mother and baby's communication link is medically cut, baby may not find the best position for descent, and it will be the same old story: "failure to progress." An epidural also requires fetal monitoring, which may produce false alarms, leading to surgical intervention. And a mother with an epidural often requires pitocin, which requires still more fetal monitoring. This technological spiral often continues all the way to the operating room.

As in the story of Jan and Tony, above, an epidural can, in some instances, help a mother avoid surgical birth by preventing or relieving exhaustion. We have, at times, witnessed this birth scenario: A mother is "failing to progress," so the doctor advises a cesarean. In preparation for the cesarean, mother has an epidural, which relaxes and recharges her, and while the operating team is preparing for the surgery, to everyone's surprise, mother pushes out her baby. Sometimes, choosing one intervention can prevent another more serious one. The use of an epidural in some medical conditions, such as high blood pressure during labor, may decrease a woman's chances of needing a cesarean birth. Because it allows the mother to rest and lowers her blood pressure, the mother's chance of delivering vaginally is increased.

After a long, drawn-out labor, I had had enough of doing it "on my own." After two days of long, close contractions with very little to show for it, I had an epidural and pitocin to dilate me to 10 centimeters. Then I had them turn the epidural off for pushing. When it wore off, it was great to feel the urge to push rather than just being told "Here's a contraction, now push."

How much does an epidural cost?

The price varies from hospital to hospital and from community to community, but in general expect to pay anywhere from $500 to $2000. Add to this fee the increased cost of technology required to monitor the safe administration of the epidural (intravenous fluids, electronic fetal monitoring, pitocin, possible cesarean), and an epidural can be an expensive proposition.

Ultimately, a satisfying birth experience does not depend on massage, music, or medication. It depends on making informed choices that you are comfortable with. Your doctor's goal is the same as yours — maximum comfort with minimum risk. Realistically, few women can have it all: medication brings risks; no medication means pain and effort. By understanding the options before you, your individual preferences, and your unique birthing circumstances, you will be able to make choices wisely and have a birth that is safe and satisfying for you and your baby.

THE EIGHTH MONTH

❖   ❖   ❖

Emotionally I feel: _____
_____
_____
_____

Physically I feel: _____
_____
_____
_____

My thoughts about you: _____
_____
_____
_____

My dreams about you: _____
_____
_____

What I imagine you look like: _____
_____
_____
_____

My top concerns: _____
_____
_____
_____

My best joys: _____
_____
_____

My worst problems: _____
_____
_____

VISIT TO MY HEALTH-CARE PROVIDER

Questions I had; answers I got: _____
_____
_____
_____

Tests and results; my reaction: _____
_____
_____
_____

Updated due date: _____

My weight: _____

My blood pressure: _____

Feeling my uterus; my reaction: _____
_____

How I feel when I feel you kick: _____
_____
_____

What Dad feels when he feels you kick: _____
_____
_____

What I bought when I went shopping: _____
_____
_____

Reactions of your brothers or sisters when they feel you move: _____
_____

How I feel when I think about the pain of labor: _____
_____

I'm going to try these ways to ease the pain: _____
_____

Things I'll try with this birth that I didn't try with my last birth: _____
_____
_____

photo at eight months

Comments: _____
_____
_____
_____
_____
_____
_____
_____
_____
_____
_____
_____
_____
_____

Ninth-Month Visit to Your Health-Care Provider (34–40 weeks)

The frequency and content of health-care–provider visits during the final month depend greatly on your particular obstetrical situation. Your provider may wish to see you weekly. During this month's visit you may have:

- examination of the size and height of the uterus
- palpation of your uterus to determine position of your baby
- an internal exam, if indicated
- weight and blood-pressure check
- an ultrasound exam to determine the size and position of your baby, if indicated
- urinalysis to test for infection, sugar, and protein
- an opportunity to discuss when to call your practitioner if labor begins
- an opportunity to discuss the difference between Braxton Hicks contractions and the "real" ones
- an opportunity to discuss signs that labor has begun
- an opportunity to discuss when to go to the hospital or birth center
- an opportunity to discuss your birth plan, including labor assistants, avoiding an episiotomy, or special birth requests
- an opportunity to discuss your feelings and concerns

If your weekly or twice-weekly visits drag on, your health-care provider may discuss what to do when you're "overdue." You may have weekly ultrasound examinations to assess the volume of the amniotic fluid, or discussion of possible induction of labor at some point. If you are overdue, your health-care provider will counsel you on worrisome signs to watch for.

The Ninth Month — Labor Month

YOU WILL SPEND most of your ninth month in labor. Though this extended labor will not be as powerful as the labor you will experience on the day or so leading up to delivery, it's more obstetrically correct to talk of "labor month" rather than "labor day." Throughout the weeks prior to delivery, your mind and body will get ready for one of the most memorable events in your life — the birth of your baby.

HOW YOU MAY FEEL EMOTIONALLY

Take all the emotions you've felt over the past eight months, intensify them, and you've got an idea of what you can expect emotionally during month nine. You may be tired of being big, tired of being tired, and very ready to get the pregnancy over with. Your preoccupation with the upcoming birth and change in your lifestyle can mean more emotional ups and downs, but the inevitability of what's ahead may make it easier for you to cope. Here's how most women report they feel:

More eager. Now that you're in the home-stretch, you are more anxious than ever to meet your baby. You are probably also eager to silence the nattering of your friends ("What, you're *still* pregnant?"). For many women, month nine is the longest month of the pregnancy. Several told us they wished they could just fast-forward to D day.

Two weeks till my due date and I am huge. My maternity clothes barely fit. Today I was hauling my almost two-year-old around on my hip at the church picnic. I was cranky, I was hot, and it seemed like every friend I saw thought I should have delivered yesterday. They've all had babies — they should know better.

We suggested earlier that you tell yourself, friends, and relatives a due date sufficiently vague or purposely extended a week or two. Continue to let yourself be pacified by this generous "due time." It will reduce your impatience if (when) baby doesn't show up "on time." Impatience destroys your harmony and upsets your husband and children. And who will argue with the pleasant surprise you would get if baby did come earlier? The only persons who need to be in on your little se-

Sometime during your ninth month of pregnancy, we recommend you read the opening chapters of one of our other books, called *The Baby Book: Everything You Need to Know About Your Baby — From Birth to Age Two.* In this book, we share our experiences raising our own eight children, as well as what we have learned in our pediatric practice from successful parents during the past twenty-five years. The opening chapters of this book will give you the tools to develop a style of parenting that works for you and your child, based on the temperament of your baby and your own lifestyle. You will find useful information on choosing a doctor for your baby, getting the right start with your newborn, making postpartum family adjustments, caring for your newborn's needs, and getting connected to your baby. You'll also learn about shaping up after childbirth, preventing and overcoming postpartum depression, and nesting-in with your baby to help you make a happy transition into parenthood. We also include a thoroughly illustrated section on breastfeeding and address many other common concerns that you will have about your baby during those early weeks.

cret are your mate, labor support person, and the one who will be with you at home during the first few weeks if she needs to make arrangements.

More ambivalent. Yes, you're eager to hold your baby. And you can't wait to be unpreg-

nant, to get your body back to yourself. You're probably even looking forward to lying on your stomach! Yet, you may also be feeling fleeting pangs of regret over giving up the specialness of being and looking pregnant. Many women do not want a pregnancy to end. You have a unique and special closeness with your baby now. No one else shares this experience with baby, and you will never again feel this same intimacy with this child. The good news is that this intimacy will soon be replaced by an even more special kind of closeness.

Ambivalence over no longer being pregnant can lead to anxiety about making the transition from pregnancy to parenthood, especially if you are a person who doesn't handle transitions well. You may keep looking for some definitive way to say good-bye to your old, freer lifestyle, and long for some symbol or ritual that will signify your readiness to move on to a new level of adulthood. Take heart. You'll be amazed at how quickly you forget both the pains and the pleasures of pregnancy once you hold your precious baby in your arms. Yet realize that grieving the loss of your pregnancy is a very real need. Give yourself the time and space to do it now — you'll be too busy once baby comes.

I found myself dwelling on kicks, talking to my baby, and hugging my tummy during the last month, trying to imprint these very special feelings on my brain forever. But once the baby came, I realized that while pregnancy was beautiful and I loved sharing my body with my son, having him as a separate person was even more fulfilling. Being pregnant was amazing but being a mom really blew me away!

One day I projected my life into the future, imagining what my life would be like when it was "normal" again. Then I realized that motherhood is now my normal life.

Craving solitude. While you won't become a recluse, most women in their final month turn their hearts toward home. You may become more meditative. Your social calendar will probably be filled with little until due day. Your desire and ability to entertain dwindles. Suddenly outside events don't seem so important. You couldn't care less about world events. You are also appreciating the fact that you now have the best excuse (and will have for months to come) for saying no to any requests for your time and energy that would take you away from your nest.

I decided as I entered my ninth month to cultivate the quiet and rest my mind and body needed. I wanted to be both fit and rested for labor, and I also realized there would be no time between that experience and being the mother of a newborn. I saw from watching my friends how exhausting that would be. So I knew this would be my only chance to stockpile energy. I rested up.

More sensitive. Anticipate being more touchy this month and bothered by well-meaning but insensitive comments. You may feel more irritable toward your spouse, impatient with your children, and provoked by little things that normally wouldn't faze you. Have your self-soothing activities firmly in place (see page 339) so these negative moods can't take hold, zap your energy, and interfere with the harmony in your home. Advice-giving friends who have saved all their pearls of parenthood wisdom dump on you in the final few weeks. It's normal to be irritated and overwhelmed by all this advice and to wish people would just leave you

alone and let you have (and rear) your baby your way. This is another reason that most mothers-soon-to-deliver become very private in the final few weeks — they don't enjoy being the target for unwelcome advice. You may find yourself becoming very protective of your peace. This is nature's way of protecting you from outside influences that may distract you from the higher-priority event that is soon to come, conserving your energy for what's ahead. If a bit of advice is headed your way, go ahead and temporarily zone out. Nod your head if you wish, to be polite, but there's no need to pay real attention to the advice giver. Even better, stay away from people who make you nervous. You have hard work to do in the next few months, and only you can do it.

More concerned. You've made all your plans and bought all the infant clothing. You sometimes lie awake at night going over everything in your head. In your desire to be superprepared, you make lists so you won't have to worry about forgetting anything, but then you worry about what you may have forgotten to put on the list in the first place. (Keep a pad and pencil next to your bed so you can jot items down and relax back to sleep.) Go over the last-minute checklist on page 337 and then settle down and let your mind and body do what they need to do — rest! Anything you have forgotten will probably turn out not to be so important after all.

More scared. Even if you've prepared for this event for the past nine months and feel toned up and read up, it's normal to have second thoughts. Can you really go through with labor? Obviously, there is no turning back, and billions of women before you have gone through labor, including your mother. If this is your first baby, fear of the unknown naturally leads to dread. Let your mind work through these thoughts early in the ninth month before your body is asked to do a very strenuous job. The more you trust that your body knows what to do, the more your mind will relax.

More nesting instincts. Birds do it, bees do it, even pregnant women do it — prepare their nests for "hatching." Don't be surprised if you feel a sudden, compelling urge to clean the house from top to bottom, windows, blinds, and all, or to undertake a big project such as putting ten years' worth of loose photos in albums.

Two weeks before delivery day I started washing walls. I never wash walls.

Nature may provide you with a nice burst of energy to go along with the urge to prepare your home for the important newcomer. A day of yielding to this energy spurt may provide you with a healthy diversion from the boredom of those endless last weeks. It puts you in control and gives you a sense of accomplishment. But don't overdo it. Even though this nesting instinct may be common among females of the animal kingdom, human mothers don't really need a clean and sanitized nest. You don't have to have everything perfectly decorated and in place before baby is born. Many a well-appointed nursery goes unused for the first few months (or years!) anyway. Don't let yourself get carried away; you'll end up overtired. This is not the time to use up energy. Many of these tasks can be done by someone else or done gradually after D day, with baby snuggled in a baby sling sleeping peacefully. Even though you may think that labor day is two or three weeks away, don't count on it. During the ninth month, rest as if the next day may be "it."

The midwife said the baby would be born soon, but I didn't realize how soon. I shopped all afternoon with my four-year-old, then came home, stripped the sheets off the bed, sorted the laundry into piles in the hall, cooked a big chicken dinner, and finally realized I was in labor. The kitchen was a mess, the bedroom was in complete disarray, and this was going to be a home birth! The baby was born late that night, but it was three days before the kitchen got cleaned up.

HOW YOU MAY FEEL PHYSICALLY

More changes occur in your body during labor than at any other time in your whole life. Most of these changes occur automatically. And as millions of women have realized, your "delivery system" will instinctively know how to perform. Yet by preparing for and understanding what happens in your body during this month, you can influence the delivery process for the better, so that you'll be more likely to have a safe and satisfying birth experience. Here's how you're likely to feel in these last weeks of waiting as your body prepares for active labor. Soon you'll also be watching for definite signals that the big day has finally arrived.

Feeling bigger. Now you are big — really big. You may find the muscles in your abdomen hurt from working so hard to support your belly, or that your crotch and thigh bones ache when you walk. You may find it a chore to waddle even as far as your car. Bigness is an all-over feeling. Even your legs feel heavy. In the first week or two of the ninth month, enjoy your bigger silhouette in the mirror because your baby will soon be drop-

Prebirth Checklist

In the last few weeks before birth day, you will have many last-minute things to do and people to call, so don't leave your agenda to labor day. Here are some tips to jog your memory:

☐ Arrange care for your other children.
☐ Tie up loose ends at work.
☐ Preregister at hospital.
☐ Tour birth place.
☐ Compose birth plan and discuss with health-care provider.
☐ Send copy of birth plan to hospital.
☐ Notify labor assistants of updated due date.
☐ Pay bills.
☐ Be sure you understand when to call health-care provider, when to go to the hospital.
☐ Finish outfitting baby's layette.
☐ Buy last-minute comfortable clothing: gowns and nursing bras.
☐ Buy baby's car seat and be sure it fits properly in car.

Here are items to pack for the birth:
Labor-Saving Devices
☐ your favorite pillows
☐ cassette player with favorite music
☐ massage lotion or oil (unscented)
☐ snacks, your favorites (e.g., lollipops, honey, dried and fresh fruit, juices, granola), plus sandwiches for father
☐ hot water bottle

☐ special aids that you have been accustomed to during your labor, such as a birth ball

Toiletries
☐ hairbrush, dryer, setting equipment
☐ soap, deodorant, shampoo, conditioner (avoid perfumes; may upset baby)
☐ sanitary napkins (also supplied by hospital)
☐ toothbrush, toothpaste, lip balm
☐ glasses or contact lenses (or both — you may not feel like dealing with contacts in labor)
☐ cosmetics

Homecoming Clothes for Baby
☐ socks or booties
☐ one undershirt
☐ sleeper with legs (to fit into car seat)
☐ receiving blanket
☐ bunting with legs and heavy blanket if cold weather
☐ cap
☐ diapers

Other Items
☐ insurance forms
☐ cameras (video and still)
☐ fistful of change for telephone calls
☐ hospital preadmittance forms
☐ one or more copies of your birth plan
☐ "birthday" gift(s) for baby's sibling(s)
☐ favorite book and magazines
☐ address book (for telephone numbers)

ping lower into your pelvis, and the bulge will change. You may wonder how you are going to lug yourself around for another month.

More tired. Many mothers find themselves physically exhausted this month. You may be tired of dragging a top-and-front-heavy body up and down stairs. Even getting up off the sofa can leave you out of breath. While some women enjoy being busy almost up until labor day, most feel they must either slow down or quit their jobs in the final month. Most moms-to-be admit frustration this month over not seeming to be able to get enough sleep; no matter how tired they are, they don't sleep well and never feel quite rested. This is because of the physical and emotional drain of the ninth month. It is not only due to lack of sleep. First-time moms will be getting used to a pattern they've never experienced before — light sleep. This becomes, and remains, a familiar and practical mode for mothers at night. Nursing the baby, seeing that older children are covered with blankets, comforting them during nightmares, sitting up through their illnesses, reassuring a wakeful one — all these things dictate light sleeping for a number of years.

My five children are spread out over eight years, the youngest two being twins. Fourteen years after the birth of my first child, I slept soundly without interruption one night. When I woke, I remembered this as my prebaby sleep pattern. Over the years, I'd gotten very used to waking at night to check on little ones. My ears were always listening for coughs or cries.

Some days I walk around like a zombie, probably because I'm up half the night going to the bathroom. My mom says this sleeplessness is a rehearsal for when the baby comes. I'm afraid if I'm this tired after the baby's born, I'll do something stupid like leave him in the grocery store.

I've practically been falling asleep at work, so I quit my job this week (three weeks early) and can't get over feeling guilty for not contributing to the family financially. I haven't been without a job for twelve years, and I wonder if I'll feel less guilty once the baby comes.

Losing weight. Even though your baby may gain a couple of pounds during this month, your weight may increase only slightly, stay the same, or actually drop a pound or two. Weight loss in the final month is usually due to a decrease in the amount of amniotic fluid, as hormones begin shifting fluid around in your body. You produce less amniotic fluid, and the increased frequency of urination may lead to an overall drop in total body water, and therefore a decrease in your weight. It's just your body letting go of fluid it doesn't need.

Having difficulty getting comfortable. You may not be able to get comfortable — anywhere. You're not comfortable sitting, standing, or lying in one position for more than a few minutes at a time and have great difficulty finding the right position for sleep. You may find you are miserable at work and not getting enough rest at home, and if you're like most women, you fear you'll become too exhausted to handle labor. Short, frequent naps are a necessity this month. So are the relaxation techniques you've been practicing. Use them now to get the most rest you can before labor day.

Feeling a little better. Two of the more common annoyances of earlier months, breathlessness and heartburn, often ease during the ninth month. When baby descends lower into your pelvis (see "Dropping," page 351), your diaphragm has more room to do its job, which helps you breathe easier. And now that your stomach is less squished, you may feel less heartburn. Of course, while the annoyances at the top end of the uterus improve, an old favorite reappears at the bottom — you'll need to urinate more frequently as baby's head begins to press more on your bladder. And while the upper digestive tract may feel better, the crowded lower tract may once again feel constipated and bloated. (For ways to ease constipation, see page 69.)

Experiencing new pelvic pressures. As your baby descends into your pelvic cavity, you may find yourself prone to sharp, stabbing pains at the base of your spine or in the middle of your pelvic bone, making it uncomfortable to walk. Some women get uncomfortable twinges or "pins and needles" in the cervix itself. You may feel pressure or even a sharp pain in your pelvic area whenever you try to lift up your leg to put on your underwear or get out of bed. Sometimes these pains may radiate around to your back or down your thighs. The increased pelvic aches and pains of the ninth month are most likely due to the relaxation and stretching of your pelvic ligaments in preparation for the job to come. You can ease these discomforts by changing positions. Continue to exercise gently every day — take long, slow walks or ride your stationary bicycle. If you cannot walk or exercise without pain, a chiropractor experienced in working on pregnant bodies can give you some gentle pelvic adjustments to get your hips back in balance. It is our personal theory that chiropractic attention in pregnancy not only helps prevent or relieve back pain but also can affect your labor by preparing your back and pelvic structures better to handle the stresses of labor and birth.

Feeling different kicks. Babies move even less in the ninth month than they did in the eighth, but what these movements lack in frequency they make up for in power. You may feel hard kicks in your ribs and punches in your pelvis. Sometimes it may even feel as though baby is moving his hands or feet into your vagina — a very odd sensation.

General aches and pains. During the ninth month some women feel stiff all over, the way they imagine that arthritic, elderly people feel. Baby's head pressing against the nerves and blood vessels in the pelvis may also cause cramps in the thighs. As with pelvic aches and pains, these changes are due to the influence of pregnancy hormones on the ligaments of all of your joints. The overall loosening of ligaments has been known to cause the knees and wrists to feel weak, too, making even light lifting tricky and walking less inviting. However, movement keeps your body tuned up, and once you get started on your daily walk the aches and pains will diminish. Don't become a couch potato, or your muscular, cardiovascular, respiratory, and digestive systems will lose tone.

Self-Soothing Activities

- Read a novel.
- Watch a funny video.
- Call a positive friend.
- Soak in the tub.
- Enjoy a gourmet treat.
- Visit a museum.
- Go see a romantic comedy.
- Address birth announcement envelopes while you listen to relaxing music.
- Have your music to labor by on whenever you take a nap.
- Take a few deep breaths and stretch your arms and legs.

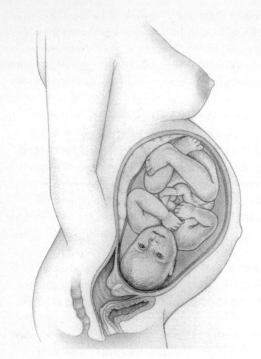

Baby at 34–40 weeks.

HOW YOUR BABY IS GROWING (34–40 WEEKS)

By term, most babies weigh between 6 and 7½ pounds and measure 19 to 21 inches. During this "finishing" stage, baby gains a tremendous amount of subcutaneous fat, filling him out for birth. His lanugo hair has disappeared, along with some of the vernix caseosa — just enough of this cheesy substance remains to lubricate him for a smoother passage during birth. By this time, your baby has pretty much run out of room and is tucked up like a little ball in position for birth. During the final weeks inside the womb, baby sucks, swallows, breathes, blinks, steps, turns his head, sucks his thumb, and grasps and clasps his hands, practicing all the movements he will need after he makes his

appearance in the world. The air sacs of his lungs are now lined with a substance called "surfactant," which keeps the lungs expanded after each breath, enabling nearly all babies born at this stage (even early in this stage) to breathe air outside the womb.

CONCERNS YOU MAY HAVE

Helping Your Labor Progress — What You Should Know

What's the worst you've heard about labor? It's painful, and it can go on for a long time. The good news is that both the intensity of the pain and the length of the ordeal are under your influence. You can help your labor progress and avoid the cycle of discouragement, that is, the scenario in which your birth attendant checks you and announces, "Nothing's happening," you become discouraged and anxious, your contractions slow even more, and you face a long, drawn-out labor. For some women, slow, steady progress is their healthy norm, but there are ways for nearly all women to get their bodies working more efficiently — and less painfully.

Be informed. During your childbirth classes you will learn a lot about the anatomy and physiology of labor, especially how the uterus contracts and how your baby turns and bends as he or she navigates the winding road of your pelvic passages. Be sure you understand the importance of relaxation, the labor-stalling effects of fear, and how your hormones work and what you can do to help them work better. At least one class will be devoted to what happens during labor. Don't miss that class.

Inform yourself before labor day about the wise use of technology and medications during labor. While technology is often life- and labor-saving, it is meant to help your labor progress, not interfere with it. A well-timed epidural, as discussed in chapter 8, can help an exhausted mother rest and get a second wind, accelerating labor in the long run. On the other hand, the wrong medication or the right one given at the wrong time can interfere with the progress of labor. Using technology that requires you to stay in bed will keep you there for a longer labor. If you need an IV, request a heparin lock, which will allow you to be mobile rather than tethered to a bedside IV pole. If you need electronic fetal monitoring, ask if it can be done intermittently. If for medical reasons you need continuous electronic fetal monitoring, request telemetry, which keeps you mobile. With this ultramodern technology, a laboring woman can have the best of both worlds — freedom to move with the safety of being monitored. (See also "A Balanced Mind-set About Pain Relief," and "New Epidurals," page 322.)

Be fit. Here's where those hours of pelvic tilts and tailor squats, daily walks, swimming, or stationary cycling really pay off. Pretoned and prestretched muscles are likely to work better for you.

Be rested. It's not only *hard* work that pushes a baby out, it's *efficient* work. The harder a job is, the more the worker will need to take breaks. Fortunately, nature provides two breaks for laboring women. The first is during early labor, when contractions are not so difficult to deal with. The second type of break is continual — those little respites between contractions. Even when labor is at its most intense, there is time between the end of one contraction and the beginning of the next. A common mistake first-time laborers make is being too busy in early labor. You may reason, "These contractions aren't so bad. I can handle them. Now is the time to vacuum or address birth announcements before the real work starts." Wrong! The real work is going to be much harder to do and much more difficult to manage if you are not rested physically and mentally. If you are laboring at home, retreat into a quiet place, take the phone off the hook, and go to sleep, or at least get some rest. Do not dwell on your to-do list. During early labor in the hospital, keep your environment restful.

Remember to rest between contractions, especially early in labor, when these breaks last five minutes or more. Click into the relaxation techniques you have rehearsed. Even during active labor, when breaks may last only two to three minutes, we have seen veteran mothers use their relaxation techniques so effectively that they are able to momentarily zone out, as if they are on another planet, and even snore between pushes in the second stage. Don't spend your time between contractions worrying about what the next one will feel like. This will make the pain worse. Fear intensifies pain perception. Rest so that you don't become worn out.

Between contractions think R-R-R: rest, relaxation, recumbency.

Be nourished. A hardworking uterus and the muscles around it need a lot of energy from food and hydration from drinks. Doctors used to discourage eating or drinking during labor in case the mother needed a general anesthetic for a cesarean delivery, relying instead on intravenous fluids to hydrate and provide energy. Since most mothers who end up with a surgical birth now elect to be awake and thus receive an epidural or spinal anesthetic, keeping an empty stomach during labor is not as important as it once was. In the unlikely event that general anesthesia is necessary for emergency delivery, the concern is that you might vomit while you are unconscious and then inhale your stomach contents into your lungs. For this reason, it is preferred that laboring women ingest small amounts of quickly digestible foods. Eating heavily is also likely to make you uncomfortable. Here's how to stay well nourished during labor:

- *Eat early.* Eat to store up energy early in labor; when labor gets hard and heavy, your stomach may not cooperate.

- *Eat often.* Grazing (eating small, frequent meals or snacks) is much friendlier to a squeamish tummy than a big meal.

- *Eat high-energy food.* During early labor, load your system with complex carbohydrates (grains and pasta) that are stomach-friendly and that will provide a slow, steady release of energy over the hours of hard work to follow. In later labor, nibble on or drink simple carbohydrates that leave the stomach quickly and provide quick bursts of energy: fruits, juices, honey. Some mothers nibble on energy bars during labor.

- *Eat foods that are stomach-friendly.* Some mothers experience nausea during labor and find eating and drinking unappetizing. Nevertheless, they need to eat. So bring along foods and drinks that were proven favorites during your early, nauseous months of pregnancy. Foods you tolerated then are the ones you are most likely to be able to digest now. Avoid fatty and fried foods,

gassy foods, and carbonated beverages — there is enough work going on inside you without making your intestines labor, too.

- *Drink, drink, drink.* Avoid becoming dehydrated, which depletes your energy, upsets your body's physiology, and slows your labor. Muscles that are underfed or underhydrated don't work efficiently. Pre-load your tank with at least 8 ounces of water per hour in early labor, and sip between contractions. Be sure to bring at least two water bottles with your favorite fluid to the hospital; place them within easy reach at your bedside. Many mothers in our practice have used a time-tested recipe they call "laborade," which is a healthy version of the familiar drink of athletes. It provides carbohydrates, electrolytes, and minerals to help keep your body chemistry balanced:

  ⅓ cup lemon juice
  ⅓ cup honey
  ¼–½ tsp. salt
  ¼ tsp. baking soda
  1–2 calcium tablets, crushed,

Add enough water to make 1 quart. You can add an additional 8 ounces of water for a milder flavor, or you can flavor this blend with your favorite juice.

Many mothers get so involved in their labor that they don't bother to quench their body's thirst. One of the jobs of a birth partner is Chief Water-Bottle Pusher.

- *Intravenous "feedings."* If you are too nauseated to eat or drink, and your practitioner feels that you are becoming dehydrated, he or she may recommend giving you intravenous fluids. This can perk up a stalled labor or an exhausted mom.

An additional benefit: more fluids means

more trips to the bathroom, which, because of the walking and squatting, are themselves labor stimulators.

Be quiet. You don't have to be like a mother cat and retreat into the closet to have your baby, but you must design a peaceful birthing environment for yourself. Birth attendants (partner, friend, nurses) need to respect your privacy during contractions, so you can concentrate on your work, and between contractions, so you can rest. This is where your mate comes in. Give him the job of peacekeeper, pledged to banish chattering, noisy, and interfering people from your labor room and to protect the privacy and the dignity of this event.

Lighten up. You'll find that during labor there is time for laughter and talking as well as peace and quiet. In fact, a little laughter is good for labor. Humor may be just what the doctor ordered to relax an anxious mother and the various helpless people hovering around her. Laughter increases the level of endorphins — your body's natural pain relievers and relaxers. Try watching a funny movie, particularly one that you already know you love. Some mothers listen to books on tape in early labor, choosing their favorite authors. It is up to you and your mate to balance the levels of quiet and levity in a way that makes you most comfortable. Create your own labor-enhancing environment: dimmed lights, relaxing music, and whatever people and things you need to manage and progress in your labor.

Be romantic. "Love makes the world go round," and it helps babies come out, too. The hormones released during lovemaking also enhance labor; endorphins create pleasurable feelings during sex and also relax mother beautifully for birth. Nipple stimulation, by the mother, by her mate, or from water splashing on her nipples during a soak in the tub, releases the contraction-intensifying hormone, oxytocin. A kiss, a caressing cuddle, a sensual massage can all get your birthing hormones working for you. These labor-enhancing hormones also counteract anxiety that may cause your labor to slow rather than progress.

You may have heard that sexual intercourse can stimulate labor because sperm contains powerful hormones called "prostaglandins," which your body makes to stimulate labor. This is true and false. True, sexual intercourse early in labor, before your membranes have ruptured and with the OK from your doctor, can stimulate labor and relax you, but this is because sex prompts mother's body to release oxytocin and endorphins. Research has determined that one man could not possibly deliver enough prostaglandins in his sperm to stimulate labor. While women seldom equate the experience of making a baby with the experience of having one, sex and birth do share the same hormones. There is no reason not to do what you can to get these natural hormones laboring for you. However, some women find their erogenous zones so sensitive during labor that they are completely off-limits (birth partners, be prepared for a sudden "Don't touch that!"). For others, nipple and genital stimulation is just OK, and some women find it pleasurable. The hormones of love are similar to the hormones of labor. Put them to work for you.

For me, giving birth is the ultimate expression of my sexuality and my femininity. So the setting was very important for me. I wanted soft music, dim lights, and a private atmosphere. The right environment for birth is like the right environment for sex.

Be positive. A negative birthing environment is no help to a laboring mother. Banish negative people from the delivery room. You don't want to hear someone else's war stories, comments about how they couldn't progress either, or their labor-strategy comparisons in which you are the clear loser. Listen to negative people and you are likely to become a member of the Club of Dragging Labors. The more we are around the labor scene, the more we appreciate the powerful mind-body connection at work in the labor room. Invite only positive people to your birth.

Be comfortable. Pamper yourself with as many labor-enhancing amenities as you can think of (and that will fit in your bags). Bring along your favorite music (see "Bring Music to Birth By," page 314). Take a shower, soak in the tub, nibble on delicacies you reserved just for labor day, keep your masseur busy with the touches you need, prop yourself up with pillows — do whatever you need for your peace and comfort. If for medical reasons you will need to spend a lot of time in bed, bring a foam-rubber pad contoured like an egg carton. (Check ahead of time to see if your hospital provides one; if not, purchase one in the bedding department of a discount or department store.) These pads are very soothing to the skin and to muscles that have to lie down a lot. Labor is your license to luxuriate. If your hospital offers them, take advantage of the new birthing beds, which can be adjusted to support you in comfort and in your style of labor and delivery.

Be progressive. The more labor tools you bring to your birth, the better progress you are likely to make. If your hospital lags behind in labor-assisting devices, bring your own. Top labor aid is a professional labor assistant. (See "Choosing a Labor Support Person," page 273.) Several women whose births we attended brought along their own collection of 3″ × 5″ cards containing encouraging quips to relax and empower them. If you like this idea, collect memorable lines from birth books, verses from poems or scriptures, or humorous limericks. You may want to read these yourself, or you can let your birth partner read them to you. Hearing a lovely verse read by your lover may be just what you need to help you relax between contractions. For other labor aids, see pages 314 to 316.

With my first two babies, the hospital considered me a sort of fanatic when I brought along my own professional labor support person, homemade tapes of my favorite music, and my favorite foods. With my third baby, the nurses really raised their eyebrows when the rented labor tub was delivered to my room. With my fourth baby, they actually welcomed all the stuff I brought with me. I think they realized that a mother like me bothers them less, and because I bring my own stuff, I probably save the hospital money. I hope my hospital will take the hint when they're designing and equipping their birthing rooms. They should ask the real experts what should be in these rooms — the mothers who are going to use them.

Be vocal. Reserve your etiquette for dinner parties; you needn't be embarrassed about the sounds you make in labor. After all, you are not laboring in a library or church. When asked how a laboring woman should act, veteran birth attendants — especially those who have delivered babies themselves — respond, "Any way she wants." Many women find power and comfort in letting go with a yell, a prolonged moan, or gutsy grunt when the going gets tough. These sometimes involuntary gut sounds vocalize your release of tension and are a powerful way of mustering up inner energy to get through a really tough contraction. They are in fact similar to the sounds athletes make during a particularly grueling event or one that requires tremendous concentration. Of course, some sounds help labor, some hinder. Low-pitched, long groans (gut sounds called "sounding") are releasing and energizing. High-pitched, sharp, sudden yells are body-tensing and frightening to you (and to the woman laboring in the next room). Be sure to prepare your partner that you are likely to let loose with strange sounds; otherwise he may misinterpret these scary noises as a sign that you are losing control and will want to do something to fix and quiet your noises.

I'm a trained singer, and I found making noise to be very releasing during labor. I bundled up the pain of the contraction and let it go in the sounds I made. My voice was tired after the birth but not hoarse. Proper singing requires relaxation. Relaxing my body kept me using good vocal techniques during labor.

Be mobile. Included in every laboring mother's Bill of Rights is the freedom to move during labor and the freedom to improvise whatever birthing positions work best for her. In order to take advantage of your body's natural ability to guide you to the best positions for labor and delivery, however, you may have to first go through a bit of cultural deprogramming. Scratch from your memory the on-your-back scenes from the movies; they are leftovers from birthing's painful past. In fact, studies show that women who

are not culturally locked into the horizontal birthing mind-set tend to assume any of eight different positions during the course of their labor, and most of these are upright, semi-upright, or moving.

If you confine yourself to a bed during your labor, you are likely to labor a lot longer. Walking is especially helpful in early labor, both to ease discomfort and speed progress. As we have previously mentioned, if you need tests and technology, ask for newer technology that allows even the most monitored mother to be on the move.

Be upright. Most women, if left to their own devices, labor in an upright or semi-upright position. When you're upright, gravity helps baby descend. Laboring on your back makes no physiological sense for mother or baby. Not only does gravity pull the baby toward mother's back, but her uterus is forced to push baby uphill. What's worse, the uterus can compress major blood vessels that run along the spine, reducing blood flow to the uterus and causing the contractions to become less efficient. Laboring on the back is also more likely to cause severe backache. Research has shown that laboring upright increases uterine efficiency, shortens labor, and dilates the cervix better. In our birth-watching experience, mothers who spend the most time in the horizontal position are

Labor Tip: Ask your birth helpers not to sit around and stare at you. Remember the saying "A watched pot never boils." Go about your usual business as much as possible. Being watched closely and being hovered over can build anxiety and cause you to feel there is something to watch out for.

the most likely to suffer long, agonizing labors.

Laboring vertically rather than horizontally also widens the pelvic passage, giving baby an easier way out. When you are upright, your pelvic joints, relaxed by the hormones of pregnancy, are better able to shift and accommodate the little passenger with the large head and broad shoulders. Being upright also allows a more natural stretching of the birth-canal tissues, making tears less likely.

It may be easier to stand up (literally and figuratively) for your birthing rights if you know how the horizontal birth position became so fixed in our collective mind-set. Horizontal laboring is a carryover from the days of anesthetized and forceps births, when women were so heavily drugged during delivery that they couldn't stand up or help push their babies out. Because mother couldn't give birth herself, someone had to take the baby from her. In time, baby-catchers became quite comfortable sitting at the foot of the delivery table to help baby out, and soon they decided it was "safest" just because it was easier for them. Actually, a baby can be safely delivered in just about any position, as long as mother or an attendant can "catch" baby.

Upright laboring does not mean that you are standing, leaning, walking, or squatting during the entire labor. Here is the best

---

How Far Along?

"How far along am I?" You'll want to know. It helps to understand the labor language your birth attendants use and how this translates into what's happening in your body. Your birth attendants will gauge your progress by three measurements: effacement, dilatation, and descent.

"Effacement," or "being effaced," means your cervix is thinning, changing from a thick-walled cone to a thin, wide cup under baby's head. During an internal exam your birth attendant measures how far effaced you are.

- "0 percent effaced" means your cervix has not yet started thinning.
- "50 percent effaced" means it is halfway there.
- "100 percent effaced" means your cervix is totally thinned out and ready to open for your baby to be born.

The cervix of a first-time mother may need to be completely effaced before it begins dilating. With subsequent pregnancies, effacement and dilatation can occur together. During an internal exam, you may hear your birth attendant announce that your cervix is "ripe," which means that your cervix is soft enough to begin effacing and dilating.

"Dilatation" refers to how far open your cervix is. During an internal exam, your birth attendant uses his or her fingers to estimate your degree of dilatation in centimeters. In the prelabor stage or very early in labor, you may be 1 or 2 centimeters dilated; as labor intensifies, you may reach 5 centimeters dilated; when your birth attendant gives you the good news that you are 10 centimeters dilated, your cervix is completely open. Obstetrically speaking, being "in labor" position-changing routine for helping your labor progress most efficiently:

- labor upright *during* contractions
- recline and rest *between* contractions

Working Out Your Best Birthing Positions

I realized when I was lying in bed and my obstetrician came to visit that I had suddenly become a patient. When she saw me walking around my room, strolling in the halls, or laboring in the arms of my husband, she perceived that all was going well, I was managing nicely, and there was no need to intervene. Lying in bed, I was clearly a target for intervention. I guess my being in bed made me seem dependent and sick, and the doctor felt obliged to do something.

You should have seen the look on my obstetrician's face when I asked her to kneel and catch the baby from below while I pushed in the squatting position with my husband supporting me from behind. (I'm sure this birth position has not yet made it into the obstetrics textbooks.) But it worked great, and the next time someone asks, I bet she'll be all ready — with knee pads!

Just as there is no single right position for making love, there is no "right" position for

means your cervix is progressively dilating.

"Descent" means how far down baby's presenting part (usually the head) is in the pelvis. During an internal exam, your birth attendant will determine to what "station" baby has descended. Station zero is the middle of the pelvis. Each centimeter above or below zero marks another station. The highest station is "floating," meaning the baby's head is above the pelvic inlet, and not engaged. If your birth attendant announces, "Your baby is at minus four," that means that he is floating four centimeters above station zero. If your birth attendant announces, "Your baby is at plus four," your baby's head has descended all the way through the pelvis and your birth attendant can get a glimpse of your baby's head.

Besides effacement, dilatation, and descent, another factor in labor progress is baby's changing position. Baby not only has to come down the birth canal, his body has to turn to navigate the path of least resistance through the pelvis. Sometimes during labor the degree of dilatation and descent stays the same for an hour (or more) while your baby and your body work to change baby's position, affording him an easier way out. Although this change won't be charted on your dilatation and descent notes, it is "progress" all the same.

Don't be discouraged if your birth attendant announces, "You're still four centimeters . . ." Obstetricians generally regard "normal" or "usual" progress in active labor as a rate of 1-centimeter dilatation per hour and 1-centimeter descent per hour (1.5 for subsequent pregnancies), but these are only obstetrical rules of thumb. They may not necessarily be the rules followed by your uterus. A labor that progresses more slowly than usual is not necessarily abnormal. Your uterus and your pelvic passages may simply not be "average."

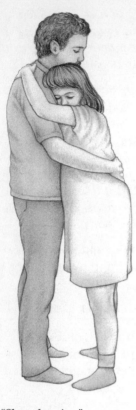
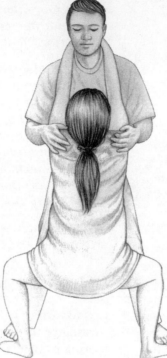
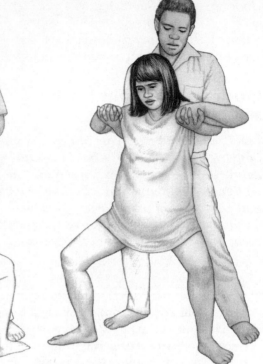

"Slow dancing."

Dangling squat.

Supported squat.

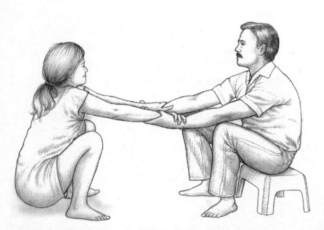
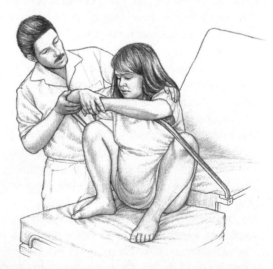

Supported squat.

Using a squat bar.

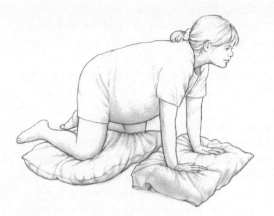

On hands and knees.

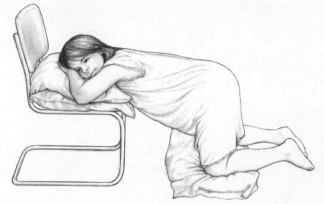

Leaning on a chair.

pushing out a baby. Knowing what positions to try and having the freedom to experiment is what laboring efficiently is all about. Try these labor-tested favorites:

Squatting. You may wonder why you should squat when you could be lying comfortably on your side in bed. Squatting benefits mother and baby. It widens the pelvic opening, relieves back pain, speeds the progress of labor, relaxes perineal muscles so that they are less likely to tear, improves oxygen supply to the baby, and even facilitates delivery of the placenta. If you have practiced squatting a lot during pregnancy, it will be easier during labor.

If you try squatting down right now, you can probably feel where your upper leg bones, the femora, are attached to your pelvic bones. When you squat, your leg bones actually act like levers to widen your pelvic outlet by 20 to 30 percent. Squatting gives your baby a straighter route through a wider passage, creating the easiest path for moving baby through your pelvis. When you labor horizontally instead of squatting, your uterus must work baby through a narrower and

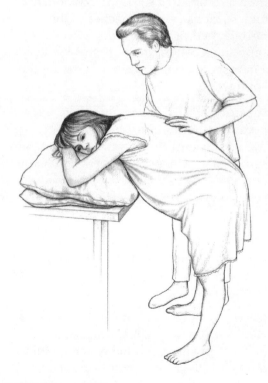

Leaning on a table.

curvier tunnel, which is usually harder and more painful work to do. (Women who have short second stages will choose not to squat.)

Squatting tips:

- Unless it helps your earlier labor progress, reserve squatting for the second stage of labor, when your cervix is fully dilated and you want to get the maximum efficiency out of your contractions. Squatting is seldom necessary during the first stage of labor if your contractions are not overwhelming and your cervix is dilating. It's better to avoid tiring your legs until your contractions really get serious.

- The urge to push is your signal to squat. As soon as a contraction begins, pull yourself from a resting to a squatting position. Ask for a squat bar, which attaches to the birthing bed, or use someone's neck for support (see illustrations, page 348). Rest in a more comfortable position between the contractions.

- Squatting makes contractions more intense because it positions baby's head to put pressure against the cervix — that's why squatting accelerates your progress. If you find squatting in the active phase makes your contractions overwhelming, modify what you are doing.

- To avoid slipping and tiring, place your feet at least shoulder width apart and squat gradually. Don't bounce, as this strains your knees.

- As you squat, release your abdominal muscles so that you look like you are eleven months pregnant. Tensing your abdominal muscles is likely to increase your pain.

The dangling squat (see illustration, page 348) is a natural "releasing" position, reminding your body to let go, release the tension, and birth the baby. Positioning your body this way will also send your mind surrender messages.

Kneeling. Kneeling is helpful to ease overwhelming contractions, relieve back pain, or turn a posterior baby. It is also a position that helps you improvise and can lead to the kneel-squat, kneeling on all fours, or the knee-chest position.

Sitting. The sitting position widens the pelvis, but not as much as squatting does. The most labor-efficient position is sit-squatting on a low stool. Alternatives are to sit astride a toilet seat, a chair, or a birth ball (see page 315) you may have practiced on. If you must stay in bed because you've had pain medication, sit astride the birthing bed.

Standing and leaning. Since your labor is likely to progress more quickly and efficiently if you walk a lot, you may find yourself upright during an intense contraction. Try stopping and leaning against the wall or your birth partner, or resting your head against pillows on a table.

Side-lying. Even though moving and being upright helps your labor progress, it is not humanly possible to be upright during your whole labor. Your hardworking body will need some rest, and if you don't get it, it may stop doing its job so well. Best to be upright, in varying positions, during active labor contractions, but to rest as much as possible during early labor and between contractions. Lie on your left side as shown in the illustration on page 225.

How often and how much you remain on your side depends upon your labor. If you want to ease a hard and fast labor, use the side-lying position, especially during a strong contraction. If you want to speed up a dragging labor or increase the efficiency of contractions, kneel or squat during the contractions and then return to side-lying be-

Labor Tip: All the suggestions given in "Managing Pain in Childbirth," page 299, also help labor progress. Pain and progress in labor are interrelated, often inversely: the more pain, the more exhaustion, the less progress. Be sure to study the section in chapter 8 on pain relief for tips on helping your labor progress.

tween them. We cannot overemphasize the importance of the three R's — relaxation, rest, and recumbency — between contractions.

Some mothers feel so comfortable lying on their side that they deliver their babies in this position. If you wish to use this position, have one of your birth attendants help you hold your top leg up to widen your pelvis.

Be sure to rehearse these positions during your childbirth classes and at home. Remember to think "upright" during contractions and "rest" between them. In labor, keep experimenting until you find the positions that help you manage your discomfort and help your labor progress.

LABOR AND DELIVERY

During your ninth month your eagerness to deliver yourself of this bulge and hold in your arms the precious life you have been growing may make you think every twinge from your uterus is "it." It usually isn't "it," and days or weeks will have to pass before you get to touch your baby. Some mothers start their labor with a bang — suddenly, undoubtedly, powerfully — and progress fast. Others ease into labor slowly, sometimes unconvincingly,

and progress gradually, yet efficiently. Some tired moms will have a labor that starts, stops, goes in spurts and pauses, and drags on for days. It's easy to be confused by all the terms: "false labor," "real labor," "prelabor"; the list goes on. While every mother's labor and delivery are as individual as her pregnancy, there are typical stages most women go through when delivery time is approaching.

Prelabor: Labor Day Is Near

What You May Experience

In a manner of speaking, most of your final month is labor, as many things are happening to get your body ready to give birth. Here are clues that labor day is near:

Dropping. Sometime during the final few weeks you may notice that your baby has moved down lower in your abdomen. Most first-timers notice their babies dropping within two weeks of delivery, though some mothers "drop" as many as four weeks before D day. Many second-time mothers find their babies do not drop lower until labor begins, because mom's pelvic muscles have already been stretched, and no warm-up is needed. Baby's head settling into the pelvis is also called "lightening" (because the lower-riding load seems smaller and lighter) or "engagement" (since baby's head engages the pelvic opening). Whether baby "drops," "lightens," or "engages," you will feel and look different. Your breasts probably no longer touch the top of your abdomen. You might be able to sense baby's head resting just beneath the middle of your pelvic bone.

Frequent urination. Now that baby's head lies closer to your bladder, you may be going to the bathroom more often.

When to Call Your Health-Care Provider

"Oh, my gosh, this is it!" You awaken your mate, whose reflexes tell him to summon the doctor for further instructions. Hold the phone call for now — you have some homework to do first. When to make that long-awaited call depends on your individual obstetrical situation, but here are some general guidelines to ease your apprehension and give your hardworking health-care provider a few more hours of sleep:

• During one of your ninth-month prenatal visits, ask for specific instructions on when to call. You may have some particular obstetrical needs that require you to call earlier than most mothers. Your doctor or midwife will also give you some "numbers" to keep track of before you call, such as timing how far apart your contractions are and how long they last. He or she will also review the signs of true labor (discussed on page 354). If this is not your first baby, when to call will also depend upon whether your previous labors were fast and furious or slow and draggy.
• Review the difference between prelabor and labor contractions (page 354) to be sure that you are in progressive labor.
• Before calling, make an at-home contraction chart, as shown on page 355.
• Once the information on your contraction chart matches the guidelines from your practitioner, place that call. You should also call your practitioner if there are signs that a

problem may be occurring (see below) or if you are worried, scared, or unsure of what to do. Never feel you have to apologize for false alarms. Especially if this is your first baby, it's normal to need some assurance as to what to do when. (Second-time moms may need some reassurance, too.)

Here are signs that a problem may be occurring and that you should call your doctor immediately:

• You have excessive vaginal bleeding (fresh blood, and more than your usual menstrual period).
• Your membranes rupture and you notice thick, green fluid coming from your vagina. This is meconium, the baby's first stool, and it could be a sign of fetal distress.
• Your instinct sets off an internal alarm, even if you have no concrete reason to think a problem may be occurring. Trust your mother's instinct.

Be sure you let your doctor know how you're managing. If you are doing well at home and would like to stay in your nest as long as possible, state your case. If you're having trouble focusing and would like some help, ask if it's OK to get to the hospital a bit earlier than usual, if for no other reason than to be checked, reassured, and sent home if that course of action seems best.

Low backache. As baby gets heavier and drops lower, count on some aches or pains in your lower back and pelvis as your uterine and pelvic ligaments stretch even more.

Stronger Braxton Hicks contractions. You may notice that your warm-up contractions (see page 223) go from feeling uncomfortable to being rather painful, like menstrual cramps. Even though these prelabor contractions are not as strong as labor contractions, they are strong enough to be starting the work of thinning out, or effacing, your cervix from a thick-walled cone to a thin-walled cup. While these contractions will get even stronger just prior to labor, they can continue this way, on and off, for a week or two before labor starts. They become less intense when you change position or start walking. Remember to practice your relaxing techniques during these contractions. (See the differences between prelabor and labor contractions, page 354.)

I felt like I had a belt inside my abdomen that tightened and released and tightened again. This went on for two weeks before my "real" contractions began.

Diarrhea. Birth hormones acting on your intestines may cause abdominal cramps and loose, frequent bowel movements — nature's enema, emptying your intestines to make more room for baby's passage. Those same hormones can also make you feel nauseated.

Increased vaginal discharge. You may notice more egg-white or pink-tinged vaginal discharge. This differs from the "bloody show" described below.

"Bloody show." The combination of baby's head descending into the pelvic cavity and the prelabor contractions thinning the cervix can "uncork" the mucous plug that previously sealed the cervix. The consistency of this mucus varies from stringy to thick and gooey. Some women notice the one-time passing of an obvious mucous plug; others simply notice increased blood-tinged vaginal discharge. Some of the tiny blood vessels in your cervix

break as your cervix thins, so you may see anything from a pink-tinged to a brownish red–tinged teaspoon of bloody mucus. If your discharge shows more blood than mucus — like a menstrual period or a lot of bright red blood — report this to your practitioner immediately.

Once you notice a "bloody show," you are likely to begin labor within three days, but some mothers hang on for another week or two.

Bag of waters breaking. Only one in ten mothers experiences her bag of waters breaking prior to labor. For most mothers this doesn't happen until they are well into labor. If your water breaks before labor has started, plan on your labor starting intensely within the next few minutes or hours, or at least within the next day.

The signs listed above tell you that labor is going to happen, but not necessarily when. Some women experience some or all of the signs within a few days of delivery; others notice them a week or two before. When these cues occur and to what degree varies from woman to woman. Many women are not aware of these changes as they happen. If you experience a number of these signs, it's best to get some rest, because chances are great that you will be delivering within a few days.

What's Happening in Your Body

Even though labor has not yet begun, your body is beginning the job of delivering your baby. Your hormones are changing; progesterone levels decrease; estrogen, oxytocin, and prostaglandin levels increase. These birth hormones relax your pelvic ligaments even more than in previous months and cause your vaginal tissues to become more stretchable. The hormones begin working on your cervix to get it "ripe," meaning softer, thinner, and ready to dilate.

"Prelabor" may last from a few hours to a few weeks. Typically, your baby is descending lower into your pelvis during this time, while your cervix is thinning (becoming partially effaced) and opening (dilating) 1 or 2 centimeters.

What You Can Do

Rest, rest, rest. Do not try to work at your job during this time, if at all possible. You have a lot of hard work ahead of you. Now is a good time to pack your bag, tie up loose ends, and go through your prebirth checklist (see page 337). Nourish your body by eating lots of complex carbohydrates to store up energy; nourish your mind by studying and rehearsing the following:

- relaxation techniques (see page 305)
- pain-relieving techniques (see page 299)
- techniques for helping your labor progress (see page 340)

Be as rested up, energized, and rehearsed as you can be for the more intense work that is soon to come.

Labor Is Beginning: How to Tell

You're officially in *active labor* (see page 355 for a description of phases) when your cervix is 4 centimeters dilated. Some women can stay just shy of this stage of dilatation for days or a week or two before they experience consistently regular, hard contractions. So we will arbitrarily say your labor has begun when your contractions become regular and increasingly intense. When this happens you are likely to see your baby within a day.

We do not find the terms "true labor" and "false labor" helpful or accurate, since there is no such thing as a "false" labor contraction. As discussed, all those prelabor Braxton Hicks contractions you've had for weeks and months have been toning the uterus, adjusting baby's position, and effacing your cervix, all preparing for the day when you're going to labor a baby out. Instead, we find it helpful to divide contractions into prelabor contractions (which prepare the passage for baby) and labor contractions, which deliver the baby. Many women, especially first-timers, can't pinpoint the exact moment labor contractions begin. Labor contractions can seem like prelabor contractions at first. After the fact, of course, mothers can look back and say, "Oh, yes, that was when they started." Once active labor is well under way, you'll no longer doubt that this will end with the delivery of your baby. Here's how to tell the difference.

Prelabor contractions (also known as "false" contractions):
- Are irregular, following no discernible pattern for more than a few hours.
- Are nonprogressive; they don't become stronger, longer, or more frequent.
- Are felt most in front, in the lower abdomen.
- Vary from painless to mildly uncomfortable; they feel more like pressure than pain.
- Become less intense and less uncomfortable if you change position or walk, lie down, or take a hot bath or shower.
- Make your uterus feel like a hard ball.

Labor contractions (also known as "real" or "true" contractions):
- Follow a regular pattern (though timing is seldom precise to the minute).

Labor Tip: If you are in doubt about whether you are experiencing prelabor or labor contractions, apply the 1–5–1 formula: if your contractions last for at least 1 minute, are 5 minutes (or less) apart, and continue for at least 1 hour, you are probably in labor.

This is a good time to begin at-home contraction charting as follows:

Time of Onset	How Long?
10:02 P.M.	60 seconds
10:06 P.M.	65 seconds
10:10 P.M.	50 seconds
10:13 P.M.	40 seconds
10:17 P.M.	65 seconds
10:22 P.M.	60 seconds

- Are progressive; they become stronger, longer, and more frequent; the contractions get longer and the intervals between them shorter.
- Are felt most in the lower abdomen and radiate around to the lower back.
- Vary from uncomfortable pressure to a grabbing, pulling pain that can usually be managed, even lessened, by conscious release of tension in the rest of your muscles.
- Don't change if you lie down or change position; may be intensified by walking.
- Are usually accompanied by a "bloody show" (see page 353).

Unless you are experiencing danger signs (see page 352), there's no need to call your health-care provider unless it's during regular office hours and your curiosity just won't let you wait. Your practitioner can do an internal exam to tell whether you are in prelabor or progressive labor. If your cervix is softening,

thinning, effacing, and possibly dilating, you will feel encouraged.

Now that you (and perhaps your health-care provider) have determined that this is the real thing, it's time to look for the signs of each phase of labor. No one's labor ever matches up precisely with a nice, neat outline. Nevertheless, labors have these stages and phases in common:

1. First stage of labor
   - early or latent phase
   - active phase
   - transition phase

2. Second stage of labor
   - resting and pushing phase
   - crowning and delivery phase

3. Third stage of labor
   - delivering the placenta

For some women the phases of the first stage are distinct; for others they blend together. And bear in mind that the length and intensity of these phases vary tremendously from woman to woman and from labor to labor in the same mother. The descriptions that follow contain general guidelines; your labor will have its own unique duration, timing, and intensity.

The First Stage of Labor: Early Phase

What You May Experience

The first phase of labor is called the "early" or "latent" phase because active labor is soon to follow, even if now it seems as if little is going on. Some women may not even realize they are in labor or may think they're just experi-

Labor Tip: This is a good time to use a birth watch. These devices, which are available through childbirth catalogs (see page 401), are specialized stopwatches that record the length of and interval between contractions. Most dads like this toy; it makes them feel useful to be measuring something. A warning to fathers: don't let gadgets and charts prevent you from focusing your attention on your laboring partner.

encing stronger Braxton Hicks contractions. For most women the latent phase is the easiest part of labor; it's also the longest. In this early phase, contractions can range from five to thirty minutes apart and last from thirty to forty-five seconds. They are not usually strong enough to prevent you from moving around your home doing business as usual, and most women feel calm and in control. You may feel like chatting, enjoying company, or taking a walk. You may be excited that the time is really here, yet apprehensive about what labor will be like and how you will cope. You may have an attack of nesting instinct, and you may experience several of the bodily signs discussed in the section on prelabor above (diarrhea, low backache, increased vaginal discharge, menstrual-like cramps, "bloody show," frequent urination). During this phase some mothers leak amniotic fluid or the membranes may rupture, although this usually does not happen until the next phase, the active phase of labor. The early phase of labor lasts an average of eight hours for first-timers, but it can vary from a few hours to a few days. Some women sleep through this phase when it occurs at night.

What's Happening in Your Body

During early labor your cervix thins out, becoming from 50 to 90 percent effaced. It also dilates, reaching 3 to 4 centimeters by the end of early labor.

What You Can Do

Your body can play tricks on you in this phase of labor. You may feel euphoric, chatty, or get a sudden burst of energy and feel like keeping busy — the desire to retreat into a quiet place may not click in yet. If you feel excited and full of energy, you may not feel like resting — but you *must*. Many first-timers waste so much energy during this early phase of labor that they are tired by the time the harder work begins, and they often run out of energy. Although you need to rest and sleep, mental excitement and mild bodily annoyances may make you restless. Ask your mate for a relaxing back rub, take a warm bath or a shower, read, or watch television. Try to sleep or at least rest — do whatever you can to conserve your energy for the work to come. If you simply cannot stay still, take a leisurely walk. The upright position and gentle movement will allow gravity to help baby descend into your pelvis and to keep your contractions progressing. Be careful not to click into fear mode, which can happen if you had a difficult previous labor or if you distrust your body. Fear can cause you to resist your labor mentally and physically. If you feel yourself becoming anxious, try to talk it out with someone (hopefully your labor support person or a trusted friend) who can help you manage.

As your contractions get stronger, begin to use your relaxation techniques and natural pain-relief methods. Experiment with different positions during contractions. Try resting in the side-lying position between contractions. If a backache becomes more intense, try spending some of your resting moments in the all-fours position. As latent labor becomes more active and intense, you will find yourself spending more and more of your contraction time leaning against someone or something for support.

Most women spend this early phase of labor in the comfort of their home. (Some hospitals have a policy that says you must be in active labor to be admitted to labor and delivery.) Be sure to eat frequently (see page 341) to store up energy. Keep your bladder empty, as this helps your labor progress. Above all, keep your mind and body as relaxed as possible.

Your mind or your body will tell you when you are nearing the end of the latent phase. Toward the end of this early phase your contractions will increase in frequency (around five minutes apart) and intensity. One common sign of the onset of active labor is that you come down from your euphoria and become introspective, wanting to tune out what's going on around you and retreat into a quiet place. This emotional change is often a clue that it's time to notify your health-care provider that you are in labor. Listen to your emotional and physical signs and act on them. (See "When to Call Your Health-Care Provider," page 352, and "When to Go to the Hospital," page 359.)

Tips for Dad During the Early Phase

Be a gofer. Encourage your wife to rest in whatever nest she has prepared while you serve her food and drink. Offer massages and back rubs and whatever physical and emotional support she requests.

This can be a scary time for you. Long before you accompanied your partner to childbirth classes, you encountered movies and books about dangerous labors in which women were screaming in pain and men were pacing about frantically outside the delivery room; this may have conditioned your unconscious to be fearful in this situation. These old pictures are bound to surface when labor begins. Suddenly you are afraid that your lovemaking nine months ago has put your beloved in danger. You feel responsible for her increasing discomfort and powerless to alleviate her distress. Back rubs, cheery words, even kisses and caresses seem only mildly helpful, especially if the work of labor is making your wife distant or irritable. You have fears about what life will be like after the baby comes — whether your wife will ever enjoy romantic evenings again, whether you can make enough money to meet the medical or educational needs of your new addition, whether you'll be a good father, and on and on. Most of all, it's hard to imagine how that watermelon can ever get out of your wife's vagina.

Most men don't like hospitals, pain management, or blood, so the next forty-eight hours may not look appealing, despite careful preparation. Be brave. You can do it. Your love and concern for your partner will carry you through. What she needs most is for you simply to stand by her and share the hours ahead. This is a stressful time, but you will be so thrilled and so proud when you hold your very own son or daughter that you will forget the fear and worry. This little person and his mom will be very dependent on your steady, calm, supportive presence in the weeks and months to come. You and your life will be enriched beyond measure by the most important gift your wife will ever give you — your child.

The First Stage of Labor: Active Phase

What You May Experience

As a general guide, once your contractions are intense enough to stop you in mid-sentence — you can't talk through them — you are in active labor. During the early phase of labor you may have been lulled into thinking, "These aren't so bad, I can handle them." Now, as your contractions come on harder and faster, last longer, and demand your total attention, you may change your tone: "Wow! This is tough!" Typically, contractions in the active phase occur every three to five minutes and last forty-five to sixty seconds. You may be walking along and find a contraction stops you dead in your tracks, all but taking your breath away. You can no longer manage these pains by distraction only; you need to call on your previously rehearsed relaxation and pain-relieving techniques.

Women often describe active labor contractions as waves starting at the top of the uterus and going to the bottom, or from the back radiating around to the front. These waves reach peak intensity midway through contractions, then gradually ease off. In active labor your whole body seems to be involved in the contractions. You may feel intense pulling and stretching right above your pubic bone, along with a deep backache or deep pelvic pressure. This is also the phase of labor when your membranes are most likely to rupture and produce a gush of fluid (for what to do when your water breaks, see page 353).

You may find your emotions changing even before your body tells you that you are in active labor. Just prior to or at the onset of active labor, many mothers instinctively seek out a more peaceful place to do their work. Partners and others who are caring for the laboring woman should recognize this signal of the mother's need to turn inward and adjust their routines accordingly.

This active phase of the first stage of labor lasts three to four hours, but this is just an average. Your uterus has its own timetable. Many women experience active labor in bursts and pauses; labor is intense for a while, a lull follows, and then contractions intensify again.

What's Happening in Your Body

During this active phase, your cervix completely effaces, and you dilate from 4 to 8 centimeters. Baby's head descends lower into your pelvis, which often breaks the membranes and releases the amniotic fluid with a gush. Your brain responds to your increased discomfort by releasing endorphins, your body's natural pain relievers.

What You Can Do

Employ your relaxation techniques and self-help pain-relieving techniques (see page 299). Also, remember the suggestions for helping your labor progress (see page 340). Early in the active phase of labor is the time many women opt for medical pain relief (see "A Balanced Mind-set About Pain Relief," page 322). Remember these important keys to easing the discomfort and enhancing the progress of labor:

- Rest between contractions to recharge your body.
- Relax and release during a contraction. Take a deep breath as it begins. Breathe slowly and rhythmically in through your nose and out through your mouth. Once it's over, take another deep breath to let go of any tension that may have built up.
- Change positions frequently. Improvise; do whatever works for you.

- Empty your bladder every hour.
- Consider immersing yourself in water.

During this phase of labor there may be periods when your mind seems to escape to another world. You may feel this zoning out sensation during or between contractions. Don't be afraid — you're not losing your mind. Your body is doing just the right thing to help you handle your pain.

Tips for Dads During the Active Phase

It's important for all who are on the labor scene to respect the mother's desire for mental peace by providing a peaceful environment and a peaceful presence themselves. Ask nurses and other hospital personnel to cut the chatter and unnecessary noise so the laboring woman can do her work in peace.

When to Go to the Hospital

You may picture yourself rushing frantically to the hospital or birth center, only to deliver your baby in a taxi cab. Maybe you worry that your mate-turned-midwife will have to do an emergency bedroom delivery because you waited too long. Despite what you see in the movies, this rarely happens. Most soon-to-be-mothers, with a little coaching from their birth attendant, time their hospital entrance just fine. During one of your last prenatal visits or during a phone call to your practitioner during early labor, you will receive specific instructions as to when to go to the hospital. (If you have a specific obstetrical problem for which it is deemed safest to go early, do it.) Here are some general guidelines:

- A rule of thumb that works for most first-time mothers is to go to the hospital when you reach 4-1-1: contractions 4 minutes apart, lasting 1 minute, and occurring consistently for 1 hour or more.
- Leave for the hospital if contractions are strong enough to stop you in your tracks,

prevent you from speaking, or require you to muster up serious comfort techniques.
- Follow your inner voice. If it says, "It's time to go," go.

Unless your practitioner instructs you otherwise, be sure your labor is well established before going to the hospital. Try to labor in the comfort of your own home as long as possible. Most women are most comfortable in their own surroundings during early labor. Arriving at the hospital too early can often cause your labor to stall. Arriving too late may not be the most comfortable thing to do, either.

Don't worry about what the birth attendants at the hospital will think if your arrival is a false alarm. They are used to this happening. They won't patronize you, snicker, or embarrass you with questions like, "What are you doing here so soon?" If this is your first baby you are not expected to know what labor is like. Nor can you check your own cervix to determine how far along you are. If this is not your first time, you have every reason to believe that labor will happen faster.

Now is the critical time to make sure you don't fall victim to the fear-tension-pain cycle. Watch closely for signs of fear, tension, and pain and do whatever you can to diffuse the anxiety and tightness. Speak reassuringly and calmly. Watch your own voice and body language for fear and tension. Remind her all is well, that she's doing great. Start using relaxation techniques with her when the active phase begins. It may not occur to her to do it, and she will gradually lose the ability to relax if she doesn't start soon enough.

The First Stage of Labor: Transition Phase

What You May Experience

Transition means you are moving from the first stage of labor — stretching the pelvic passages open — into the second stage, pushing baby out. Transition is the most intense phase of your entire labor, but the good news is it's also the shortest, usually lasting only fifteen minutes to an hour and a half. Many women do not experience more than ten or twenty contractions during transition. Transition contractions are more frequent than those of active labor — one to three minutes apart — and will last at least a minute to a minute and a half. They may also have more than one peak. They come on fast and furious, so that you have little time to rest and recharge between them.

As baby rounds the curve from womb to vagina, you may feel more backache and very intense pelvic and rectal pressure. In addition, the overpowering nature of the contractions may cause nausea, vomiting, belching, heavy perspiration, hot and cold flashes, and shaking all over, especially in the legs. Your thighs may ache intensely.

Many women feel overwhelmed during transition. The relentless contractions seem unmanageable. It's normal to think (and say), "I can't go on" or "I don't want to do this anymore" or "Get me an epidural — now!" Even if you have been managing your labor well to this point, keeping on top of your contractions, you may not be able to relax through these. They come on like tidal waves, and there is very little respite between them. You may yell and groan, or make whatever earthy, from-the-gut sounds you need to make to do the work you have to do.

When you reach the point where you begin to feel you cannot possibly go on, remind yourself you're now almost over the hump, so to speak. Feeling like you can't do it anymore is a sign that you won't have to do it much longer. Once transition is over, it is literally downhill from there. While the pushing that's ahead is hard work, most women find it much less painful and more rewarding.

What's Happening in Your Body

Your cervix dilates the final few centimeters during transition. At the end of this phase you'll hear those magic words: "Good news! You're fully dilated." The reason transition is so intense is that your uterine muscles are now doing double duty to reach total dilatation: still pulling your cervix up over baby's head and beginning to push baby's head through. In addition, baby's head squeezing through the cervix puts tremendous pressure on your rectum and pelvic bones, accounting for the overpowering sensations you feel during transition. Fortunately, your brain also recognizes the intensity of transition and continues to release endorphins.

What You Can Do

Because transition is so strenuous, you will need to muster up all the relaxation and pain-relieving tools you brought to your birth. Try the following:

- Change positions to find what works: kneeling, sitting, on all fours, side-lying, squatting. Your body will tell you when it's time to shift position.

- Stay off your back.

- Use a labor tub or shower to regain your relax-and-release mode.

- Rest completely between contractions; don't think of the last one or the next one.

- Focus on releasing; visualize your opening cervix as it is pulled up over your baby's head.

- Overcome any urge to push by blowing out air over and over. If you allow yourself to bear down too much before your cervix is fully dilated, you can cause your cervix to swell, and it will take longer to be pulled up over baby's head. Resisting the urge to push too soon is very hard to do. Let your birth attendant know if you feel an urge to push so he or she can check your cervix and give you the green light to go ahead and push.

Mothers who have chosen not to have an epidural often change their minds and request one during transition. Don't feel disappointed if your birth attendant tells you that it is too late; by the time the epidural is placed and takes effect, transition is likely to be over.

Tips for Dads During the Transition Phase

Remember, there are no rules for how a laboring woman is supposed to act. Transition is not a romantic time. Your loving, but labor-ing, mate may turn on you and her other helpers and become hostile. She will probably be unable to tell you how you can help. She will be too preoccupied to think of anything you might do to make things better; she will also be too impatient and exhausted to explain her needs. Don't be hurt if she yells, "Don't do that" or "Stop it!" Certain touches can be distracting in this phase. If she snaps at you to "get away," back off but stay with her. Reassure her, praise her, and try to keep her breathing on track by breathing slowly and deeply with her. If you are using a professional labor assistant, this will be a time when you will be glad to lean on her experience (or that of the labor support person or the labor nurse). Your wife will need both of you.

When your wife is at her worst, you need to be at your best. Be a tower for her to lean on, an anchor to steady her. You don't have to fix anything — just be there. Love her. She'll appreciate it more than you know, but don't expect her thanks until later.

The Second Stage of Labor: Pushing Baby Out

What You May Experience

The two most welcome features of the pushing stage are: it's usually much less difficult than transition, and it ends with the birth of your baby. Your contractions may now be less painful and further apart, around three to five minutes from the beginning of one to the beginning of the next.

A blissful rest. Between the pain of transition and the beginning of the urge to push, many women get a ten- to twenty-minute lull in their labor called the "time of peace" by childbirth educator Helen Wessel Nichol, or the "rest and be thankful" phase by childbirth educator Sheila Kitzinger. If you have this brief break in the action, *rest.* Most women also experience a burst of energy, a sort of second wind for the pushing stage.

The urge to push! Once your cervix is fully dilated, baby's head begins to descend into the birth canal. You may feel an uncontrollable urge to bear down.

This was an irresistible, overpowering feeling, almost like having the most intense bowel movement of my life (but then again, not at all like that). It was the most earthy feeling I've ever experienced, and it felt wonderful compared to transition.

As you push your baby through the birth canal you may feel an alarming sensation of tearing momentarily as your vaginal tissues stretch to accommodate baby's head. Remember, your vagina is designed for this stretching. In minutes the pressure of baby's head against the vaginal walls will numb these sensations.

Some lucky moms deliver their baby with a few hard pushes; others labor strenuously for a couple of hours more. The average length of the pushing stage is from one to one and a half hours in first-time moms. (Second-pregnancy pushing usually goes much faster.) As with most of labor, there is wide variation in the length of the pushing stage, and it may be longer than nature intended if an epidural anesthetic lessens your urge and ability to push. This is why many women and their birth attendants decide to turn the epidural down or off during transition, allowing the mother to participate fully in the pushing phase. Depending on the strength of the medication, it may take up to an hour for the drug to wear off completely.

What's Happening in Your Body

Your cervix, fully dilated after transition, allows baby's head (or buttocks, if breech, see page 294) to enter the birth canal. As baby's head stretches the vaginal and pelvic-floor muscles, microscopic receptors in these tissues trigger the urge to bear down, called the "Ferguson reflex." This reflex also signals your system to release more oxytocin, the hormone that stimulates uterine contractions. These two natural stimulants work together to push baby out. One tells you to push with your whole body, while the other tells your uterus to contract and help push baby down. In the previous stage your uterus did all of the work; now it's up to your abdominal and pelvic muscles to help finish the job. When you push (bear down), your abdominal and pelvic muscles put pressure on the uterus, adding to the effort of that great muscle, moving baby down and out.

What You Can Do

Knowing when and how to push will help you get to hold your baby sooner and with less work. These are some pushing pointers we have learned from our own births and from veteran mothers who learned how to use their body most efficiently during this strenuous but most rewarding stage of labor.

Try self-regulated pushing. Bear down when your instincts tell you to, not when someone else yells, "Push!" This is a more physiological way of pushing. To get baby out in the shortest time with the most efficient effort, your uterus and pushing muscles must work together. As soon as you have the overwhelming urge to push, bear down. This urge may come at the beginning of a contraction or well into a contraction. Sometimes you may feel one long, continuous urge during the contraction; other times you may feel several pushing urges per contraction. Push when and how your body makes you push. Use any position and spurt of emotions that work for you.

Avoid staff-directed pushing. Birth attendants, like fans cheering a runner at the end of a race, like to urge the mother on with encouraging words during the pushing stage. This cheerleading needs to be peaceful and supportive. Inform any overbearing "coaches" that they are disturbing your inner rhythm by yelling, "Bear down harder!" "Hold your breath!" "You can do it — try harder!" "Push! Push!" This directed pushing is a carryover from the days when mothers were so medicated and immobile that they could neither feel when to push nor push efficiently when they tried. These well-meaning, but counterproductive, taskmasters are often responsible for tired mothers and torn perineums.

Letting a mom push when, as long, and as strong as each contraction indicates is like allowing the contracting uterus to conduct the symphony of birth. (childbirth educator Sheila Kitzinger)

Sometimes a more peaceful kind of directed pushing is necessary — if, for example, you don't feel the urge to push, or if this reflex is masked by medication. The labor and delivery nurse or labor support person, perhaps with one eye on the electronic fetal monitor, will help you know when to push (perhaps by placing your hand on your uterus so you can sense the coming contraction). When the contraction begins, your director may offer instructions: "Take a deep breath, round (don't arch) your back, tighten your tummy muscles, relax your bottom, and bear down. Gradually, blow out your breath while you push and imagine you are opening

and releasing your baby . . ." (See the related section "The Timing of Epidurals," page 324.)

Push properly. Erase from your memory any movie scene in which a purple-faced mother is lying flat on her back pushing until her eyes practically pop out. Unlike the physiological pushing we described above, "purple pushing," urged on by a loud and anxious cheering squad, is usually not helpful for mother and can be harmful for baby. After all, this is not an Olympic weight-lifting contest. When a mother bears down and holds her breath for a long time, pressure within her chest increases. This slows blood return to her heart, drops her blood pressure, and can slow blood supply to her hardworking uterus. The longer the breath-holding and the bearing down, the more likely it is these circulatory disturbances will happen. Studies link prolonged breath-holding and pushing beyond six seconds to changes in the fetal heart rate, suggesting that baby may not be getting enough oxygen.

Research validates what many mothers do instinctively: short, frequent pushes conserve your energy, preserve blood vessels in your face, deliver more blood to your uterus, enhance contractions, and deliver more oxygen to baby. In fact, studies show most mothers push properly without anyone telling them how. Besides being healthier for baby and less exhausting for mother, proper pushing also decreases the likelihood of perineal tissues tearing and decreases the chances of your getting an episiotomy.

So what's the best way to push? Push with as much effort as you can without overdoing it. Short (five to six seconds) and frequent (three to four per contraction) pushes will not tire you unduly and will keep the oxygen level in your blood constant. After five or six seconds of bearing down to your maximum

Avoiding an Episiotomy

Soon episiotomy will join the list of outdated obstetrical procedures that aren't done routinely anymore, along with such delights from the past as perineal shaving and enemas during labor. For an episiotomy, the doctor, using a local anesthetic to numb the tissue, makes an incision into the skin and muscles of your perineum and vaginal canal just before your baby crowns, in order to make the opening larger.

Myths about episiotomies. Routine episiotomy is a holdover from birthing's past, when most women delivered on their backs with their legs up in stirrups, a position that tenses perineal muscles and makes them more likely to tear during delivery. Forceps were used to get babies out. Women now birth their babies differently, leaving many mothers, midwives, and physicians questioning whether routine episiotomy is advisable.

Actually many obstetricians agree that routine episiotomies are not necessary, but episiotomies are still performed more often than needed, especially on first-time mothers. This is because of several myths.

- **Myth one:** A straight cut made by scissors heals better than a natural tear. *False.* Research shows that a few little tears, which may involve only the skin layer, heal better than one big incision, which goes through all the layers of skin and muscle. What nature cuts, nature heals. Of course, an obstetrician may prefer stitching up a straight-edged incision rather than a zigzaggy tear, but whose body is it anyway?
- **Myth two:** Natural tears during delivery are likely to extend into and damage the rectum. *False.* Research shows that episiotomy incisions are more likely than natural tears to extend themselves and tear even into the rectum, causing more long-term problems. Hold an old piece of cloth by the edges and try to tear it. Then make a tiny cut in the cloth and try to tear it. The cloth tears more easily where it has already been cut.

- **Myth three:** An episiotomy shortens the second stage of labor and is therefore healthier for baby. *True and false.* Episiotomies may occasionally shorten the second stage of labor, but studies have shown that this makes no difference to the health of the baby, except in emergencies.
- **Myth four:** A woman is less likely to suffer long-term pelvic floor–muscle problems, such as bladder incontinence, if she has an episiotomy. *False.* Research suggests just the opposite: women who do not have an episiotomy tend to have stronger perineal muscles postpartum.
- **Myth five:** An episiotomy keeps your vagina from stretching out of shape. *False.* Nonsense. Your vaginal canal has already been stretched to its max, and it is unlikely that cutting a few minutes off the total stretching time will make any difference long term. No surgical procedure can return the vagina to its "like new" state — after all, a baby worked its way through there! If whether or not to have an episiotomy is a sexual issue for you (perhaps you've heard that an episiotomy ensures postpartum vaginal "tightness"), you may be interested to know that recent research confirms that women who give birth without an episiotomy are able to resume sex more quickly, experience less pain during sex, and report greater sexual satisfaction. (Vaginal tightness is determined more by the strength of your pelvic-floor muscles than anything else, so do those Kegel exercises!)

Not only does new research show that routine episiotomy is unwise and unnecessary, it may even be risky. Tearing is not inevitable at birth, and episiotomies are often done when no tear (or a minimal tear) would have occurred. An episiotomy opens you up (literally) to problems: the perineum is an area of the body that often does not heal easily, and it is also likely to become infected. Many women experience months of discomfort from their episiotomy.

The episiotomy was worse than the birth. I couldn't sit for two weeks. Then I had to drag around my rubber doughnut every place I went.

There are a few obstetrical circumstances that may necessitate an episiotomy:

- Fetal distress — when it's necessary to get the baby out quickly
- Shoulder dystocia — when a shoulder is stuck
- Vaginal breech delivery
- Forceps delivery

Avoiding an episiotomy. Episiotomy is not just a little cut into trivial tissue; you should be a major part of decisions about this procedure. Since research shows that episiotomy is not necessary routinely, here are ways that you can lessen your chances of having this unkind and usually unnecessary cut:

- Practice your Kegel exercises (see page 176) at least a hundred times a day for the last six months of pregnancy. The simplest way to perform Kegel exercises is to squeeze your rectal muscles as if trying to prevent a bowel movement while squeezing your muscles of urination as if trying to stop the flow of urine. Also, don't forget to practice the *release* mode of this exercise. Relaxed tissues are more likely to stretch and less likely to tear.
- Avoid the back-lying, feet-up-in-stirrups position for delivery. This least-efficient birthing position not only narrows your pelvic outlet, but it tenses your perineal muscles, making them more likely to tear or invite an episiotomy. Studies have shown that mothers who birth in the squatting or side-lying position are much less likely to tear or "need" an episiotomy.
- Control your pushing. Pushing too hard and birthing too fast is likely to either tear your perineum or get you an episiotomy. The birth attendant sees that the perineum is not being allowed to stretch gradually, and so he cuts to avoid a tear (still not a good reason to cut, but it happens). Pushing the way that comes naturally to you stretches the vaginal and perineal muscles slowly, making them more likely to open without tearing. Childbirth educators teach the coat-sleeve analogy: If you try to shove your arm quickly through a crumpled coat sleeve, you are likely to meet resistance from a puckered-up lining. If you persist forcefully, you may even tear the lining. But if you gradually straighten the sleeve, smooth the lining, and ease your arm through gently, you meet much less resistance and are unlikely to tear the lining.
- Ask your birth attendant about perineal massage, a maneuver called "ironing." Your birth attendant gently smoothes out the tissues of the perineum as baby's head stretches them, and supports your perineal tissues with a warm compress while baby's head is crowning. You can also do perineal massage with oil at home during the last few months to increase elasticity of the vaginal opening.
- Ease into the crowning stage of delivery. Once you feel the burning sensation that goes along with the stretching of your perineal tissues as baby's head crowns, let up on your bearing down. Allow your birth attendant to support the perineal tissue, and gently ease baby out, a technique called "breathing baby out."

When your baby is crowning is not the time to initiate a dialogue with your obstetrician about the benefits of a no-episiotomy birth. Discuss the subject of episiotomy during one of your eighth- or ninth-month visits. Let your preferences be known to your doctor: unless it's absolutely necessary for the health of your baby or yourself you wish to avoid this surgical procedure (situations requiring episiotomy occur in less than 5 percent of deliveries; see possible reasons above). Be sure your wishes are recorded in your birth plan. Remind your obstetrician of your request during labor and then again at delivery.

intensity, blow the air completely out of your lungs. Then inhale quickly, filling your lungs with enough new air for the next push.

Assume the best position for pushing. Lying on your back is the worst position for pushing; upright squatting is the best. If you are lying on your back, you will be trying to push your baby uphill, the least efficient route. If you are perched on your lower backbone (your coccyx), you may prevent it from flexing outward as baby passes through, slowing the progress and increasing the pain of delivery. Squatting widens your pelvis and takes advantage of gravity so baby can move down and out faster. There are various ways to get the effect of squatting, one of which is a semi-reclined position that gets the pelvis widened by having your legs pulled back as you push. However, this arrangement takes advantage of gravity to a lesser degree than more upright squatting.

If your baby is coming down too fast, use the side-lying position with a birth attendant or labor support person supporting your perineum with a warm compress. You will need someone to hold up your top leg.

Take your time. Often mothers and birth attendants want to speed up the pushing stage of labor. You will be eager to get labor over with and to hold your baby. The "medical urge" to push babies out quickly is based upon an outdated belief that the longer baby is squeezed in the birth canal, the more he or she risks being deprived of oxygen. Current research shows that a long second stage, properly managed and properly monitored, does not adversely affect baby. New studies suggest that it is the intense and prolonged bearing down during the pushing stage that can deprive baby of oxygen, not the length of the second stage itself. Don't be alarmed if

you hear the beeps on the electronic fetal monitor slow down during your contractions, as long as they bounce back to normal after the contraction is over; baby's heart rate normally slows down during contractions and recovers between them. If these beeps worry or bother you, ask to have the sound turned off. One of your birth attendants can keep an eye on the monitor.

Rest between pushes. As much as childbirth educators and veteran mothers offer this advice, many first-timers do not take advantage of the down times in their labor. When your contraction is over, ease into a position that lets you rest. Suck on some ice chips, listen to soft music, keep your room and attendants quiet, and use whatever relaxation techniques you need to drift into your own calm world. Visualize "opening," "releasing," and "unfolding" scenes between contractions, as well as during them. Imagine the graceful unfolding of rose petals as a way to encourage your mind and body to open and release baby.

Protect your perineum. The first few urges to push may take you by surprise, prompting you to tense instead of relax your pelvic-floor muscles. Here's where your Kegel and relaxation exercises really pay off. (See related section "Avoiding an Episiotomy," page 364.)

Tips for Dads During the Second Stage

Remind your partner to relax and help her to do so. Support her desired labor position; wipe her forehead with a cool cloth; offer ice chips; offer to massage where she needs it; stroke her arms and legs. Remind her to breathe deeply and let go. Keep the birth room quiet and peaceful; banish disturbing

How Your Uterus Delivers

Ever wonder how your uterus pushes your baby out? No one knows what makes labor begin, though researchers think that prostaglandins produced by the baby, uterus, or placenta (and maybe all three) trigger labor when baby is "ripe."

Picture your uterus as an upside-down pear covered lengthwise by hundreds of rubber bands, representing muscles. These long muscle fibers fan out over the top and largest part of your uterus, called the "fundus." The lowest and narrowest part of the pear, the cervix, contains more thick and fibrous tissue than muscle, and the muscle is arranged in a circular pattern around the cervix. Think of your uterine muscles working in a push-pull motion: the upper group pushes the baby down; the lower group is pulled up over baby. In order for these groups of muscles to birth a baby, they must work in harmony with each other: the upper muscles contract and harden while the lower ones soften, relax, and open. Eventually the uterus goes from pear-shaped to tubular, allowing baby to descend. If you are tense and resisting the work of your uterus, these two groups of muscles can get out of sync, with the muscles on the top of the uterus contracting against unrelaxed muscles on the lower uterus —"Ouch!"

Another magnificent feature of uterine muscles is that, unlike any other muscle group in the body, they become shorter after each contraction. Thank goodness — otherwise your uterus would never return to its original size after its work is done!

influences and persons. Encourage her progress even though she thinks it's slow ("Great job!"). And don't forget a well-timed kiss.

Crowning: Baby's Head Appears

After you push for a while, your labia will begin to bulge — visible results of your work. Soon your birth attendant can see a puckered little scalp appearing as you bear down, then retreating when the contraction stops, to reappear with the next one. When your birth attendant announces, "Baby's starting to crown," your perineum gradually begins stretching until eventually your vaginal opening fits like a crown around baby's head. This gradual back-and-forth descent slowly eases the vaginal tissue open, protecting the perineum over which baby is birthed. Once baby's head rounds the corner and ducks under your pelvic bone, it won't be able to slip back anymore. (You can reach down and touch baby's head at this point to motivate yourself to keep going.) As your labia and perineum stretch, you will feel a stinging, burning sensation called a "ring of fire." (Grab the corners of your mouth and pull. Notice the stretching and burning sensation. Magnify this for birth.) This stinging feeling is your body's signal to stop pushing for a moment. In a matter of minutes the pressure of baby's head naturally numbs the nerves in the skin, and the burning sensation will stop.

Once baby crowns, your birth attendant may advise you not to push, but rather to ease baby's head out slowly to avoid tearing your internal tissues or your perineum. As baby's head begins to stretch the skin of your perineum, some practitioners will decide to do an episiotomy. Be sure you have made your episiotomy wishes known ahead of time (see "Avoiding an Episiotomy," page 364). A few more contractions and baby's head turns as the shoulders maneuver under the pubic bone. A few more contractions and the baby slithers out into the hands of your birth attendant or onto the bed.

Your health-care provider will suction mucus out of baby's nose and mouth if necessary, rub baby's back to stimulate a breath (you'll then hear baby's first cry!), and then drape baby over your belly tummy-to-tummy, where a quick checkup for Apgar score is done. The cord will be cut (some dads want to do the honors), and your baby is ready to meet you. Some babies may need some special care, such as suctioning meconium, stimulating respirations, or administering oxygen, in order to make a healthy transition into life outside the womb. As soon as baby's vital systems are working well, he or she will be brought to your eager arms.

The Third Stage of Labor: Delivery of the Placenta

What You May Experience

At this point you'll probably be exhausted after the work you have done and elated over the prize you have won. While you and your mate behold your baby admiringly and wonder over his tiny body, your birth attendant will go on working and so will your delivery system. You still have a small job left to do — deliver the placenta.

You may be so engrossed in your baby that you are oblivious to the placenta being delivered. But most women find their family bonding time is interrupted by mild ouches as your uterus and your birth attendant remind you that your job is not quite finished. You will feel some cramping and even a weak

pushing sensation as somewhat milder contractions help deliver the placenta. If you had an episiotomy or have a tear, your birth attendant may have a bit of stitching to do. As the local anesthetic is being injected in preparation for the suturing, it may sting a bit. The minor discomforts of the third stage of labor are overshadowed by the relief that birth is over and that you are finally holding your precious baby.

Being tired from the work you've been through and the sudden changes in your body may cause you to have chills and shiver. Uncontrollable shakes can be quite unnerving, distracting, and uncomfortable. Ask for a warm blanket. And use your deep breathing to physically relax yourself as much as possible.

What's Happening in Your Body

Your uterus continues contracting, both to expel the placenta and to clamp down on the blood vessels to stop the bleeding. If there's a problem, you may receive an injection of pitocin and ergot to help contract the uterus and stop the bleeding more quickly. A birth attendant may massage your uterus to help it contract and make sure it stays firm, since bleeding stops sooner if the uterus stays firm. This procedure is usually pretty uncomfortable. Delivery of the placenta may take from five to thirty minutes.

What You Can Do

Enjoy your baby. Hold, love, and caress this little life that you have labored for so hard. Place your baby skin-to-skin on your abdomen. The warmth of your body will help keep baby warm. (A birth attendant will cover baby with a warm towel.) Bring her up to your breast and encourage her to suck.

Is Labor Good for Baby?

You may worry that being squeezed out of the uterus and through the birth canal might not be good for your baby. Exciting new research shows the opposite. Mother Nature's design wins again.

While the process of labor and delivery is stressful for baby, the stress has positive effects. In mothers, labor brings on the release of healthy stress hormones that help a mother cope with pain and adapt to caring for a newborn. Mother's hard work also stimulates her baby's adrenal gland to secrete high levels of stress hormones called "catecholamines." This is known as the "fetal stress response." These are the same "fight or flight" hormones that are released into an adult's system in response to a stressful or life-threatening situation to help the adult quickly adapt. These hormones help baby "fight" to adapt to life outside the womb. Studies show that newborns whose mothers went through labor had higher levels of these "helper hormones" than were found in newborns delivered by scheduled cesarean without the benefit of labor. The fetal stress response helps baby make a healthy transition to life outside the womb in these ways:

- *Facilitates breathing.* These hormones increase secretion of the chemical surfactant, which helps keep the lungs expanded.
- *Helps keep baby's lungs open* to make the transition to breathing air. It also speeds the process that clears amniotic fluid from the lungs.
- *Increases blood flow to vital organs.* Stress hormones direct the blood flow to baby's heart, brain, and kidneys.
- *Increases the newborn's immunity.* Adrenal hormones increase the number of infection-fighting white blood cells in baby's bloodstream.
- *Increases energy supply to baby* by providing nutrients for baby to use during the transition from placental feeding to breastfeeding — tiding baby over until mother's milk comes in.
- *Makes bonding easier.* A high level of stress hormones helps newborns be more alert and responsive to interaction with caregivers.

The fetal stress response is yet more testimony to how mothers' and babies' bodies are beautifully designed to cope with birth and to begin a new life together.

The sucking on your nipple coupled with the rush of motherly feelings as you see and touch your baby release the hormone oxytocin, which naturally helps your uterus contract, helping to expel the placenta and stop the bleeding.

Each time you breastfeed your baby during the first week after birth, you will feel uterine cramps, called "afterpains." These are more intense in second and subsequent pregnancies than they are the first time. Don't let this discomfort discourage you from breastfeeding or put off a feeding. If the afterpains bother you a lot, ask your practitioner if you can take acetaminophen or ibuprofen. Cramping means that the uterus is returning to its normal size, as it should. The cramping will be gone before you know it. Deep breathing helps you relax through it.

Be sure dad gets to hold his new little person, preferably without his shirt on so they can be skin-to-skin for a while. If your baby must go to the nursery for routine checking or for a medical concern, send dad with your little one. Ask for baby to be brought back to you as soon as possible.

There is no reason for baby to cry after the first wails. If the nursery is busy, dad can hold your new little person and rock her until the nurses can process her. Do not leave her alone in the nursery. She'll cry because she's born with a biological need to be next to her mother. She came from a warm, secure place and needs to feel the world is safe and loving. (See page 384 for a discussion of bonding.)

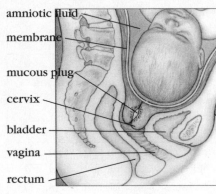

amniotic fluid
membrane
mucous plug
cervix
bladder
vagina
rectum

Prelabor.

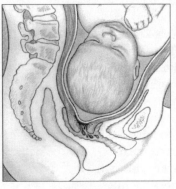

*Bloody show;
cervix dilating.*

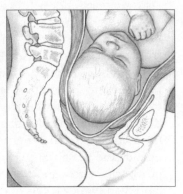

*Membranes bulging;
cervix effaced.*

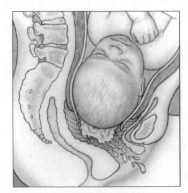

Membranes ruptured.

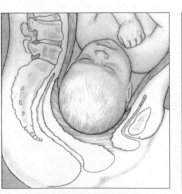

*Transition; dilatation
complete; pushing.*

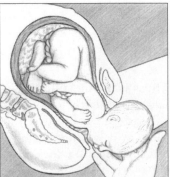

Delivery of baby.

THE NINTH MONTH

❖　❖　❖

Emotionally I feel: _____
_____
_____
_____

Physically I feel: _____
_____
_____
_____

My thoughts about you: _____
_____
_____
_____

What I imagine your birth will be like: _____
_____
_____
_____
_____

My weight: _____
My blood pressure: _____
My top concerns: _____
_____
_____

My best joys: _____
_____
_____

My worst problems: _____
_____
_____
_____

VISIT TO MY HEALTH-CARE PROVIDER

Questions I had; answers I got: _____
_____
_____
_____
_____
_____

Tests and results; my reaction: _____
_____
_____
_____
_____
_____

How I feel when I feel you move: _____
_____
_____
_____
_____
_____

How Dad feels when he feels you move: _____
_____
_____
_____
_____
_____

How I felt when labor began: _____
_____
_____
_____
_____
_____

photo at nine months

Comments: _____
_____
_____
_____
_____
_____
_____
_____
_____
_____
_____
_____
_____
_____
_____

The Tenth Month — Postpartum

FOR WEEKS after your baby's birth, your mind and body will remind you of the intense work you've just completed and of the major changes that are now taking place in your life. You have two tasks to complete: recovering from the birth and adjusting to motherhood. Even though holding the prize of your labor in your arms will more than compensate for the aches and pains throughout your body after birth, there are a few annoyances to cope with.

HOW YOU MAY FEEL EMOTIONALLY

If you thought pregnancy was an amazing emotional experience, prepare yourself for the whirlwind of postpartum feelings. All of a sudden your life is no longer your own — you jump at your baby's every sound. Your body is going through another set of changes, and your hormones are shifting radically. In a month or two, you'll feel more in control, but for now you may feel joyful and fulfilled one moment and frightened and worried the next. Here's a sampling:

Thrilled and excited. You've just survived the rigors of birth, and your baby is finally here. This is a big moment in your life, a natural high. You may find it hard to sleep, hard to think of anyone but your baby. You and your partner may feel compelled to tell your birth story to anyone who will listen. If events occurred during your labor and delivery that led to a less satisfying birth than you hoped for, talk them over with your doctor and midwife so you don't blame yourself for situations that were beyond your influence.

Overwhelmed. The full-time care of a tiny baby is a critically important twenty-four-hour-a-day job, and it's yours now, even though you may have had no previous training. The job begins when you're already worn out from labor and birth, and it may be months before you get more than three or four hours' sleep at a stretch. Of course you feel overwhelmed.

Let down. Lows often follow emotional highs. For months you've been preparing for your baby's birth day, and now the big event is over. It's natural to feel a bit of a letdown, especially with the new challenges you're fac-

374

ing. You may also feel a twinge of sadness about no longer being pregnant. You are no longer the center of attention — your baby is. And even though you are his primary caregiver, you now have to share the baby with your partner, family, and friends.

Weepy. "Baby blues" are a fact of life for many postpartum mothers. They strike a few days after the birth. You may feel very sad and depressed, and not even know why. You may feel anxious and worried about your ability to care for your baby, and you may feel guilty about having all these feelings.

Baby blues are probably the result of sudden changes in your life and in your hormones. Fatigue is also a factor. Experts estimate that baby blues occur in approximately 50 percent of mothers postpartum. You should feel better soon, especially if you are being well cared for and have lots of support. If you arc unable to shake your depression, seek professional help.*

HOW YOU MAY FEEL PHYSICALLY

Feeling "beat-up." You've just been through the most strenuous work of your life. Nearly every muscle, joint, and organ of your body has worked overtime to push the baby out. It's no wonder you feel the effects from head to toe. Depending on the length and intensity of your labor and whether you had a vaginal or surgical birth, expect your body to feel the effects of delivery for at least a few weeks. Your eyes may be bloodshot due to broken blood vessels from intense pushing. You may

also have popped a few blood vessels in your face. Your baby's face may have similar marks, but on baby's face, these "spider marks" will clear up within a few days; yours may take a few weeks. In the days after birth, you may look and feel washed out, pale, and exhausted.

During the first few days, or longer, you may feel bone-deep exhaustion and overall achiness and stiffness. Walking may be a chore. Even taking a deep breath may cause those overworked chest muscles to ache. Besides the benefit of time, try these remedies for your postpartum soreness:

- Rest.
- Soak in a warm bath.
- Get frequent massages, especially on sore muscles.
- Replenish your body's need for fuel by eating and drinking nutritious foods.
- Hold your baby a lot to get your mind off your body.

Feeling faint. For a day or so after delivery it's usual to feel light-headed and dizzy, especially when changing position from lying to sitting or from sitting to standing. You may feel woozy and wobbly when you walk. The end of pregnancy brings a sudden shift in blood volume and total body fluid; it takes a while for your cardiovascular system to adapt and compensate for changes in position. Move from lying to sitting or from sitting to standing gradually. Until this light-headed stage subsides (usually after a day), you may need to seek assistance when getting out of bed or walking.

Shivers and shakes. Immediately after delivery many women experience chills and whole-body shakes, probably due to a reset-

---

* *For more on postpartum depression, see* The Baby Book, *by Sears and Sears (Little, Brown, 1993).*

ting of the body's temperature-regulating system after a long bout of hard work. Rest and ask for warm blankets to cover yourself. These chills should subside within a few hours after delivery.

Bleeding and vaginal discharge. For days or sometimes weeks after birth, your uterus continues to discharge leftover blood and tissue, called "lochia." In the first few days the lochia is usually red, in an amount comparable to a heavy menstrual period, and it may contain a few clots. Toward the end of the first week the amount of lochia usually decreases and becomes reddish brown and thinner. In the next few weeks this discharge changes from reddish brown to pinkish, then to yellowish white, and you will find yourself changing fewer pads. Any activity that increases the emptying of the uterus, such as standing, walking, or breastfeeding, will also increase the amount of discharge.

Continued vaginal bleeding can be frightening if you are not sure what's normal and what's not. Here are signs of possible trouble — situations in which you should call your doctor:

• Bleeding continues to be bright red and copious. With each day postpartum, the amount of your vaginal discharge should decrease, and its consistency should become less bloodlike. If after the first few days you are still soaking a sanitary pad with blood every hour for more than four hours at a time, call your doctor.

• You pass large clots or continuous gushes of bright red blood. Many women will experience an occasional gush or golf ball–size clot after breastfeeding, but the bleeding should soon stop. Passing clots the size of a grape is normal for the first few days.

• The lochia has a persistent foul-smelling odor. It should either have no odor or smell like menstrual blood.

• You're experiencing increasing faintness and paleness, feel cold and clammy, and your heart is racing.

If the bleeding worries you, don't hesitate to call your doctor. As you are healing postpartum, it's your job to notice the changes in your body; it's your health-care provider's job to determine whether or not these changes are normal.

If you experience heavy and worrisome bleeding, lie flat and place an ice pack over your uterus just above the center of your pubic bone while waiting for a return call from your doctor or while en route to the emergency room. Or place the ice pack against the episiotomy site if the pain and bleeding seem to be coming from there. Usual causes of bleeding are failure of the uterus to contract sufficiently, retained fragments of placenta, or infection. Your doctor will examine you to see if any of these problems have occurred or if what you are experiencing is just normal postpartum vaginal discharge.

Afterpains. Even after you've given birth, your uterus must continue contracting to get back to its original size. Uterine contractions also help to pinch off the blood vessels in the uterine lining to control postpartum bleeding. For a few hours after delivery, these contractions may be regular and intense. They will decrease in frequency and intensity over the next few weeks. Afterpains may resemble menstrual cramps or the Braxton Hicks contractions you experienced in the final few months of pregnancy. They intensify during breastfeeding, since sucking stimulates the release of the hormone oxytocin, which contracts the uterus and stops bleeding. Many birth attendants suggest mothers encourage their baby to suck right after delivery to help the uterus contract.

Afterpains are not usually very intense following a first delivery, but they will be quite noticeable after subsequent births. To cope with the discomfort, use whatever relaxation techniques worked for you during labor. This will help make breastfeeding more comfortable. Ask your doctor about taking pain relievers to relieve the discomfort; most of these medications are safe to take while breastfeeding.

Difficulty urinating. During the first day postpartum you may feel no urge to urinate, have difficulty passing urine when you do feel the urge, or feel a burning sensation while urinating. The bladder and urethra are right next to the delivery path, so it's no wonder these tissues are feeling squeezed, stretched, and bruised. Bladder function is suppressed by epidural anesthesia and may not recover until the effects of the drug wear off. An episiotomy or even a small tear can make it difficult to urinate, since the raw skin burns when urine touches it. You can see why it may take some time before you feel at ease in the bathroom. Urinary retention is so common after delivery that the nurse will repeatedly ask you, "Have you urinated yet?" And be prepared for the nurse to try to check your bladder through the abdominal wall to see if it's distended. Here are ways you can get your urinary system working again:

• Drink lots of fluids, at least two 8-ounce glasses of liquid (water or juice) immediately after delivery.
• Run the water in the sink. Hearing running water gives your system the same idea.
• Relax your pelvic-floor muscles.

• Be upright. Stand or walk. Allow gravity to help you urinate.
• Try to relax your pelvic-floor muscles as you try to urinate. Try to relax your whole body.
• Soak your bottom in a warm tub, and urinate right there if that's more comfortable for you.
• The nurse may massage your bladder (if it's enlarged) to get it going.
• If your perineum has raw spots from a cut or a tear, ask for a "peri-bottle" (a plastic squeeze bottle). Fill it with warm water and squirt it onto your perineum as you urinate. The water will dilute the urine and lessen the burning.

Sometimes the bladder becomes full but won't empty despite all the effort from you and your nurse. If you haven't urinated by eight hours after delivery, your doctor may recommend a urinary catheter to empty your bladder and relieve the discomfort of its fullness. Retaining urine too long sets you up for cystitis, an infection of the bladder.

Problems with urinary retention end after a day or two, but expect a week or two of frequent trips to the bathroom. This is your body's normal way of getting rid of the extra fluid it accumulated during the past nine months.

Leaking urine. It's normal, but annoying, to leak a few drops of urine when you cough, sneeze, or laugh. This "stress incontinence" is a temporary nuisance that occurs while your bladder and pelvic organs are rearranging themselves back to their prepregnancy positions. Wear a sanitary pad for a few weeks until this annoyance subsides.

Profuse sweating. Another way your body gets rid of the excess fluids accumulated during your pregnancy is by perspiring more, especially at night. For the first night or two wear cotton clothing to absorb the perspiration, and cover your sheet and pillow with a towel to absorb the night sweats. Excessive sweating or "hot flashes" is most prominent during the first week and gradually subsides by the end of the first month.

Painful perineum. Your sensitive perineum has been stretched to the limit and it may have been bruised or torn. If it has been cut into, it's bound to smart. To ease discomfort, promote healing, and prevent infection of this area, follow these guidelines:

- Do all you can to avoid an episiotomy (see page 364). Many mothers report that the discomfort during the healing of an episiotomy is worse than labor, since the throbbing at the site of the incision can sometimes last for weeks.

- Ask your nurse or health-care provider to instruct you on "peri-care." Heat increases blood flow and promotes healing; cold numbs pain and decreases swelling. Both measures are necessary to heal a traumatized perineum. The nurse will tuck an ice pack up against your perineum as soon as possible (it will feel *so* good). She will advise you about soaking in a warm bath and show you how to squirt warm or cool water over your perineum, using a "peri-bottle." Try placing cool witch hazel pads between your perineum and the sanitary pad.

- Sit or lie in whatever position is comfortable. Leaning to one side may hurt more than sitting straight on a firm surface. If no position is bearable, try a rubber surface or inflatable "doughnut" to take pressure off your perineum. To prevent infection,

change your sanitary pad every few hours and always wipe yourself from front to back to avoid dragging rectal germs across your perineum.

- Clean your perineum after urinating or having a bowel movement by squirting a stream of warm water over the area. Blot dry with a soft towel. Wiping with tissue may be painful to sensitive tissues and enlarged hemorrhoids.

- If your perineal pains persist, your doctor may prescribe an analgesic that is safe to take while breastfeeding.

Constipation. Your bowels may be as reluctant to work as your bladder is, and for similar reasons. The muscles involved in passing a stool may have been traumatized during passage of the baby. Drugs and anesthetics temporarily cause the intestines to be a bit sluggish. During labor your bowels were probably emptied naturally by the diarrhea that usually precedes birth. Besides these physical causes of constipation, many mothers have a psychological reluctance to do any pushing with their perineal muscles, either for fear of hurting these tissues or because of a desire to rest them. Yet the sooner you get your intestines moving, the better you will feel. Here's what to do:

- Walk. Moving your body is likely to move your bowels.
- Drink plenty of fluids.
- Eat and drink natural laxatives: nectar (prune, pear, apricot), fresh fruits, whole grains, and vegetables. Avoid caffeine-containing foods and beverages, such as chocolate, coffee, and colas.
- Relax. Don't worry that passing a bowel movement will pop your stitches. While straining may not be friendly to your hem-

orrhoids, you can start using your perineal muscles as you did before delivery.

Gas and bloating. The bowel sluggishness that contributes to constipation may also make you feel gassy, especially if you are recovering from a cesarean section. Drinking and eating frequently, but in smaller amounts, and getting your body moving again will ease these discomforts. Rocking in a rocking chair is especially helpful for mothers recovering from a surgical birth.

Engorged breasts. In the first couple of days postpartum you will notice only slight changes in your breasts. You may even wonder where all the milk is supposed to come from, as you produce only small amounts of the first milk, called "colostrum" (which, nevertheless, is power-packed with nutrition and immune factors). But then, around the third day, you may suddenly awaken with breasts the size of melons, and nearly as hard. You find that you've grown two cup sizes overnight. Your milk has come in, and you wonder how you are going to handle this uncomfortable swelling, and how your baby's tiny mouth is going to get a grip on a nipple shaped like a softball.

This is breast engorgement. Some mothers find that their breasts become suddenly and painfully engorged, while others, especially those whose babies have been nursing frequently and effectively since birth, experience only a gradual increase in breast fullness. Yes, it's hormones at work again: as estrogen and progesterone levels drop in the days after birth, prolactin — the milk-making hormone — takes over. As the breasts begin to do their work, the tissues swell, partly with milk and partly with other fluids. These dramatic breast changes may not have been part of the lovely, peaceful breastfeeding experi-

ence you envisioned during pregnancy. Plus, your newborn may still be struggling to learn to latch on. Try to stay calm — the best is yet to come. After your baby learns to latch on properly and your breasts settle into a comfortable balance of milk production where supply equals demand, you will be well on your way to a gratifying, nurturing experience. Realize that some breast discomfort is quite common, especially for first-time mothers, but it will pass. While some breast fullness is inevitable, you should take action to ease the discomfort and minimize the swelling. Prolonged engorgement sets you up for breast infections and other nursing difficulties.

- Teach baby to latch on properly *before* engorgement occurs. In the first couple of days, when your breasts are still soft, teach baby to open her mouth wide as she takes the breast, so that her lips and gums are placed way back on your areola, behind the nipple. She should get a big mouthful of breast. Don't let baby suck on your nipple only. You'll get sore very quickly.

- Try the "lower-lip flip." Be sure baby's lower lip is everted (see illustration, page 380) comfortably under your areola. If the lip is tucked in, you can gently pull it out with your finger or take the baby off the breast and try again. Don't let baby "tight-lip" or purse her lips around your nipple, as this is a setup for nipple soreness.

- Rather than applying warm compresses, which may increase the swelling of breast tissue, apply cold compresses or packs of crushed ice to hard, painfully swollen breasts.

- Standing in a warm shower can trigger the milk-ejection reflex and help empty your swollen breasts. Let the water flow over

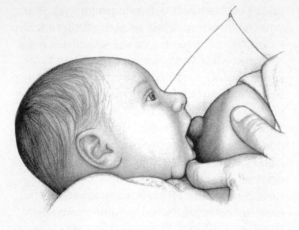

Open baby's mouth wide for proper latch-on.

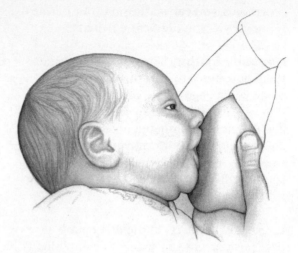

Lower-lip flip.

your breasts and try some gentle massage and milk expression.

• With engorgement, the nipple tissue flattens and the areola hardens, preventing baby from getting enough of your breast into her mouth to compress the milk sinuses, which lie behind the areola. Baby then sucks only on your nipple. He won't get much milk this way, but he will stimulate your body to produce more milk, increasing the engorgement. If your breasts seem too full for baby to latch on properly, use a breast pump or express some milk by hand to soften your areola enough that your baby can latch on to more than just your nipple.

The best remedy for engorgement is frequent breastfeeding. Nothing relieves breast fullness as quickly as a baby who is nursing well. Frequent feedings will also bring your milk supply in line with your baby's demands. Encourage your baby to nurse often. If he sleeps for long stretches during the day,

wake him up to nurse after a couple of hours go by.

The medication formerly used to "dry up" the milk of mothers who were not breastfeeding is no longer considered safe. (It wasn't all that effective anyway.) If you are not breastfeeding, you'll still need to remove enough milk from the breasts to relieve fullness and prevent infection. Your milk production will subside within a week or two.

Dr. Bill notes: When I used to make obstetrical rounds with pediatric residents, the students would call these sessions "Dr. Sears's lower-lip rounds." As we went from room to room showing first-time mothers how to get their newborns to latch on properly, I would take my index finger and depress baby's jaw and lower lip to encourage a better seal. Immediately mother would exclaim, "Oh — that feels better."

Sore nipples. Most sore nipples result from baby's not latching on to the breast correctly.

When a baby latches on and sucks effectively, your nipple goes to the back of his mouth, away from the tongue and gum action that can irritate skin. Sore nipples are not an inevitable part of breastfeeding. If your nipples are starting to get sore, you need to pay some attention to what's going on during feedings. Part of your job as a mother in the first few days is to teach your baby how to breastfeed properly. You can do this, even if you're a first-time mother. While you may want to call in some helpers for expert advice (a knowledgeable nurse, a lactation consultant, an experienced friend, or a La Leche League leader), you are the expert on your baby. Stay calm, be patient, and the two of you will soon work it out. Here's what to do to relieve nipple soreness until your baby begins to nurse more effectively:

- Be sure to break the suction before removing baby from the breast. Press down on the breast tissue, or slide your index finger inside his mouth between his gums. "Popping" a baby off the breast hurts!

- Nurse on the least sore side first. Nipple pain usually lessens as the milk begins to flow. Switch to the other side after you notice signs of the milk-ejection reflex: milk dripping from the other nipple, a tingling sensation in your breasts, a change in the baby's suck-and-swallow rhythm.

- Try stimulating the milk-ejection reflex before you put your baby to the breast, using warm compresses, massage, or gentle pumping.

- Breastfeed frequently — every two hours or so during the day. This will lessen engorgement and make it easier for baby to latch on.

- Let your nipples air-dry between feedings. Express a few drops of milk and let them dry on the nipple. The immunities in your milk will help heal your skin.

- Use a purified lanolin product (such as Lansinoh) on your nipples between feedings to keep the skin moist so it will heal more quickly. Avoid using preparations that must be wiped off (ouch!) before feeding the baby.

- Wear an all-cotton bra that fits well, or go braless under a cotton T-shirt. Avoid bras with plastic or synthetic linings that hold moisture against the skin.

- Nursing pads with plastic in them can aggravate sore nipples. If a pad sticks to your breast, moisten it with water to release it and avoid skin damage.

Most breastfeeding problems can be solved in a matter of days. If you are not getting the help you need and you believe your baby isn't getting enough milk ask your doctor to refer you to a lactation consultant or contact La Leche League International (800-LA-LECHE) for the name of a representative in your area. Breastfeeding is worth the effort.*

CONCERNS YOU MAY HAVE

Getting Back to Your Prepregnancy Weight and Shape

You will lose around half of the weight you gained during your pregnancy when you de-

---

* Consult the breastfeeding section of The Baby Book, by Sears and Sears (Little, Brown, 1993), for step-by-step diagrams of proper latch-on and how to avoid and treat breast engorgement.

liver your baby. Much of the remaining weight is in the form of retained fluid, which is gradually lost through increased urination and perspiration over the next few weeks. The rest is stored fat put there to supply calories for milk production over the next few months. How you shed the final few pounds (or more) depends on how much weight you gained during your pregnancy and how well you follow your postpartum nutrition and exercise program. Nine months of caloric overindulgence won't be shed with the delivery of the baby. You are going to have to burn it off in other ways. If you gain just the right amount of weight during your pregnancy, you may return to your prepregnant weight (plus a few pounds for breastfeeding reserves) within a few months postpartum. Most women don't return to their prepregnant weight until around nine months postpartum. Some women simply remain around five pounds heavier after becoming a mother.

How quickly you return to your prepregnant shape also depends upon how well you toned your body during your pregnancy and whether you continue your exercise program after delivery. Don't expect to stand in front of a mirror and see your prepregnant figure the day after delivery. In fact, you will still look four to five months pregnant during the first few weeks while your middle gradually slims. You will still see and feel a "pooch" in your lower abdomen while your uterus contracts to its prepregnant size — which may take around six weeks (less if you're breastfeeding). Ask your health-care provider to show you how to feel your shrinking uterus as it disappears under your pelvic bone. Immediately after delivery you can feel your uterus just below your navel. It should feel like a hard grapefruit. After a couple of weeks you probably won't be able to feel it, al-

though the uterus doesn't return to its prepregnant size for a couple of months.

Many women, especially after several pregnancies, notice their rib cage is slightly larger than it was before their pregnancies. This is a normal and often permanent change due to the demands of breathing around a uterus in full bloom.

Losing weight effectively and safely. It took nine months to put it on, so expect to take at least nine months to take off the extra weight. Here is a simple, yet safe and effective, way to lose unwanted postpartum weight:

• Figure out your daily basic caloric needs. This means the number of calories of balanced nutrition you can consume to maintain your feeling of well-being yet not gain weight. Remember, most breastfeeding mothers will need approximately 500 extra calories for lactation. Most postpartum mothers can eat around 2000 nutritious calories per day and still expect a gradual weight loss. Naturally, the number of calories you can consume daily without weight gain will also depend on how many you burn off by exercise.

• Exercise one hour a day. This could be something as simple as walking briskly while carrying baby in a sling. Brisk walking or swimming for one hour burns off around 400 calories. This exercise plus abstaining from one unnutritious treat each day (one chocolate chip cookie is around 100 calories) means you have a deficit of 500 calories each day, or 3500 calories per week — enough to lose one pound of body fat. A weight loss of one pound per week is about right. It allows a mother to still consume enough nutrition for her well-being and that of her baby. Gradual weight loss is best during breastfeeding. Burning off fat quickly is not safe because the body stores pesticides and other contaminants in fat. Quick weight loss releases these contaminants into your milk.

- Breastfeeding women often experience their greatest weight loss between three and six months postpartum, when they are producing a lot of milk for their babies. So don't get frustrated if the pounds aren't coming off at first.

- Chart your weight loss, and tailor your exercise and eating habits to reach the goal you set.

Invest in some nice, comfortable clothes that fit your postpartum figure. If you focus only on getting back into the jeans you were wearing nine months ago, you may get very depressed. And no one wants to keep on wearing maternity clothes for weeks after the birth. Some pants or leggings with an elastic waist worn with a colorful top will help you feel better about your still-changing body. Two-piece outfits that are easy to breastfeed in will make it easier for you to get out and around with your baby.

Making the Transition into Motherhood

The leap from carrying your baby in your womb to raising a child can be challenging and scary. Many women begin motherhood feeling overwhelmed and inadequate. How often during your pregnancy did you wonder, "Will I be a good mother?" If you've read a lot about babies, you may feel as if the future of civilization hinges on what you do about

every burp, whimper, and messy diaper. Parenthood is an awesome responsibility. You really can shape your child's life and personality. It's normal to feel inadequate and to worry that you won't know what to do when your baby cries. The good news is that both you and your baby have built-in mechanisms that will help you get to know one another. Every mother is naturally equipped to nurture a child, though some pairs need more help than others in getting started.

In more than twenty-five years in pediatric practice we have observed that some women have an easier transition into motherhood than others. And over the years we have recorded the secrets of their success. By practicing all or most of the following suggestions, you improve your chances of getting a good start with your baby.

Get Connected to Your Baby

How mother and baby get started with one another sets the tone for how the relationship unfolds. Getting connected means getting to know your baby, being able to read her needs and cues, discovering what works and what doesn't, responding sensitively to your baby, and ultimately getting a handle on parenting. From this foundation you will be able to get behind the eyes of your child. You will be able to shape your child's behavior toward a very simple, but important, goal — to like living with your child. Sounds good, doesn't it? But you may still wonder if you are the only woman in the whole world who does not possess that fabled "intuition" that every woman is supposed to leave the delivery room with. Don't let the concept of intuition intimidate you. True, some mothers seem to develop intuition sooner than others, but every mother has this ability. Intuition is nothing more than an accumulation of knowledge about your baby. As you store up all these facts about your baby — what makes him cry, what calms him down, how he likes to be held, how he reacts to his environment — you'll soon find that you no longer have to worry what's wrong. Your "mother brain" will work faster than conscious thought. That's your intuition.

The best way to bring out your maternal intuition is to use the attachment tools that nature provided. These tools are ways of caring for your baby that help the two of you get connected, the three baby B's: bonding, breastfeeding, and babywearing.*

Bond with your baby at birth. "Bonding" is a buzzword around obstetrical units and in parenting literature. Every parenting pamphlet and baby magazine talks about the concept of bonding as if it's a late twentieth-century discovery. "Bonding" simply means getting close to your baby and getting to know your baby, and it is what savvy mothers naturally do anyway. Baby-care specialists simply repackaged these natural mothering ways, coined the term, and sold it back to mothers. In some ways, bonding is modern medicine's way of making up for decades of detachment advice, which tended to disconnect mothers and babies.

Bonding is not like an instant glue applied immediately after birth that automatically cements the mother-infant relationship forever. Bonding at birth simply gives mothers and babies a head start. If for medical reasons you are not able to hold your baby and spend time with him right after birth, don't worry. Bonding is an ongoing process; your bond with your child will develop as you spend time with him over the next few days, weeks, and years.

Unless a medical complication prevents you, have your baby room-in with you from the moment of birth to the moment of discharge from the hospital. In this situation you are your baby's primary caregiver, and the nursery staff assume the roles of advisers and helpers. Rooming-in is the natural extension of the bonding period. It smoothes the transition from mother's womb to mother's room. Being together twenty-four hours a day is the best way to get to know one another. In our experience, babies who room-in with their mothers cry less and learn to breastfeed sooner, and mothers actually get more rest because they experience less anxiety about their babies. If you are nervous, tense, and feel you don't know how to take care of your baby, and if the first moments were not love at first sight as the childbirth classes promised, rooming-in is for you. Spending a lot of time in touch with your baby, looking into her eyes, will awaken your calm, motherly feelings.

Breastfeed your baby. You probably already know how good your milk is for your baby; you may not realize how good breastfeeding is for you. Breastfeeding is an exercise in baby-reading. Initially, you sensitively respond to baby's cries for feeding or holding. Whether baby is hungry or just wants to nurse for comfort doesn't matter — your response is the same. The breast is a source of both nutrition and comfort. Eventually, you learn to recognize baby's pre-cry signals, so he doesn't even have to cry to get his needs met.

Breastfeeding gets your mothering hormones going. Each time your baby sucks from your breast, hormones that help you feel calm and loving are released into your

---

In The Baby Book, by Sears and Sears (Little, Brown, 1993), you will find a complete description of all three of these tools.

system. These magical substances not only relax you, but they may well be the biological basis for mother's intuition. It's easier to learn about your baby and respond to his needs when you're feeling peaceful.

Wear your baby. Carry your baby in your arms or in a baby sling for at least several hours a day. This age-old custom of infant care does good things for baby and good things for mother. Carried babies cry less and are therefore more fun to be with. Snuggled securely against you, baby has no need to fuss. Instead of fussing, baby can spend more time relating with you and learning about his environment. Carrying your baby right under your eyes allows you to read your baby's needs easily. Like breastfeeding, babywearing promotes baby-reading. You learn to read baby's cues, baby learns to cue better, and the two of you get in harmony with each other — because you have set the conditions that let this happen.

Get Help

In order to get connected to your baby, you need to have time, space, and energy to let this attachment develop, without having your energy diverted into household chores. We call the opening weeks at home the "nesting-in" period, a time when the whole family pitches in and helps mother build a peaceful nest and then helps her enjoy it. If your friends, relatives, and spouse can free you of all duties except caring for your baby, all the better. If not, hire a doula, a helper who specializes in mothering the mother (not the baby) and relieving her of household chores that drain her energy away from her baby. Postpartum-care services, or doula services, are springing up all over the country, and you will find them in nearly every major city.

Be sure that whoever is helping you realizes that you will be caring for the baby while the helper takes care of the household.

Your doula is there to help you enjoy your early days of motherhood, to keep postpartum stress within manageable limits for you. Her presence should free you and empower you to respond freely to your baby's needs. If you are being cared for by someone, say, a mother or mother-in-law, who can't resist the urge to take over, you may have to set some limits, tactfully but firmly. ("The baby's crying, so I am going to nurse her. Perhaps you could make some lunch for us.") Of course, when you need to take a shower or get out for a brief walk, grandma can hold and rock the baby.

My mother came over frequently to help with the older children after our third child was born. She would sweep the floor, read books to our two-year-old, pick up toys, and, of course, enjoy hanging around the new baby. One quiet afternoon I decided it was time to grab a shower, so grandma took the baby. When I came out of the bathroom, toddler, grandma, and baby were all cuddled in the big chair, sound asleep. They all looked so happy.

Pamper Yourself

In your zeal to take perfect care of your baby it's easy to neglect yourself. Be prepared for your newborn to have an occasional high-maintenance day when she wants to be held and nursed constantly — day and night. These days are one of the "joys" of motherhood that no one ever told you about. Yet giving all to your baby and having no time or energy left over for yourself is not good for either of you. Figure out what you need most for your own well-being and create your mothering style around your needs. If you need an hour a day for yourself, take it. (Don't use it to do housework, however!) If you need more peace and quiet around the house, demand it. Learn to delegate responsibilities. Pampering yourself is also one of the best preventive medicines against postpartum depression, which often occurs when a mother exceeds her energy reserves. Next time you're on an airplane, listen to what the flight attendant says when demonstrating the proper use of the oxygen: "Should oxygen be needed, place a mask on yourself *before* placing one on your child." In other words, if you are suffocating yourself, you are no good to your baby.

Dr. Bill notes: Even after eight children, Martha still tends to get into the "my baby needs me so much I don't have time to take a shower" mode. Periodically I have to remind even this veteran mother, "What our baby needs most is a happy, rested mother." Then I take the baby while she takes a shower.

Be Open, Be Responsive

When you begin motherhood, you may not yet know very much about what parenting style you will adopt (i.e., how you want to care for your baby). And you will not yet know what the temperament and need level of your baby is. Don't start motherhood locked into rigid ideas. Be open. Be flexible. Keep working at finding a style of mothering that works for you and your baby.

Shun advisers who preach, "Let your baby cry it out." They don't know you and they don't know your baby. This advice not only keeps you from getting connected to your baby and desensitizes you to your baby's cues but also is not biologically correct. Studies have shown that when a mother hears her baby cry, the blood flow to her breasts increases, and she has an overwhelming urge to

Beware of Baby Trainers

When you have a new baby, you become a target for advice. Be especially wary of self-proclaimed experts who prescribe rigid recipes for baby care, such as, "Let him cry it out so he learns to sleep through the night," and "Get her on a schedule so she won't manipulate you," and "You're going to spoil that baby!" Listen to your instincts and your baby, not to some baby trainer who is not biologically wired to your baby and who may offer advice that may not apply to your baby. Remember, this is *your* baby; *you* are his mother.

Before following anyone else's advice about caring for your baby, consider whether it feels right intuitively, and run it past veteran mothers whose advice you trust. Shun any method that advises you to rely on the method rather than on your own internal instincts. The "let's have babies conveniently" methods create a distance between mother and baby, keep you from getting to know your baby, and destroy the mutual trust between mother and child. Babies are the most wonderful inconvenience. Even methods of infant care that seem flexible may make no allowances for the difference in temperaments among children and the varied lifestyles of parents. Become an expert on your baby. No one else can do the job as well as you.

pick up and comfort her baby. You are biologically wired to respond to your baby's cries, not ignore them. Your baby's cry is your baby's language. Respond to it; this is how your baby will learn to trust you. Start off your mothering career by giving intuitive responses to your baby's cry, and in time you and your baby will work out a communication network that allows you to gradually delay your response as baby becomes mature enough to wait for a few minutes or to comfort himself. Listening to your instincts and trusting your ability to respond to your baby lay the foundation for good parent-child communication in the years to come.

If It Isn't Working, Change It

As you're developing a parenting style that works for your whole family, be open to changing what isn't working for you. Lou and Marie were new parents who wanted to get as much information about baby care as possible. They attended a new-baby class where the teacher outlined a method of baby training that was guaranteed to get babies to sleep through the night by six weeks and fit into a convenient schedule for the parents. The method promised, for the price of a few books and tapes, that if the parents followed the instructions, their marriage would be much better because the baby wouldn't interfere that much. Because this method was presented as authoritative, these young and vulnerable parents bought into it, and from the first day, they put their baby on a rigid schedule. They fed her only when the schedule allowed and put her down and let her cry herself off to sleep. Marie found this very hard to do, and many times she had to cover her ears and restrain herself from responding to her baby. But as time went on, it seemed to become easier to tune out her baby's cries. When Baby Jessica was about three weeks of age, Mary, a veteran mother, came to visit. As they were talking in the living room, Baby Jessica started to cry from the nursery. Marie kept on talking, seemingly oblivious to her

baby's cries. Mary became increasingly bothered by Jessica's cries and said to Marie, "Go ahead and attend to the baby. We can talk later." Whereupon Marie, looking at her watch, replied, "No, it's not time for her feeding yet." Mary, a sensitive and experienced mother, pointed out to Marie that she had become desensitized to her baby. By not responding to her maternal instincts, she was losing them. Her baby's cry was supposed to bother her, but it no longer did.

When Jessica was about a month old, the family came to my office for counseling. A distance had developed between parents and child, and they knew they were getting off to the wrong start. Marie opened our conversation, "I've been robbed of a month of my motherhood." She was angry at herself for being so foolish as to follow someone else's method instead of working out her own. Fortunately, she was wise enough to discover this. I consoled these parents by pointing out to them how vulnerable all new parents are to advice, especially when it's given by an authority figure such as a doctor or a minister. I also reassured them that it's never too late to reconnect, though it would take some time. Once they began responding to Jessica's cues and seeing them as needs rather than nuisances, the whole family got along much better.

Surround Yourself with Experienced Parents

Just as you did during your pregnancy, choose your advisers carefully. Nothing divides friends like differences in child-rearing beliefs. Listen to veteran parents whose advice you value and whose kids you like. You may want to join a parent-support group, especially if this is your first baby. The oldest and largest group is La Leche League International (to find the league group in your area call 800-LA-LECHE).

POSTPARTUM

❖ ❖ ❖

First stats: _____

  Your birthdate: _____

  Time: _____

  Place: _____

  Weight: _____

  Length: _____

Who was there: _____

_____

_____

_____

_____

newborn photo

The story of your birth: _____
_____
_____
_____
_____
_____
_____
_____
_____
_____
_____
_____
_____
_____

How I felt when I first held you: _____
_____
_____
_____
_____
_____
_____
_____
_____

During those first days, we: _____
_____
_____
_____
_____
_____
_____
_____
_____

Appendix A: If You Get Sick

ERE'S A PARENTING PEARL that we've found to be true: TAKE GOOD CARE OF YOURSELF SO YOU CAN TAKE GOOD CARE OF YOUR BABY. This advice applies already in pregnancy, but even mothers who pay close attention to their health do get sick at times.

TAKING MEDICATIONS DURING PREGNANCY

If you get sick while pregnant you will naturally be concerned about your baby. The worry is twofold: Will your illness harm your baby? And will any medications you take harm your baby?

There is good news in answer to both questions. The great majority of illnesses in the pregnant mother, if properly treated, do not harm baby, and the great majority of medicines that pregnant mothers need to take do not harm their babies. Nevertheless, you don't have a blank prescription to take any medication you see on the drugstore shelf. You must consult your doctor first. Most medications are safe, some are safe with reservations, and a few are definitely unsafe.

Your fears about taking medicine during your pregnancy can work to your and your baby's advantage — and disadvantage. Wanting to avoid medicines forces you to practice preventive medicine (you minimize your exposure to infectious diseases, pollutants, and allergens and you eat well) and learn about safe alternatives to taking drugs. But your fears about taking medicine may also cloud your reason. Sometimes not taking the medicine is riskier than taking it. Getting mother healthy again may be what's best for baby. Sometimes the effects of the disease on mother and baby are worse than the effects

> Be sure to check with your doctor before taking any medication while you are pregnant. The information in this book is up-to-date at the time of writing. New studies may prove that a drug previously thought harmless is not safe to take during pregnancy. The information in this section is meant to help you make informed choices, but it should always be used in consultation with your doctor.

of the drug. Sometimes waiting too long to get proper medical care requires the mother to take a stronger drug for a longer time with more side effects; this might have been avoided with earlier medical intervention. Consider these dos and don'ts when taking medicines while pregnant:

- Do take the medicine in the exact dosage and for the length of time your doctor recommends. Taking more is not better and is often worse.

- Don't take a lower dose than your doctor prescribes without consulting your doctor. The lower dose may do you no good, yet baby may still get the effects of the drug.

- Don't read the *PDR (Physician's Desk Reference).* The information in the *PDR* about drugs during pregnancy is there to protect the manufacturer rather than to inform the consumer. The warnings are needlessly scary and are often based upon research in which huge doses of a drug are given to experimental animals; the research may have little application to humans. Oftentimes there is very little broad-based research available about using a drug during pregnancy, so it's safer for the manufacturer just to advise women not to take any of the medicine while pregnant. (With this advice on the record, the manufacturer is at less risk of a lawsuit.)

- Don't take medicines, even over-the-counter ones, without consulting with your doctor.

- Don't take over-the-counter remedies that contain several drugs unless advised by your doctor (e.g., cold remedies may contain mixtures of antihistamines, decongestants, aspirin, etc.). Because mixtures are difficult to study, it is hard for researchers

or doctors to provide reliable information about the safety of the combined drug.

- Do consider safer alternatives to medicines. For example, if you're treating a cold, what alternatives are there to taking the medicine?

- Don't panic if you've taken a drug that you later read may be unsafe. Odds are greatly on your baby's side that no harm was done. Very few drugs taken as a one-time dose will harm your baby. Most drugs must be taken for extended periods or in large doses to produce harmful effects.

- Do compromise. While some medications pose some risks to baby, a sick mom is not good for baby either. For example, depriving yourself of oxygen because your breathing passages are clogged or letting yourself get dehydrated from vomiting and diarrhea would be risky for baby. You would be better off taking medicines for these conditions. For example, if your nasal passages are so clogged you can't breathe, one dose of a decongestant spray, such as Afrin, for a day or two, has been shown not to have any harmful effects on the fetuses who were studied.

- Do think about the effect of the drug on your baby. Because your baby's liver and kidneys are immature, he cannot eliminate the drug as you can, so the drug may stay in baby's system longer and at a higher level.

- Don't use medicines if you are trying to conceive, especially in the first month. The first month of fetal organ development is a high-risk period for the effects of drugs. The "flu" you're experiencing may turn out to be early pregnancy nausea.

- If you are already taking physician-approved medications while pregnant, check with your doctor before taking an additional drug. Also, when your doctor gives you a prescription for a new medication, be sure to tell him or her about any other medications you are taking. Certain drugs may be safe if taken individually but not in combination with others.

COMMON ILLNESSES DURING PREGNANCY

During pregnancy the discomforts of common illnesses are magnified. You're already tired, your nutrition may be marginal (at least in the early months), and your energy reserves are already devoted to growing a baby. Being sick upsets an already tenuous balance. The following are the most common illnesses mothers experience while pregnant, along with safe treatment regimens that will work for most pregnant mothers most of the time.

Nasal Congestion and Sinusitis

The mucous membranes in the nasal passages of the sinuses often swell and become congested during pregnancy, probably due to the same hormones that cause vaginal membranes to become congested. Some women feel they have a persistent "cold" or sniffles throughout pregnancy. Women who are already prone to allergic rhinitis, or hay fever, may find this nuisance worsens during pregnancy (others find that it improves). Because of the extra person and the extra tissues you are growing, the need for oxygen greatly increases during pregnancy. To meet these increased demands, pregnant women must inhale and exhale more air per breath. This requires clear nasal passages.

Because the sinuses are an extension of the nasal passages, nasal congestion can lead to sinusitis. Swollen nasal membranes trap secretions in the sinuses, and fluid that can't drain, like water in a stagnant pond, becomes infected. Signs that you may have developed a sinus infection are feeling fullness or pain in the sinuses, alongside the nose, or over the eyebrows; snotty nasal discharge; increasing tiredness; or the feeling that you have a cold that just won't go away.

Keeping nasal secretions thin and moving. Here are ways to keep your nasal secretions uncongested, and thus prevent them from being infected:

What to Ask Your Doctor

Remember, taking good care of yourself requires a partnership between yourself and your doctor. Make sure you understand why and how you are to take medications, what the effects are, and what alternatives are available. Ask your doctor these questions:

☐ How necessary is the medicine? Am I likely to get worse without it? Could not taking the medicine jeopardize my health, my baby's health?

☐ What are the possible harmful side effects, if any, to me or my baby?

☐ Are there safer alternatives that I could try instead of or in addition to the medicine?

☐ How often and for how long should I take the medicine? (Be sure you clearly understand these instructions.)

Many medicines, even those in the "yellow light," or caution, category (see page 396), can be safely taken while pregnant as long as you follow your doctor's instructions.

- Avoid unnecessary exposure to nasal allergens and pollutants, such as smog and cigarette smoke.

- Drink even more water each day.

- Flush your nasal passages with saltwater (or saline) nose drops several times a day. These are available without prescription, or you can make your own: ¼ teaspoon of salt to 1 cup of water.

- Use a facial steamer (basically a hot-mist vaporizer attached to a face mask) to "steam clean" your nasal passages and sinuses. Treat your nasal passages to this steam treatment for ten to twenty minutes. (You can watch television or read a book at the same time.) Facial steamers are available in cosmetic departments, beauty supply stores, or in some pharmacies. You can make your own steamer by boiling water in a wide pot, removing the pot from the stove, and breathing the steam from the water with your head covered with a towel to form a steam tent. A long, warm shower is another way to loosen up nasal congestion.

Treating sinus infections. Sinus infections can be treated with decongestants or antihistamines.

Decongestants. In theory, medicines that constrict the blood vessels of the nose may enter the bloodstream and constrict the blood vessels of the uterus or placenta; therefore, decongestants should be used only under a doctor's supervision, and only in the dosage and frequency your doctor recommends. Women with decreased placental circulation should be particularly careful about taking any form of inhaled or oral decongestants. Some nasal sprays are safer than others, but don't use any except for saltwater (or saline) nasal spray without first consulting your doctor. If your nasal passages are so clogged that you feel miserable or have difficulty getting enough air, the benefits of decongestants to you, and therefore to your baby, far outweigh the risks. Many nasal decongestants are probably safe if used once a day for one or two days. Suggestions of a harmful effect of decongestants on a developing baby were based on situations in which these medications were used many times a day or for many days. In consultation with your doctor, consider the following nasal decongestants:

- Afrin (oxymetazoline) when used only twice a day and for a couple of days has not been shown to cause harmful effects on the developing baby.

- Inhaled nasal steroids (Vancenase, Beconase) are in the "probably safe" category, especially when taken only a couple of times a day and for a short period of time. Best to stick with the lower-potency inhaled steroids unless advised by your doctor.

- Nasal or oral decongestants that contain the following compounds have been shown to be possibly harmful to the developing baby and should not be taken unless all other alternatives have been tried and your doctor judges that the benefits outweigh the risks: ephedrine, phenylpropanolamine, Neo-Synephrine, phenylephrine. The main worry with these decongestants is that because they constrict the vessels in the airway passages, they may also constrict the blood vessels delivering blood to the baby.

Antihistamines. Some antihistamines, such as chlorpheniramine and tripelennamine, are categorized as safe to take during pregnancy ("green light"; see page 396). Others are recommended only with reservation ("yellow light"), such as those containing brompheniramine, diphenhydramine, terfenadine, and clemastine. In a rare finding these were implicated in causing eye damage in premature infants if taken in the last two weeks of pregnancy. Unless you are certain your congestion is due to allergies and it is compromising your breathing, it's best to use the medical and nonmedical methods of clearing nasal passages listed above and avoid the antihistamines in the yellow category.

Other medications. If you were taking allergy shots before becoming pregnant, your doctor may advise continuing these shots during your pregnancy, but because reactivity to these injections may change during pregnancy, your doctor may elect to change the dosage. It is unlikely that your doctor would advise starting allergy shots during a pregnancy.

Cromolyn (Intal) is safe to take during pregnancy. It is not a decongestant, a steroid, or an antihistamine, but rather a medication that when taken over a long period of time lessens nasal congestion due to allergies. It is especially helpful during seasonal allergic rhinitis or hay fever. It is not helpful during an acute attack of a stuffy nose.

Cough syrups should be taken with caution while pregnant and are best limited to nighttime use or to severe coughs. Avoid cough syrups that contain iodine or alcohol. Studies have shown no link between guaifenesin and fetal defects. For annoying coughs, especially those that interfere with your sleep, treat yourself to a facial-steamer treatment before bedtime.

Asthma

Like most chronic allergic problems, asthma may get better for some women during pregnancy and worse for others. Because the airway is already working overtime during pregnancy (the amount of air you move with each breath increases), asthma can be particularly worrisome at this time. If your airway is compromised and you're not getting enough oxygen, your baby may not be getting enough oxygen either. So, for your health and your baby's health, it's particularly important to take care of asthma during pregnancy. Try these ways of managing your asthma:

- Early in your pregnancy (or, even better, when you are planning to conceive), consult your family physician or allergist and your obstetrician to review your current asthma management program. Determine what self-help regimens you can use and which medications you can take while you're pregnant. Depending on the frequency and severity of your asthma, it may be wise to repeat this consultation later in your pregnancy. Some medications cause different problems at different stages of pregnancy.

- Avoid unnecessary exposure to allergens, primarily cigarette smoke and other pollutants. Pay particular attention to your sleeping environment. You may need an air filter in your bedroom during your pregnancy, even though you may not have needed one before (a HEPA-type is the most effective).

- Keep your nasal passages and sinuses clear using the methods suggested on page 392. As veteran asthmatics know, keeping nasal passages and sinuses clear is one of the best preventive measures against asthma.

- Seek medical attention and treat your asthma *early,* before the attack escalates to compromise your breathing. While pregnant, many women find it's necessary to call the doctor earlier and to treat their asthma more aggressively than before they were pregnant.

Medications for asthma. If you have chronic asthma and are on a treatment regimen that has been working for you, do not stop or change your medication before checking with your doctor. Don't let the fear of taking medicine set you up for an asthma attack, which may be more harmful to your baby than the medication. Albuterol, the mainstay of asthma treatment, is the most common medication used in pocket inhalers and home nebulizers. Because albuterol can elevate the heart rate in mother and baby, raise maternal blood pressure, and cause changes in maternal and fetal blood sugar, it must be used exactly as prescribed by the physician. Even though albuterol is generally considered safe during pregnancy and is an example of a medication in which the benefits usually outweigh the risks, it still is in the "yellow light" category, meaning it needs to be used with caution. Cromolyn is in the "green light" (safe) category as a maintenance medication for chronic asthma. Epinephrine-containing products should be avoided unless recommended by your doctor; they are usually used only in severe asthmatic attacks. Despite the "yellow light" rating, inhaled steroids are considered safe for treating asthma as long as they are used under a physician's close supervision and in the dosage and frequency advised by the doctor.

Urinary Tract Infections (UTIs)

A full bladder competes for pelvic space with a growing uterus. Urinary tract, bladder, or kidney infections may result. Many women will have at least one episode sometime dur-ing their pregnancy. The symptoms of a urinary tract infection (UTI) or bladder infection (cystitis) include painful urination, burning on urination, increased urgency and frequency of urination, lower abdominal or pelvic pain, and possibly blood in the urine. Sometimes the infection can spread upward into the kidneys (called "pyelonephritis"), causing severe back pain, fever, chills, rapid heart rate, vomiting, and a generally very ill feeling. Urinary tract infections are treated with a combination of self-help methods and medicine prescribed by your doctor. Here are ways to lessen your chances of getting a UTI.

- Drink extra fluids. Cranberry juice in particular is thought to kill bacteria in the urine.
- Don't hold on to your urine; go as soon as you feel the urge.
- Empty your bladder thoroughly at each urination by triple voiding: urinate once, wait about ten seconds, urinate again, and then a third time.
- Empty your bladder before and after intercourse.
- Wear loose-fitting underwear, panty hose, and slacks.
- Keep your regularly scheduled prenatal appointments, at which your doctor will routinely check your urine for signs of infection.
- If you suspect you have a bladder or kidney infection, have your urine checked immediately. Oftentimes, your doctor can detect a UTI immediately with routine urinalysis; sometimes an overnight culture is needed. Some women will grow bacteria in their urine even without symptoms (called "asymptomatic bacteriuria"), and this condition increases the chances of getting UTIs. To screen for this, your doctor may perform frequent urine cultures as part of your prenatal care.

Taking Medications Safely While Pregnant*

Green Light: Go Ahead
These medications, if used in the dosage and duration prescribed by your physician, have not been shown to be harmful for mother or baby.†

Acetaminophen
Antacids (Tums, Rolaids, Mylanta, Maalox, Tagamet, Zantac, Pepcid)
Antibiotics
   Penicillin
   Cephalosporin
   Erythromycin
   Clindamycin
   Nitrofurantoin
   Sulfa (first 6 months only)
Aspartame (Nutra-Sweet)
Cromolyn

Doxylamine (Unisom)
Dramamine
Emetrol
Ibuprofen (first 6 months only)
Insulin
Naproxen (Aleve; first 6 months only)
Phenacetin or Chlorpheniramine (an antihistamine)
Prednisone
Pyridium
Stool softeners
   Lactulose (laxative, short-term use only)
   Mineral oil laxative (occasional, short-term use only)
Tripelennamine (an antihistamine)

Yellow Light: Use Caution!
Drugs in this category should be taken only when the physician decides that the health benefits to the mother (and usually, therefore, also to the baby) outweigh the potential risk to the baby. Most of the drugs in this category are available only with a prescription and should be taken only under the supervision of your doctor, and only in the dosage and duration prescribed. Some drugs are in this category because animal studies have shown potential risk to the fetus. Others should be used with caution

* *See* Drugs in Pregnancy and Lactation: A Guide to Fetal and Neonatal Risk, *4th ed., by Gerald G. Briggs et al. (Williams and Wilkins, 1994). A consultation service staffed by pharmacists for answering questions about safe drugs in pregnancy and while breastfeeding is Rocky Mountain Drug Consultation Center (1-900-370-3784).*
† *The "green light" category is based on evidence available at this writing. Because newer information may show otherwise, even medications in this category should be first approved by your physician.*

If you have a urinary tract infection, your doctor will prescribe an antibiotic that is safe for you to take while pregnant. The type and the duration of the antibiotic will depend upon the severity of your UTI and your stage of pregnancy. It's important to be vigilant about following your doctor's instructions in treating UTIs. Improperly treated UTIs increase the risk of having a problem pregnancy or premature delivery.

Intestinal Disorders

The intestinal flu can strike the already queasy stomach of pregnancy. An infection of the intestinal lining is called "gastroenteritis." It is recognized by the symptoms of nausea, vomiting, diarrhea, crampy lower abdominal pain, and often fever. While you don't have to worry that the infection affects your baby, the resulting loss of fluids and body salts (electrolytes) could cause you to become dehydrated, jeopardizing your health and that of because there are not enough human studies available to determine whether or not the drug is safe.

Acyclovir
Albuterol‡
Antibiotics
  Chloramphenicol
  Cipro
  Flagyl
  Gentamicin
  Isoniazid (INH)
  Rifampin
  Vancomycin
Anti-emetics (Compazine, Tigan, Phenergan)
Benadryl
Codeine-containing analgesics (first 6 months only)

Decongestants containing ephedrine, phenylephrine, phenylpropanolamine
Guaifenesin-containing cough syrups (probably safe if taken short-term)
Lomotil
Percodan
Prozac
Pyrethrins (for scabies)
Terfenadine (antihistamine)
Vaccines (killed only)
Zoloft

Red Light: Stop!
These drugs have been shown to pose a risk to the fetus and are recommended only when a safer alternative cannot be used or when mother's

health is seriously in jeopardy.

Accutane
Anticoagulants
Aspirin (third trimester)
Codeine (third trimester)
Ergot
Iodine-containing medications (cough syrups)
Phenobarbital-containing drugs
Sulfa-containing antibiotics (third trimester)
Tetracycline (last half of pregnancy)
Trimethaprin (third trimester)
Vaccines, live (measles, rubella,§ mumps, yellow fever)
Valium

‡ *An asthma medication in which the benefit to the mother usually outweighs the potential risk to the fetus and that is considered safe as long as taken in the dosage and duration recommended by mother's physician.*
§ *Don't worry if you were given the rubella vaccine before you knew you were pregnant. Infants of mothers to whom this has happened have not been shown to have a higher incidence of congenital defects.*

your baby. So, your main goal if you have any intestinal disorder that causes vomiting and/or diarrhea is to keep yourself adequately hydrated.

• Go to bed and rest as many hours a day as you can.

• Prevent dehydration. Sip on fluids all day long. Small, frequent sips are best. You may need to drink an additional quart of fluids in addition to your already increased fluid intake. To be sure you're replenishing adequate electrolytes, try oral electrolyte solutions (Pedialyte, Resol, Rehydralyte, Ricelyte), available over the counter. Commercially available oral rehydration fluid has the proper balance of sugar and electrolytes to promote adequate absorption of fluids from inflamed intestines. Many homemade mixtures contain either too much sugar or not enough sodium. Too much sugar in the solution can actually increase the diarrhea. You can make your own solution: to 1 quart of juice (orange, grape, apple, or pineapple) add 2 teaspoons of table salt.

- Because of nausea and vomiting you may find it easier to retain fluids taken in the form of juice bars or ice chips.

- Unless you really can't keep them down, it's important to eat some solid foods; otherwise the diarrhea may worsen and your nutrition may be inadequate. Try these easy-on-the-intestines foods: rice, baked potatoes, bananas, and yellow vegetables.

Medications for vomiting. Some medicines to treat vomiting (called "antiemetics") are safe, some are not. Emetrol (basically a cola syrup) is a safe and sometimes helpful medication for nausea and vomiting. One tablespoon taken several times a day may relieve stomach upset. Phenothiazines (Compazine) and Trimethobenzamides (Tigan), despite the "yellow light" category, are generally considered safe for pregnancy, especially in the short term used for the treatment of occasional vomiting from gastrointestinal disorder or severe morning sickness.

Antidiarrheal medications. No antidiarrheal medications (even those obtained over the counter) should be taken without your doctor's advice. Increased intestinal motility and consequent diarrhea is the body's natural way of getting rid of harmful bacteria and toxins in the intestines. Medicines that slow down intestinal motility or cause the infected material to remain longer in the intestines may actually be dangerous because they prolong the time the bacteria and toxins remain in the intestines. Unless there is severe discomfort or the woman is in danger of dehydration, most doctors suggest their patients not use antidiarrheals. The combination of kaolin and pectin (Kaopectate), even though

it is safe to take during pregnancy, is not very helpful. Imodium A-D is a more effective antidiarrheal and is reported to be safe to take during pregnancy. Still, it may be better to allow the intestines to rid themselves of bacteria and toxins naturally, so we have put these two medications in the "yellow light," or caution, category. However, if your doctor feels that it would be better in your situation to slow down the diarrhea, Imodium A-D may be the best choice. Pepto-Bismol contains salicylate (similar to the drug found in aspirin), which may cause bleeding in mother and/or baby; Bismuth has been linked to birth defects in experimental animals. Neither of these medications is regarded as safe to take while pregnant.

If you are in danger of becoming dehydrated from vomiting and/or diarrhea, and your illness does not seem to be self-limiting, your doctor may choose to rehydrate you with an intravenous solution that can be administered over several hours while you are an outpatient in the doctor's office or in an emergency room. For many women, intravenous rehydration is the quickest way to prevent dehydration, and most report they feel better immediately after the treatment.

Medications for treatment of gastroesophageal reflux or heartburn. Medications that block gastric acid secretion (called "H^2-receptor antagonists"), such as Tagamet, Zantac, and Pepcid, seem to be safe to take while pregnant and fall into the "green light" category. However, even these medications should not be taken without a doctor's advice. Over-the-counter antacids, such as Tums, Mylanta, Mylecon, Milk of Magnesia, Maalox, and Rolaids, are all safe to take during pregnancy and are also in the "green light" category. Because it contains aspirin (see page 399), Alka-Seltzer is not safe to take during pregnancy, although Alka-Seltzer–brand compounds that do not contain aspirin are safe. Phenobarbital-containing antispasmodics (Donnatal) are in the "red light" category, since phenobarbital has been reported to harm fetal development.

Fever

During pregnancy, a woman's body temperature increases by approximately 1° anyway due to the hormones of pregnancy and also because of her stepped-up metabolism. High fever, however, is both uncomfortable for mother and potentially harmful to baby. Both animal experiments and studies in pregnant women have shown a statistical increase in spinal column abnormalities in mothers who had prolonged, elevated temperatures above 102° F (39° C) in the first trimester, especially between the third and fifth week of pregnancy. These studies looked at women whose body temperatures were elevated from extended hot tub exposure; the up-and-down fever pattern associated with most infections is less likely to harm baby. Nevertheless, it's prudent to treat a fever aggressively while pregnant. Here are safe measures to lower fever:

• **Dress for the temperature.** Don't overdress or underdress yourself. Putting on too many clothes retains your body's heat; underdressing encourages shivering, which produces more heat. Wear lightweight, loose-fitting clothes that allow the air to circulate over your skin. Change your clothes frequently if you are perspiring profusely.

• **Keep cool.** Open a window, turn on the air conditioner, go outside. Cool, fresh air removes the heat from your body.

• **Drink lots of fluids.** Sweating and fast breathing cause your body to lose fluids that need replacing. Carry around a water bottle and sip all day long.

• **Feed the fever.** The extra heat you produce burns up fuel that needs replacing with nutritious calories. Calorie-filled, cool smoothies combine the need for food and fluids.

• **Take a cool dip.** Soak in a lukewarm bath or shower that is cool enough not to be uncomfortable or make you shiver. Then step out of the tub while still wet and allow your body to cool as the water evaporates. Rubbing yourself vigorously with a towel increases the circulation to the skin and accelerates heat loss.

Medications for pain and fever. Aspirin is not the preferred fever-reducing medication to take while pregnant, because there are safer and equally effective alternatives. Don't worry if you have taken a couple of aspirin on a couple of occasions. This is unlikely to harm your baby. The main concern with aspirin is that prolonged high doses, especially in the third trimester, may cause bleeding in mother or baby (aspirin is an anticoagulant) or interfere with the normal onset of labor (aspirin inhibits prostaglandins). Obstetricians sometimes use low-dose aspirin to prevent pregnancy-induced hypertension, eclampsia, and other intrauterine problems. The jury is still out on whether prolonged use of aspirin in the first trimester is associated with congenital defects, but the evidence seems to favor no link between taking aspirin during the first trimester and congenital defects.

Ibuprofen (Motrin, Nuprin, Advil) is safer than aspirin during pregnancy, but it should be taken only with a doctor's advice. No studies link ibuprofen taken during the first and second trimesters with congenital defects, placing ibuprofen in the "green light" category for the first two trimesters. Ibuprofen does not have the anticoagulant effect of aspirin and is therefore unlikely to cause bleeding in mother or baby when taken in the third trimester. However, because, like aspirin, it also inhibits prostaglandins (natural hormones that influence labor), it must be used with caution during the third trimester. Because of its antiprostaglandin effect, ibuprofen can also interfere with the normal blood flow within the heart and blood vessels of the baby during the third trimester. These effects are likely to disappear when the drug is stopped, though, and have not been shown to harm baby. Thus, ibuprofen is considered an effective fever-lowering medication, safer than aspirin, and safe to take in the first two trimesters — but only under a doctor's supervision.

Acetaminophen is safe to take throughout all stages of pregnancy. It is an effective fever-reducer and an analgesic for pain. Even though acetaminophen is in the "green light" category, if high doses are needed over a prolonged period of time, it should be taken under a doctor's supervision. (This is true of all medications.) Studies have shown that high doses of acetaminophen throughout pregnancy may be harmful to mother and baby. Acetaminophen, if used in the proper dosage and for the usual two-to-three-day illnesses associated with fever, is considered safe for both mother and baby.

Appendix B:
Additional Resources

The American College of Obstetricians and Gynecologists. This organization of physicians dedicated to improving women's health care provides women the most up-to-date scientifically accurate information about preconception, prenatal, and postpartum care. It distributes a variety of pamphlets, books, and videos on special concerns during pregnancy and all aspects of women's health care. Contact the Resource Center at 409 12th Street SW, PO Box 96920, Washington, DC 20090-6920 (202-638-5577).

Briggs, Gerald G., Roger K. Freeman, and Summer J. Yaffe, eds. *Drugs in Pregnancy and Lactation: A Guide to Fetal and Neonatal Risk*. 4th ed. (Williams and Wilkins, 1994). This classic reference book is a useful source for the most up-to-date information on which medications are safe to take during pregnancy and lactation and which are not.

Childbirth Graphics. This large catalog of informative and useful products for the pregnant couple along with books, charts, and pamphlets on just about every concern expectant parents could have are available at

PO Box 21207, Waco, TX 76702-9718 (tel: 800-299-3366, ext. 287; fax: 817-751-0221).

Erick, Miriam. *No More Morning Sickness: A Survival Guide for Pregnant Women* (NAL-Dutton, 1993). Written by a nutritionist who specializes in the dietary needs of pregnant women, this book provides an understanding of morning sickness and offers lots of helpful hints and stomach-friendly foods.

Flanagan, Geraldine Lux. *Beginning Life: The Marvelous Journey from Conception to Birth* (Dorling Kindersley, 1996). This useful book is a photographic and narrative commentary on fetal development month by month. The stunning photographs give expectant couples a deeper understanding of the marvels that are taking place in the woman's body.

The Miracle of Life. This one-hour 1986 video photographed by Lennart Nilsson and produced by Swedish television in association with WGBH takes you on an incredible voyage through the human body as a new life begins, showing fertilization and fetal development in a dynamic way. It is available through childbirth supply catalogs and infant product stores.

Nilsson, Lennart. *A Child Is Born* (Delacorte, 1990). This book is a masterpiece of fetal photography from one of the world's leading medical and scientific photographers. It takes expectant couples on a photographic journey from fertilization to delivery and helps them appreciate the miracle that is happening inside the woman's body.

Sears, William, and Martha Sears. *The Baby Book: Everything You Need to Know About Your Baby — From Birth to Age Two* (Little, Brown, 1993). This useful companion to *The Pregnancy Book* begins with information about the postpartum period and is especially helpful in getting parents off to the right start with their newborn.

Sears, William, and Martha Sears. *The Birth Book: Everything You Need to Know to Have a Safe and Satisfying Birth* (Little, Brown, 1994). This book discusses in more depth than *The Pregnancy Book* the events leading up to and surrounding birth and contains many birth stories to illustrate a wide variety of labors.

Shapiro, Howard I. *The Pregnancy Book for Today's Woman: An Obstetrician Answers All Your Questions About Pregnancy and Childbirth and Some You May Not Have Considered* (HarperCollins, 1993). This useful book by an obstetrician discusses thoroughly the most common medical problems that pregnant women are likely to encounter. It has especially good sections on environmental and occupational hazards and on medications during pregnancy.

Appendix C: Emergency Delivery

AT HOME

Sometimes babies don't follow the usual signals to let you know how far along you are. Suddenly you realize, "My gosh, it's coming!" and you know you are not going to make it to the hospital in time. Remember, this scenario has happened thousands of times this year, and mothers and babies are almost always fine.

- Recognize the signs that delivery is imminent: You feel a sudden, uncontrollable urge to push, and these urges get increasingly intense; you feel like you're going to have a huge bowel movement; you feel the head in the vagina, and it is coming down further with each push.

- Call your doctor or midwife immediately. Describe your feelings and ask for further instructions. If your health-care provider advises you to stay home, he or she may guide you through the delivery process by phone. If possible, put your consultant on speaker phone and turn the volume up loud.

- Call 9-1-1, especially if you haven't been able to reach your doctor or midwife imme-

diately. If this is the first call you make, ask the 9-1-1 receptionist to call your doctor and notify your intended hospital. Then get back to the business of birth.

- Prepare your nest, usually your bed. To avoid soiling the mattress, place waterproof materials between the mattress and the sheet (e.g., garbage bags, a shower curtain, several thicknesses of newspaper, or a plastic tablecloth). Place a clean sheet over this.

- Warm your makeshift birthing room to between 70° and 75° F. Open the shades to allow natural sunlight to warm and light the room.

- Designate a gofer, preferably someone other than your spouse, who is suddenly drafted into the role of both labor coach and baby-catcher. This person (e.g., neighbor, teen, or friend) should boil two large pots of water to sterilize instruments and let one pot cool to lukewarm to be used to cleanse mother after delivery. Into the pan of boiling water, put the scissors and two foot-long pieces of string (or two shoe strings) to tie baby's cord. Have ready the following: a dishpan to catch the placenta; at least three clean, large towels; warm, clean blankets or towels for baby (warm them in the dryer).

- It's likely that your bag of waters has already broken or you wouldn't be this far into labor. If it has not, don't purposely break it, as it will break at the appropriate time.

- Place towels on the floor at the side or end of the bed, wherever your birth attendant is going to sit. It's dangerous to be maneuvering around on a slippery floor.

- Lie on your bed in whatever position is the most comfortable: back, side, hands and knees. Usually squatting is the best position for delivery, but in an emergency home delivery, you don't necessarily want to speed things up.

- Do not deliver your baby in the position you've seen in the typical hospital delivery in the movies, with the woman's buttocks perched just on the edge of the bed. Babies are slippery and can shoot right through the baby-catcher's hands and onto the floor. As a precaution, place yourself far enough back on your bed so that baby will be delivered onto it. Position yourself for your comfort and the safety of your baby, not to make it easier for the baby-catcher.

- The one who is going to catch the baby should wash his or her hands with alcohol or an antiseptic soap. If you are alone and have to ease your baby out by yourself, be sure to wash your hands first.

- Use physiological pushing (see page 363), and don't try to force a fast delivery. It's safest if baby is allowed to twist and turn to find the easiest path out.

- As the head emerges, expect to see and feel it more with each push, and then it will go back up an inch or so between pushes.

- As baby's head is crowning (i.e., at least half of the head is out), don't push. Don't pull on the head, but let it ease gently out into the hands of your birth attendant and onto the bed. The umbilical cord is often looped once or twice around baby's neck. Gently lift it over baby's head.

- As baby's head suddenly turns, the delivery of the shoulders begins. When baby's head is out but the shoulders have not yet been delivered, protect your perineum from tearing by supporting it with your hands on a towel just above the anal opening as the shoulders emerge.

- If you have a suction bulb, your birth attendant should suck the mucus out of baby's nose and hold baby's head downward for a few seconds to allow the mucus to drain away from baby's throat.

- If baby's shoulders have still not been delivered, as your birth attendant holds baby's head in both hands, push to deliver the shoulders. The upper shoulder and arm will usually appear first. Then your birth attendant should support baby's head and shoulder and lift gently upward in the direction of your navel to ease the bottom shoulder out.

- Once baby is totally delivered, place baby immediately tummy down on your abdomen. Blot excess fluid from baby. It's not necessary to wipe off the cheesy coating on baby's skin. Cover baby's back and head with a warm towel.

- All babies look blue for the first few seconds to a minute. The easiest place to feel baby's pulse is just where the cord enters baby's navel. With your thumb and forefinger gently placed, you should feel a pulse that is almost too fast to count and at least greater than 100 (counting fast "one-thousand-one, one-thousand-two, one-thousand-three"). If baby's pulse is at least 100 and not falling, you can be assured baby is breathing whether or not baby cries. If baby does not seem to be breathing on her own, or if the pulse seems to be steadily declining, stimulate baby's breathing by rubbing her back vigorously. It is not absolutely necessary to make baby cry, but once baby cries she should "pink up" and you should feel the pulse increase. Usually by this time the emergency medical squad has arrived and can administer oxygen or any breathing assistance baby may need.

- If baby's lips look blue (remember, hands and feet are blue for five to ten minutes in most newborns), you do not see baby breathing, and you are feeling a pulse certainly below sixty (counting slowly "one-thousand-one, one-thousand-two," etc.), administer half a dozen gentle mouth-to-mouth breaths. Cover baby's nose and mouth with your mouth.

- If trained medical help is en route to your home, it is not necessary to cut the cord or to deliver the placenta. Just let baby lie on you skin-to-skin, and be sure to keep baby's body and head covered with warm blankets or towels. If you do not cut the cord and the placenta is not delivering automatically, you and baby should lie side to side (but still tummy-to-tummy), so that baby remains at the same level as the placenta, thus allowing just the right amount of blood to go from placenta to baby.

- If your phone consultant advises you to cut the cord or if there is no medical help en route and you need to do so, wait a few minutes after birth, until the cord becomes thinner and paler (meaning the blood being transferred between the placenta and baby through the cord has stopped). Then tie one string tightly around the cord about an inch above its insertion to the navel and another knot an inch above that. Cut *between* these two knots.

- Don't pull on the cord to force the placenta out. Have baby suck on your nipple to release the hormones that naturally constrict the blood vessels to prevent excessive bleeding and stimulate delivery of the placenta. Usually the placenta will follow the baby within five to thirty minutes.

- Allow baby to continue sucking at your breast until trained help arrives or until you and your baby are stable enough to go to the hospital, or do whatever your health-care provider advises. This will ensure that your uterine muscles stay clamped around the open blood vessels from the placenta, so that you don't bleed too much.

- Because you will likely be weak after delivery, remain lying in bed or walk only with assistance.

- You and your baby should keep warm and quiet until help arrives or until your doctor or midwife gives further instructions.

- After delivering the placenta, gently massage the uterus just above the pelvis to help it continue contracting and normally compress the blood vessels.

EN ROUTE TO THE HOSPITAL

- Drive safely. This is not such a medical emergency as to risk the lives of all the passengers, including the little one being born.

- If you have a car phone, notify the hospital that you are en route. Put on your hazard lights. Let mother recline on the backseat. Protect the seat covers with newspaper, sheets, towels, or clothing. Be sure to keep baby and mother warm en route.

- Slow or stop the car for the moment of delivery. As soon as baby is delivered (follow the procedures above), continue on to the hospital.

Glossary of Obstetrical Terms

This glossary includes common concerns, problems, tests, and terms that you'll encounter during your pregnancy. Less common problems are also listed here rather than in the main part of the book, so as not to worry you with unusual problems you might, but probably won't, encounter during your pregnancy.

Abruptio placentae (placental abruption). In this condition the placenta partially or completely detaches from the uterine wall before or during labor. Placental abruption occurs in varying degrees in slightly less than 1 percent of pregnancies; it is most common during the third trimester. An early sign of placental abruption is the sudden onset of profuse bleeding, which is often accompanied by severe back or abdominal pain. When examining you, your doctor may notice that your uterus is unusually tender. An ultrasound may detect the separated placenta, but often does not. Premature separation of the placenta may be a medical emergency requiring emergency delivery if the blood supply to baby is compromised or the bleeding continues. If this condition is suspected, your doctor will probably put you in the hospital and monitor your baby's well-being and your

blood loss. If the bleeding stops, you are not in labor, and baby is in no distress, your doctor may recommend bed rest at home to help your pregnancy continue to term or to a point where a preterm delivery would be relatively safe. Depending on the degree of separation, you may or may not need a cesarean. There is a 10 percent risk of placental abruption recurring in subsequent pregnancies, so your doctor will monitor you extra closely in the later months of your next pregnancy.

Acquired Immune Deficiency Syndrome (AIDS). Caused by the human immune deficiency virus (HIV), this infection weakens the body's immune system and is eventually fatal. Most women with AIDS can successfully complete a pregnancy, and many of them go on to deliver a healthy baby. However, up to 50 percent of HIV-positive women and as many as 70 percent of women who have active AIDS transfer the virus to the fetus through their bloodstream, so this ultimately becomes a fatal disease for baby, too. Don't be offended if your doctor offers the blood test for AIDS as part of your prenatal care. Many health-care providers routinely test for

407

AIDS, even in women who have no apparent risk factors.

Amnioinfusion. If the amniotic fluid volume is insufficient for baby's well-being in the final weeks of pregnancy, your doctor may inject a saline (saltwater) solution into the uterus. This procedure is especially valuable in preventing or correcting fetal distress due to cord compression during contractions.

Amniotic fluid. Inside the womb babies float in a special fluid designed to protect them from infection and cushion them in a free-floating environment. Amniotic fluid begins forming around the fourth week of pregnancy, and for most of the first trimester mother makes all of the necessary fluid. Around eleven weeks baby's kidneys start to produce urine, adding to the fluid. After twenty weeks, baby's urine provides most of the amniotic fluid, and mother makes up the rest. The amniotic fluid completely replenishes itself every day. Babies swallow the fluid and pass it out again through their digestive tract. They also breathe in the fluid through their developing air passages. Amniotic fluid is basically nutrient-enriched saltwater, containing proteins, fatty acids, amnio acids, fructose, glucose, and many other nutrients. The volume of amniotic fluid peaks between thirty-four and thirty-eight weeks and slightly diminishes during the final two weeks of pregnancy.

Amniotomy. Also called "artificial rupture of membranes." In this procedure the doctor inserts a tiny hook through your cervix to catch and break the amniotic membrane — your water bag. This procedure is painless and is done to jump-start a stalled labor, induce an overdue labor, or to make it possible to insert an internal fetal monitor during labor. The amniotic membrane is ruptured only if necessary, because an intact bag of waters allows the force of contractions to be more evenly distributed during the stretching of the lower uterus and cervix and protects baby's cord when the head is coming down. Rupturing the membranes before baby's head has dropped into the pelvis may result in the umbilical cord's being caught and strangled between baby's head and the pelvic bones. Premature rupture of membranes also increases the chance of germs entering the uterus and infecting the baby. Your doctor should discuss with you the benefits and risks of artificial rupture of membranes before doing the procedure.

Apgar score. At one and five minutes after birth, a birth attendant assesses your newborn's heart rate, breathing effort, skin color, muscle activity, and response to stimulation and "rates" each one of these physiological signs of health with a score from 0 to 2. If each one of these functions makes the grade, baby's score adds up to 10. It's important that parents and professionals keep the Apgar score in perspective. A baby who scores a 10 is not necessarily healthier than a baby who scores an 8. Because most babies temporarily have blue hands and feet, few score a 10, even though they are healthy. A baby who is calm at birth and does not cry will also lose points, but this does not mean he is any less healthy. The Apgar score is not a newborn fitness test, nor was it ever meant as a rating to be given to parents. It was originally devised as a quick screening test to see which babies need more observation, since some take longer than others to make the transition from intrauterine living to breathing air.

Artificial rupture of membranes (AROM). *See* **Amniotomy.**

Biophysical profile (BPP). The BPP is used in the last few weeks of pregnancy to monitor fetal well-being during high-risk or post-term pregnancies. The procedure is performed in the doctor's office and combines the results of a non-stress test, an ultrasound assessment of fetal activity, and an evaluation of the quantity of amniotic fluid present in the uterus. The doctor uses the results to make decisions as to the safest mode and timing of delivery. This test is risk-free and pain-free to both mother and baby and takes a little less than an hour to complete.

Chicken pox. Chicken pox exposure during pregnancy causes some concern if you are not already immune to the disease. Most women are immune to chicken pox even though they may not remember having had the illness as a child. If you are uncertain about whether or not you are immune, your health-care provider can order a blood test to check your level of immunity. If you are immune to chicken pox, you don't have to worry, and no treatment is needed. If you are not immune, the chances are in your favor that neither you nor your baby will contract chicken pox, even if you are exposed. However, there is a small chance that a baby may develop a birth defect as the result of chicken pox exposure during the first trimester. Exposure to chicken pox during the final month of pregnancy is of greater concern. If a mother becomes ill with chicken pox more than fourteen days prior to delivery, she will produce enough antibodies to pass along to her baby and prevent him from getting chicken pox in the newborn period. But when a mother develops chicken pox within two weeks of giving birth, the baby will be born exposed to the virus but without the benefit of maternal antibodies. In this situation, a newborn may develop a po-

tentially serious case of chicken pox. Also, complications of chicken pox, mainly pneumonia, are more common in women who have the illness during pregnancy.

If you are not immune and have had close exposure to chicken pox during pregnancy, your doctor may recommend an injection of varicella-zoster immune globulin (VCIG) within four days of your exposure in order to provide immediate antibodies and lessen the chance of the virus passing to your baby. The same VCIG may be given in the last week of your pregnancy if you are not immune to chicken pox but are exposed. Because the currently available chicken pox vaccine is a live vaccine, it is not known whether it is safe to give it to pregnant women; the current recommendation is that it not be administered during pregnancy. For this reason, it is best to find out whether you are immune to chicken pox before becoming pregnant; you can then get the vaccine if you need it. If you are already pregnant, you should plan on getting the vaccine immediately after delivery to prevent problems in subsequent pregnancies. If you are pregnant and have other children who have not yet had chicken pox, it would be wise to consider giving them the chicken pox vaccine in order to minimize the chances of their getting the illness and passing it on to you. It is safe for other family members to get the chicken pox vaccine while you are pregnant.

Contraction stress test (CST). This test is usually done during the final weeks of pregnancy if there is concern about baby's well-being. Usually performed in the hospital, the CST is like a tiny test dose of labor to assess whether or not baby is able to tolerate the stress of contractions. While baby's heartbeat is electronically monitored, uterine contractions are stimulated, either artificially by intravenous pitocin or naturally by nipple stimulation. A negative CST is reassuring; it means that during three normal contractions baby's heart rate patterns remained normal. A positive CST is cause for concern; this means that baby's heart rate patterns were not normal during or following a contraction, suggesting that baby did not receive enough oxygen during contractions. Along with other tests, the doctor uses the CST to decide whether or not to deliver the baby by cesarean before the stress of labor contractions begins. Because the CST may trigger labor, it is not done in situations in which induction of labor could cause problems, such as prematurity or an abnormally placed placenta.

There is a high incidence of "equivocals" and false positives with the CST, which means that test results suggest baby's health is jeopardized during contractions when really it is not. This is why the doctor will use other tests of fetal well-being along with the CST in order to determine the safest mode of delivery. In many instances the CST alerts the doctor to monitor the baby more closely during labor for signs of fetal distress.

You may prefer to stimulate contractions naturally using nipple stimulation rather than having intravenous pitocin. Depending on your obstetrical situation, your doctor will advise you which one would be best. Studies show that nipple stimulation and pitocin are equally effective, yet nipple stimulation is easier and less expensive.

Couvade syndrome. "Couvade" (from the French *couver,* "to hatch") is a term applied to pregnancy-like symptoms that some men experience during their mate's pregnancy. Occurring in varying degrees in anywhere from 25 to 50 percent of fathers, the most common symptoms are food cravings, mood swings, nausea, morning sickness symptoms, weight gain, fatigue, backaches, and sleep difficulties. This syndrome most commonly appears around the third month of pregnancy, subsides during the middle trimester, and may appear again in varying degrees toward the end of the pregnancy. It is thought to represent a subconscious desire to identify with and be involved in the pregnancy, and perhaps share the attention lavished on the pregnant mother. These feelings may also be the body's reaction to an exaggerated pride in becoming a father.

Diabetes mellitus. The good news is that most diabetic women can, with proper control, have a healthy pregnancy and deliver a healthy baby. If you are diabetic, it is best to get your diabetes under control and reach your ideal weight prior to becoming pregnant. Your health and your baby's health depend upon how well your blood sugar is controlled during your pregnancy. While it is important to keep your diabetes under control throughout your pregnancy, it's especially important during the first month, when baby's organs are developing, and during the last couple of months, when the risk of prematurity is highest. Diabetes is more difficult to control during pregnancy, but control is extremely important. Your insulin requirements increase when you are pregnant because pregnancy hormones interfere with the action of insulin. Insulin doesn't cross the placenta, but your blood sugar does. So if your blood sugar is too high, baby will be overdosed and may be required to produce extra insulin. The extra sugar that gets into baby's bloodstream is stored as extra fat, accounting for the large size of babies born to mothers with diabetes. If your diabetes was controlled with oral medication prior to becoming pregnant, it is likely that your doctor will ask you to switch to injectable insulin.

Not only are oral medications usually ineffective in controlling diabetes during pregnancy, but some of them have been shown to be harmful to the developing fetus, whereas injectable insulin is considered safe. If you used one daily dose of insulin prior to becoming pregnant, you will probably need an extra dose during pregnancy. It's important to work closely with your doctor regarding adjustments in insulin dosage, exercise, and diet. Depending on how well controlled your diabetes is, your doctor may or may not elect to deliver your baby ahead of the due date, since diabetes may eventually cause the blood vessels of the uterus to become insufficient to nourish the baby. In order to minimize harmful blood-sugar swings in your baby immediately after birth, it's very important that your diabetes be well controlled within the week prior to delivery. Expect your newborn to need careful monitoring by a specialist for a few days after delivery to be sure that her blood sugar remains stable and to watch for temporary respiratory problems, which are more common in babies of women with diabetes.

Diethylstilbestrol (DES). In the '50s and '60s the artificial hormone diethylstilbestrol was given to pregnant women, sometimes without their knowledge, to prevent or delay preterm labor or prevent impending miscarriage. Years later this drug was found not to be beneficial to these problems and its use was discontinued. Daughters born to women who took DES during pregnancy may have uterine abnormalities or problems with their fallopian tubes, vagina, or cervix. Cervical incompetence is particularly common in DES daughters, so if you have this family history, it's important to alert your health-care provider to be especially vigilant for signs of preterm labor or miscarriage.

Eclampsia. *See* **Preeclampsia**.

F.A.C.O.G. These initials stand for "Fellow of the American College of Obstetricians and Gynecologists." This credential is awarded to an M.D. who has taken the required training in obstetrics and gynecology and has passed the exam given by this professional society.

Fetal medicine specialist. *See* **Perinatologist**.

Fetal-pelvic index (FPI). This test uses an X ray to measure the size of the pelvic outlet together with an ultrasound to measure the size of the baby. This test is particularly helpful in predicting the advisability of attempting a vaginal breech delivery. It is also used to assess the size of the pelvis in mothers who wish to try a vaginal birth after a previous cesarean. Because it considers both the size of the passage and the size of the passenger, FPI is much more accurate than an X ray of the pelvis alone, but the results of this test should not cause a mother to lose confidence in her ability to deliver vaginally, and the decision to do a cesarean should not be based upon the results of this test alone. Simple measurements cannot take into account the biological facts that the size of your pelvic outlet can increase as much as 20 percent when you squat during delivery and that baby's body rotates to accommodate different dimensions during labor as he navigates a seemingly narrow passage to find the easiest way out.

Fetal-scalp blood sampling. Fetal-scalp blood sampling is used during labor to assess if baby is getting enough oxygen. Through a thin tube inserted through your vagina and cervix, the doctor takes a few drops of blood from baby's scalp. The laboratory analyzes this sample for oxygen and other factors in baby's blood chemistry that reflect fetal well-being. Fetal-scalp blood sampling is a more accurate test of baby's well-being than changes in the electronic fetal heart rate patterns. It is often performed when the electronic fetal monitor suggests possible fetal distress.

Fifth disease. This viral infectious disease (so named because it was the fifth of the viruses discovered to cause fever and rash) is a common childhood viral illness that is very contagious but seldom harmful to children or adults. It is characterized by fever, a red rash on the cheeks (looking like "slapped cheeks"), and a lacy red rash on the legs and trunk of the body. Sometimes adults with this illness may also have sore joints, and people with types of hemolytic anemia may experience a flare-up during this disease. Fifth disease is contagious for up to a week before the facial rash appears, so people are often exposed to the virus unknowingly. Although this virus is usually harmless to children and nonpregnant adults, there are special concerns for pregnant women. If you are not already immune to this virus (most adults are) and are exposed during the first trimester of your pregnancy, you have a slightly higher risk of miscarriage (1 to 2 percent higher than normal). Infection of the baby during the latter part of pregnancy can break down baby's blood cells, causing anemia. If you have been exposed to Fifth disease, your health-care provider may perform a blood test to see if you are already immune. If you are, you do not need to be concerned. If the blood test shows that you are not immune to Fifth disease, or another blood test shows that you have recently been infected with the virus, your health-care provider may monitor your baby for signs of severe anemia, often detected by repeated ultrasound.

Forceps. Forceps are a salad-tong–like device that can be used to help pull the baby's head out of the birth canal. A small risk of injury to either the baby or the mother exists from the use of forceps, but properly applied, they are generally safe and can help prevent a cesarean if the mother is unable to push the baby out or if the baby is experiencing fetal distress.

Group B streptococcus (GBS). Group B streptococcus is a common bacterial inhabitant of the vagina. It is a different strain of the bacteria that causes strep throat. Many women unknowingly carry GBS and have no symptoms, yet run the risk of passing this bacteria to their baby during delivery. GBS can cause a serious, and possibly fatal, neonatal infection. For this reason, many health-care providers will routinely perform vaginal, rectal, or urine cultures to see if mother is a carrier of GBS. Several cultures may be needed because a woman may carry strep one month and not the next. If a mother is shown to carry strep near the time of delivery, she is often treated with antibiotics so that she does not pass this dangerous germ on to her baby. If you are experiencing preterm labor, or if your membranes ruptured more than twenty-four hours ago, or if you show a fever around the time of delivery, your doctor may be especially vigilant about testing for GBS. Even though GBS is a potentially serious disease for the newborn, most babies of GBS-infected mothers do not contract the disease, especially since today health-care providers are on the lookout for this bacteria.

HELLP syndrome. HELLP stands for the combination of symptoms characteristic of severe preeclampsia: *h*emolysis, (the breakdown of red blood cells); *e*levated *l*iver enzymes; and *l*ow *p*latelets (the blood cells that are involved in blood clotting). Left untreated, this is a serious condition that puts both mother and baby at risk.

Hepatitis B. The hepatitis B virus is transmitted by sexual contact or by receiving infected blood or blood products. Women can carry this virus during pregnancy but not have symptoms, and thus not know they are affected. The main concern is with transmitting the virus to the baby during delivery. Not only is there a high chance of an infected mother infecting her baby, but many of these infected babies become hepatitis B carriers and go on to develop chronic liver disease. The good news is that with the use of properly administered vaccine, newborns can be protected against hepatitis B infection. Your doctor may recommend testing for hepatitis B infection as part of your routine prenatal tests. If you are infected, your baby will be given hepatitis B immune globulin and the first dose of the hepatitis B vaccine immediately after birth. Follow-up doses of hepatitis B will be given at one month and six months of age. Later, the baby will be tested to be sure the vaccination program has prevented infection.

Incompetent cervix. When the cervix begins to dilate and thin out prematurely, there is a risk of miscarriage or premature delivery. This may occur as a result of a congenital weakness in the cervix or due to extreme stretching from previous deliveries or cervical surgery. Incompetent cervix occurs in varying degrees in 1 to 2 percent of all pregnancies, yet with proper diagnosis and management, most mothers go on to deliver healthy babies. Cervical incompetence may be diagnosed during a miscarriage, during a routine examination for spotting or bleeding, or after premature passing of the mucous plug. If cervical incompetence is suspected, your doctor may elect to perform a cervical cerclage, which involves suturing the cervix to keep it closed. This is usually done around the eighteenth or twentieth week of pregnancy, and the sutures are removed close to the due date. In addition to performing a cerclage, your health-care provider may recommend bed rest and medication should contractions begin prematurely. About 25 percent of women with cervical incompetence will deliver prematurely, but the majority of these babies are healthy.

Intrauterine growth retardation (IUGR). IUGR is arbitrarily defined as a term baby weighing less than 5 pounds (less than 2500 grams). Babies with intrauterine growth retardation have not achieved their full growth potential, usually due to a variety of conditions that compromise uterine blood flow, such as maternal smoking, high blood pressure, or a chronic condition, such as kidney disease, malnutrition, drug or alcohol use, or intrauterine infections. Oftentimes, IUGR is due to placental insufficiency for no apparent reason. Your doctor may suspect that your baby is not growing optimally based on measurements of the growth of your uterus during routine prenatal visits. The suspicion can be confirmed by ultrasound. Depending on the cause and severity of IUGR, your doctor will carefully monitor baby's growth during the third trimester. Because of the increased risk of problems with IUGR babies, your doctor may take special precautions, such as careful fetal monitoring and a preterm induction or cesarean if baby's well-being seems to be in jeopardy. Due to reduced body fat, these babies have difficulty maintaining their body temperature right after delivery. They are also prone to blood-chemistry disturbances, such as unstable blood sugar. Oftentimes, babies with IUGR will need a few days in a special care nursery, or at least close monitoring in mother's room.

Macrosomia. Macrosomia means an oversized baby, which is arbitrarily defined as more than 9¾ pounds (4500 grams). While most large babies are simply the result of family genes, some babies put on excess weight because of unhealthy maternal nutrition or diabetes that was not well controlled during pregnancy. Besides being more difficult to deliver, an oversized baby is more prone to birth injuries. In some cases, an obstetrician may feel it is safer to deliver an oversized baby by cesarean.

Non-stress test (NST). The non-stress test is used to assess fetal well-being when a pregnancy seems to be progressing past term. It is free of pain and risk to both mother and baby. The NST is performed in a doctor's office. While baby's heart rate is being recorded, the doctor asks mother to signal when she feels the baby move. The heartbeat of a healthy baby accelerates by about fifteen beats per minute with movement. If baby's heart rate does not increase during a forty-minute test period, this suggests baby's well-being may be in jeopardy. While a reactive NST correlates well with a healthy infant, a non-reactive NST (no increases in the heart rate) may be a false alarm more than 75 percent of the time. Baby may be sleeping or just not in the mood to raise his heart rate during the testing. Usually the doctor will choose to repeat the NST before worrying the mother or proceeding with more invasive testing of baby's well-being.

Pelvimetry. A radiologist can take X rays to measure the dimensions of your pelvic passage. Comparing these measurements with "normal" dimensions can determine if your pelvic passage is large enough for baby to pass through safely. Because of questions of safety and accuracy, X-ray pelvimetry alone is being used less and is gradually being replaced by the more accurate fetal-pelvic index (see above). Even though X rays have not conclusively been shown to be harmful to the fetus, especially in the last few weeks of pregnancy, they are recommended only when the benefits outweigh the risks. The accuracy of X-ray pelvimetry is also in question because the size of the pelvic outlet may increase during labor, especially in the squatting position. The "still shot" obtained in prelabor X rays may not reflect the true size of the passage. Also, pelvimetry alone does not consider the size of baby's head, and thus fails to take into account the "fit" between passage and passenger.

Percutaneous umbilical blood sampling (PUBS). This is a method of obtaining samples of fetal blood by inserting a needle through mother's abdominal wall into a blood vessel in the umbilical cord, using ultrasound guidance. It is similar to the procedure used in performing an amniocentesis. Percutaneous umbilical blood sampling is done in major medical centers between the sixteenth and thirty-sixth week of pregnancy when it is necessary to obtain fetal blood for diagnosis of blood, genetic, or metabolic disorders that cannot be detected by analyzing amniotic fluid samples obtained through amniocentesis. Because the risk of miscarriage is around twice that of amniocentesis, this procedure is performed only when the information that will be obtained is absolutely necessary in making decisions for the health and well-being of the baby. The results of the blood sampling are usually available more rapidly than the results obtained by analyzing the amniotic fluid.

Perinatologist. A perinatologist is an obstetrician who has extra training in caring for mothers with complicated pregnancies or anticipated problems at birth. He or she practices at a major medical center and usually sees patients referred by primary health-care providers. Oftentimes the perinatologist will co-manage a mother's labor and delivery along with her regular obstetrician.

Pitocin. Pitocin is a synthetically produced oxytocin that is used to enhance contractions of the uterus. It is given intravenously (in a "pit-drip"), and the rate of its infusion is regulated by a bedside pump. It is used to induce labor and to jump-start a stalled labor. Because pitocin-induced contractions are much more intense than natural contractions, mothers receiving pitocin may require epidural anesthesia. Your doctor may also recommend electronic fetal monitoring when pitocin is given intravenously because the contractions peak more quickly and may be more stressful for the baby. Discuss with your doctor the benefits and risks of artificially stimulating your contractions. While pitocin is likely to help your labor progress, you may have to remain in bed because of the epidural anesthesia and electronic fetal monitoring. Thus you risk losing the freedom of movement that may also help your labor progress and help baby find the safest path out. When pitocin is properly timed and administered, it can help a labor progress; when improperly used, it can increase the chances of surgical birth.

Placenta previa. Sometimes a normal placenta develops in an abnormal location and partially or completely covers the cervix. This is called placenta previa. A placenta that covers the cervix is prone to sudden and possibly life-threatening hemorrhage before or during labor. This condition occurs in approximately one in two hundred deliveries. Sometimes it is suspected if a woman has painless bleeding anytime during the second half of pregnancy, especially during the final month. Sometimes the woman has no signs of bleeding and placenta previa is discovered on diagnostic ultrasound. The goals of treating placenta previa are to prevent bleeding and lessen the risk of premature delivery. Your doctor may prescribe bed rest or limited activity if there is a danger of bleeding. Depending on the degree of the placenta previa, baby may or may not have to be delivered by cesarean. With modern technology, placenta previa can be detected before the health of mother and baby are in danger, and given proper medical treatment, most mothers go on to deliver healthy babies.

Preeclampsia. Preeclampsia can occur in the last half of pregnancy and is characterized by swelling of the face and hands, high blood pressure, and protein in the urine, found during routine urinalysis. Occurring in around 7 percent of all pregnancies, preeclampsia is most common in first pregnancies and is more common among women carrying multiples or who have a chronic disease, such as high blood pressure, kidney disease, or diabetes. Many women initially have no symptoms, and the first signs of preeclampsia may be high blood pressure and protein in the urine detected during a routine prenatal visit — one of the reasons that routine prenatal visits are so important. A sudden spurt in weight gain (more than 2 pounds in a week or 6 pounds in a month) due to excessive retention of fluids may also indicate preeclampsia. Some women will notice swelling in their face and hands, diminishing vision, and headaches. Preeclampsia, if left untreated, can become serious enough to compromise the health of both mother and baby; the high blood pressure is dangerous for mother, and the insufficient blood supply to the uterus will affect the growth of the baby. The primary goal in treating preeclampsia is to keep the rising blood pressure under control. This is usually done by a combination of bed rest and, if symptoms are severe, hospitalization and medication to reduce the blood pressure and increase uterine blood flow. Depending on the severity of the preeclampsia, the doctor may recommend preterm delivery, often by cesarean section, if it is in the best interest of the mother and baby. If the mother had preeclampsia in one pregnancy, she has an increased chance of having it in subsequent pregnancies. This condition used to be called "toxemia" because it was erroneously thought to be due to a toxin in the bloodstream. In most cases, the cause of preeclampsia is not known, but with modern obstetrical management, it is nearly always successfully treated, leading to the safe delivery of a healthy baby.

Prostaglandin gel. This is a synthetically produced cervical softener that is similar to the natural prostaglandins that are produced during labor. Your doctor may choose to apply prostaglandin gel to "ripen" your cervix in order to increase the progress of labor.

Rh incompatibility. If your blood type is Rh negative and baby's father's is Rh positive, you need to be concerned about Rh incompatibility. Your baby could have Rh-positive blood, and some of the baby's Rh-positive blood may leak into your circulation during pregnancy, at birth, or following a miscarriage. Your body will produce antibodies against the Rh factor in baby's blood. This sensitization does not present a problem in the first pregnancy, but in the next pregnancy with an Rh-positive baby, your antibodies will cross the placenta and attack the baby's blood, causing anemia. If you are Rh negative, your doctor will give you an injection of RhoGam immediately following delivery, a miscarriage, an abortion, or an amniocentesis. This reduces the chances of your body becoming sensitized to the Rh factor. Some physicians also give RhoGam injections at twenty-eight weeks to prevent early sensitization. If you have Rh antibodies in your blood, you may be monitored closely during your pregnancy and after birth in case early delivery or a blood transfusion becomes necessary.

Shoulder dystocia. Occurring in 0.15 to 1.7 percent of deliveries, shoulder dystocia means that the baby's shoulder is too large or in the wrong position to pass through the inlet to the pelvic bone. This is a true medical emergency that requires skillful manipulation by experienced hands in order to prevent damage to the baby. Shoulder dystocia is more likely to occur in babies weighing over 9 pounds. There are two things a mother can do to lessen the chances of her baby's shoulder getting stuck during passage through the birth canal: practice healthy nutrition to avoid excessive weight gain and an excessively large baby; and work with her body during labor using different positions to help the baby twist and turn to find the easiest way to pass through the pelvic canal.

Toxemia. *See* **Preeclampsia.**

Transcutaneous electrical nerve stimulation (TENS). TENS is a pain-easing device that is often used in pain centers to relieve postoperative pain. It operates basically like electrical acupressure. The laboring mother holds the TENS unit, about the size of a deck of cards, in her hand. Wires from the unit are taped to the skin above the area where her back hurts. When mother senses a back pain coming on, she presses a button to send electrical current into the skin and muscle around the pain site. She can adjust the level of stimulation as desired. TENS is believed to work by stimulating the tissue to produce local pain-relieving hormones, endorphins.

Vacuum extractor. This suction-cup device, resembling a plumber's helper, is an alternative to forceps as an aid to assisting a resistant baby through the birth canal. A soft rubber or plastic cup is placed on baby's scalp during pushing and is connected to tubes running to a vacuum generator tank that applies gentle suction. The doctor gently pulls on the handles connected to the suction cup and helps baby down the birth canal. Another benefit of the vacuum extractor over forceps is that episiotomy is not required for the use of the vacuum extractor; forceps require more room in the vagina. Once the baby is born, you will notice a harmless swelling of baby's scalp where the suction cup was applied. It may take several months for the swelling to subside.

Index

Page references in boldface type refer to main discussions.